Atlas of Clinical Endocrinology and Metabolism

This updated text is a pictorial atlas of endocrine and metabolic disorders. Each chapter focuses on providing multiple illustrations as well as a thorough discussion of the diagnosis and management of a variety of endocrine diseases with their appropriate treatment plans. Using updated guidelines, it provides a comprehensive discussion of the latest therapies, including diabetes technology. Presenting a large number of clinical images, including imaging of thyroid ultrasounds, DXA images, bone scans, and new technologies in diabetes mellitus, this atlas aims to provide the reader with the information needed to make accurate diagnoses, making it an updated source of highly illustrated information for endocrinologists, clinicians, residents, fellows, and trainees. With new chapters on transgender medicine and obesity, this textbook will be a valuable resource for the contemporary endocrine practitioner.

- Features new chapters such as transgender medicine and inborn errors of metabolism
- Aims to be an invaluable aid for endocrinologists, internal medicine specialists, family practice clinicians, residents, fellows, and trainees
- Explores diabetes technology with updated guidelines

T0225324

Atlas of Clinical Endocrinology and Metabolism

Edited by
Pauline Camacho

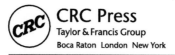

CRC Press
Taylor & Francis Group
Boca Raton London New York

CRC Press is an imprint of the
Taylor & Francis Group, an **informa** business

Cover images provided by author.

First edition published 2024
by CRC Press
6000 Broken Sound Parkway NW, Suite 300, Boca Raton, FL 33487-2742

and by CRC Press
4 Park Square, Milton Park, Abingdon, Oxon, OX14 4RN

CRC Press is an imprint of Taylor & Francis Group, LLC

© 2024 Taylor & Francis Group, LLC

Library of Congress Cataloging-in-Publication Data
Names: Camacho, Pauline M., editor.
Title: Atlas of clinical endocrinology and metabolism / edited by Pauline Camacho.
Description: First edition. | Boca Raton, FL : CRC Press, 2024. | Includes bibliographical references and index.
Identifiers: LCCN 2023022854 (print) | LCCN 2023022855 (ebook) | ISBN 9780367608354 (hardback) | ISBN 9780367608330 (paperback) | ISBN 9781003100669 (ebook)
Subjects: MESH: Endocrine System Diseases--diagnostic imaging | Endocrine System Diseases--therapy | Metabolic Diseases--diagnostic imaging | Metabolic Diseases--therapy | Atlas
Classification: LCC RB147 (print) | LCC RB147 (ebook) | NLM WK 17 | DDC 616.3/900222--dc23/eng/20231030
LC record available at https://lccn.loc.gov/2023022854
LC ebook record available at https://lccn.loc.gov/2023022855

ISBN: 9780367608354 (hbk)
ISBN: 9780367608330 (pbk)
ISBN: 9781003100669 (ebk)

DOI: 10.1201/9781003100669

Typeset in Times
by Deanta Global Publishing Services, Chennai, India

Contents

Editor

Dr. Pauline Camacho is a professor of medicine at Loyola University Medical Center and directs the Loyola University Osteoporosis and Metabolic Bone Disease Center. She is also the program director for the endocrinology fellowship at Loyola.

She obtained her medical degree from the University of the Philippines College of Medicine and completed her internal medicine residency at Rush University Medical Center and endocrinology fellowship at Loyola University Medical Center.

Her clinical practice and research focus on osteoporosis and other metabolic bone diseases such as vitamin D deficiency, primary hyperparathyroidism, and other calcium and mineral disorders. She has been on the editorial board of endocrine journals and has published numerous papers and five endocrinology textbooks. She is the lead author of the 2020 AACE/ACE Postmenopausal Osteoporosis Treatment Guidelines. Camacho is a past president of the American Association of Clinical Endocrinologists (AACE) and past chancellor of the American College of Endocrinology.

She lives in Chicago with her husband and has three daughters.

Contributors

Marriam Ali, MD
Assistant Professor
Division of Endocrinology
Loyola Medicine
Maywood, Illinois

Francis Q. Almeda, MD
Chief of Cardiology
Non-Invasive Cardiology
UChicago Medicine Ingalls Memorial
Harvey, Illinois

Rod Marianne Arceo-Mendoza, MD
Associate Professor of Medicine
Division of Endocrinology
Loyola University Medical Center
Loyola Stritch School of Medicine
Maywood, Illinois

Ezra Baraban, MD
Assistant Professor of Pathology
Department of Pathology
Johns Hopkins Hospital
Baltimore, Maryland

Gerald Charnogursky, MD
Professor of Medicine
Director, Division of Endocrinology and
   Metabolism
Loyola University Medical Center
Maywood, Illinois

Rhoda H. Cobin, MD
Clinical Professor of Medicine
The Icahn School of Medicine at Mount Sinai
New York, New York

Mary Ann Emanuele, MD
Professor of Medicine
Loyola University Medical Center
Maywood, Illinois

Maria Fleseriu
Professor Medicine and Neurological Surgery
Director Pituitary Center
Oregon Health & Science University
Portland, Oregon

Jason L. Gaglia, MD, MMSc
Associate Professor of Medicine
Joslin Diabetes Center
Boston, Massachusetts

Jeffrey R. Garber, MD
Associate Professor of Medicine
Harvard Medical School
and
Chief of the Division of Endocrinology
Atrius Health
Boston, Massachusetts

Pruthvi Goparaju
Central Michigan University
Mount Pleasant, Michigan

Pranav Gupta, MD
Pediatric Endocrinologist
Division of Pediatric Endocrinology
Emory University School of Medicine
Atlanta, Georgia

Amir H. Hamrahian, MD
Associate Professor of Medicine
Division of Endocrinology, Diabetes and
   Metabolism
Johns Hopkins University
Baltimore, Maryland

Ikram Haque, MD
Endocrinology Fellow
Division of Endocrinology and Metabolism
Loyola University Medical Center
Maywood, Illinois

Natasha S. Kadakia, DO
Endocrinology Fellow
Loyola University Medical Center
Maywood, Illinois

Sarah Kanbour, MD
Endocrinology Fellow
Division of Endocrinology, Diabetes and
    Metabolism
Johns Hopkins University
Baltimore, Maryland

Fatima Kazi, MD
Endocrinologist
Franciscan Physician Network
Munster, Indiana

Alexander J. Langerman, MD
Associate Professor
Otolaryngology, Head and Neck Surgery
Vanderbilt University Medical Center
Nashville, Tennessee

Norma Lopez, MD
Professor of Medicine
Division of Endocrinology
Loyola University Medical Center
Maywood, Illinois

Alalah Mazhari, DO
Professor of Medicine
Loyola University Medical Center
Maywood, Illinois

Reza Pishdad, MD
Clinical Fellow
Johns Hopkins University School of Medicine
Baltimore, Maryland

Caroline Poku, MD
Endocrinology Section, Medical Service
Edward Hines VA Hospital
Hines, Illinois
and
Assistant Professor of Medicine
Loyola University Health Care System
Maywood, Illinois

Louis G. Portugal, MD
Professor of Surgery
University of Chicago
Chicago, Illinois

S. Sethu K. Reddy
Professor of Medicine
Division of Endocrinology and Metabolism
Central Michigan University
Mount Pleasant, Michigan

Sobia Sadiq, MD
Assistant Professor
Division of Endocrinology and Metabolism
Loyola University Medical Center
Maywood, Illinois

Shanika Samarasinghe, MD
Professor
Division of Endocrinology and Metabolism
Loyola University Medical Center
Maywood, Illinois

Mary O. Stevenson, MD
Division of Endocrinology, Metabolism and Lipids
Emory University School of Medicine
Atlanta, Georgia

Mark Walsh, MD
Division of Plastic and Reconstructive Surgery
Emory University School of Medicine
Atlanta, Georgia

Howa Yeung, MD, MSc
Division of Dermatology
Emory University School of Medicine
Atlanta, Georgia

Thyroid Disorders

1

ABSTRACT

Thyroid disorders are characterized by either abnormal function or structure. The first section is an overview of thyrotoxicosis, hypothyroidism, and thyroid nodules, most of which are benign. The latter section is devoted to thyroid malignancy.

THYROTOXICOSIS, HYPOTHYROIDISM, THYROID NODULES

Jason L. Gaglia and Jeffrey R. Garber

Normal Thyroid

Anatomy

During development, the thyroid gland originates as an outpouching of the floor of the pharynx. It grows downward, anterior to the trachea, with the course of its downward migration marked by the thyroglossal duct. The thyroid sits like a saddle over the trachea with the two lateral lobes of the thyroid connected by a thin isthmus, which sits just below the cricoid cartilage. Normally, each lobe is pear shaped, 2.5–4 cm in lengthlong, 1.5–2 cm in widthwide, and 1–1.5 cm in thickness; the gland typically weighs 10–20 g in an adult depending upon body size and iodine supply. A pyramidal lobe may extend upward from the isthmus on the surface of the thyroid cartilage and is a remnant of the thyroglossal duct.

The thyroid gland has a rich blood supply with the two superior thyroid arteries arising from the common or external carotid arteries, the two inferior thyroid arteries from the thyrocervical trunk of the subclavian arteries, and a small thyroid ima artery from the brachiocephalic artery at the aortic arch. The venous drainage is via multiple surface veins that coalesce into superior, lateral, and inferior thyroid veins. Blood flow is about 5 mL/g/min, but in hyperthyroidism, this may increase 100-a hundredfold. Other important anatomic considerations include the relative proximity to the parathyroid glands and the recurrent laryngeal nerves.

Thyroglossal duct cysts can occur during the embryologic descent of the primordial thyroid through the foramen cecum of the tongue and through the thyroglossal duct near the hyoid bone to its final position in the midline pretracheal inferior neck. Thyroglossal duct cysts may present as a midline neck mass that elevates with tongue protrusion due to the extrinsic action of the genio-glossus muscle, which inserts muscle fibers into the hyoid bone (see Figure 1.1). Surgical excision of thyroglossal duct cysts often requires removal of a portion of the hyoid bone.

DOI: 10.1201/9781003100669-1

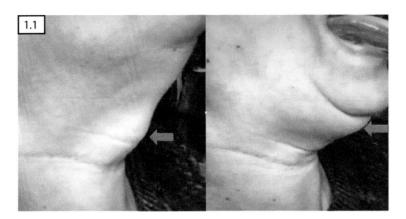

FIGURE 1.1   Thyroglossal duct cysts may present as a midline mass that elevates with tongue protrusion due to the extrinsic action of the genio-glossus muscle, which inserts muscle fibers into the hyoid bone.

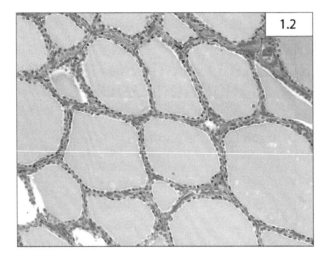

FIGURE 1.2   Normal thyroid. The thyroid gland consists of a collection of follicles where thyroid hormones are produced and stored. Each follicle consists of a central colloid surrounded by one layer of follicular cells. (Courtesy of Dr. James Connolly.)

Histology

The thyroid gland consists of a collection of follicles of varying sizes. These follicles contain a protein-aceous material called colloid and are surrounded by a single layer of thyroid epithelium (Figure 1.2). These follicle cells synthesize thyroglobulin, which is extruded into the lumen of the follicle. The biosynthesis of thyroid hormones occurs at the cell–colloid interface. Here thyroglobulin is hydrolyzed to release thyroid hormones. In addition to the follicular cells are other light-appearing cells, often found in clusters between the follicles, called C-cells (Figure 1.3). These cells are derived from the neural crest via the ultimobranchial body and secrete calcitonin. In adults, the C-cells represent about 1% of the cell population of the thyroid.

Thyroid Hormone

Thyroid hormone synthesis requires iodide, the glycoprotein thyroglobulin, and the enzyme thyroid microsomal peroxidase (TPO). Synthesis involves several steps including: (1) active transport of I$^-$ into the cell via the Na/I symporter; (2) iodide trapping with oxidation of iodide and iodination of tyrosyl residues

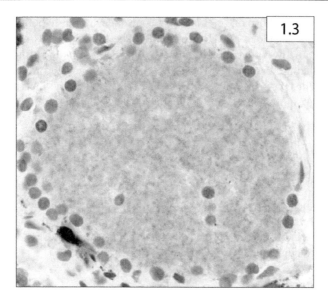

FIGURE 1.3 C-cell is demonstrated in the classic parafollicular location with calcitonin staining in brown. (Courtesy of Dr. James Connolly.)

in thyroglobulin catalyzed by TPO, forming monoiodotyrosine (MIT) and diiodotyrosine (DIT); (3) coupling of iodotyrosine molecules to form triiodothyronine (T3) from one MIT and one DIT molecule, and thyroxine (T4) from two DIT molecules; (4) proteolysis of thyroglobulin; (5) deiodination of iodotyrosines with conservation of liberated iodide; and (6) intrathyroidal 5′-deiodination of T4 to T3, particularly in situations of iodide deficiency or hormone overproduction.

Thyroid hormones are transported in the serum bound to carrier proteins. It is the much smaller free fraction that is responsible for hormonal activity (typically 0.03% for T4 and 0.3% for T3). The three major thyroid hormone transport proteins are thyroxine-binding globulin, albumin, and transthyretin (thyroxine-binding prealbumin), which carry 70%, 15%, and 10%, respectively. A number of conditions and medications can affect carrier protein concentration or binding (Table 1.1). Peripheral deiodinases convert T4 to the more active T3 or inactive reverse T3.

TABLE 1.1 Factors Influencing Total Thyroid Hormones Levels

Increased Binding Globulin
• Congenital
• Hyperestrogen states (pregnancy, ERT, SERMs, OCPs)
• Drugs: methadone, heroin, 5-fluouracil, mitotane
• Illness: acute hepatitis, hypothyroidism (minor)
Decreased Binding Globulin
• Congenital
• Drugs: androgens, glucocorticoids
• Illness: protein malnutrition, nephrotic syndrome, cirrhosis, hyperthyroidism (minor)
Drugs Affecting Binding
• Phenytoin
• Salicylates
• Furosemide
• Heparin (via increased free fatty acids)

ERT, estrogen replacement therapy; OCP, oral contraceptive pill; SERM, selective estrogen receptor modulator.

The production of thyroid hormone is normally controlled by the hypothalamic–pituitary–thyroid axis. Thyrotropin-releasing hormone (TRH) produced in the hypothalamus reaches the thyrotrophs in the anterior pituitary via the hypothalamic–hypophysial portal system and stimulates the synthesis and release of thyroid-stimulating hormone (TSH). TSH acts upon the thyroid to increase thyroid hormone production. Negative feedback, primarily via T3 (which may be locally generated from T4 via type 2 iodothyronine deiodinase), inhibits TRH and TSH secretion.

Thyrotoxicosis

Definition

Thyrotoxicosis occurs when increased levels of thyroid hormone lead to biochemical excess of the hormone at the tissue level. Increased levels of thyroid hormone leading to thyrotoxicosis may result from the overproduction of thyroid hormone (termed 'hyperthyroidism'), leakage of stored hormone from the gland, or exogenous thyroid hormone administration.

Etiology

Many cases of thyrotoxicosis are from autoimmune antibody-mediated stimulation (Graves' disease), gland destruction (thyroiditis), or autonomous nodular disease. Other less frequent causes of thyrotoxicosis include stimulation of the TSH receptor by high human chorionic gonadotropin (hCG) levels, TSH-secreting pituitary adenomas, pituitary-specific thyroid hormone resistance, struma ovarii, functional metastatic thyroid carcinoma, thyrotoxicosis factitia, neonatal Graves' disease, and congenital hyperthyroidism.

Iodine-containing drugs, such as iodinated contrast agents, or iodine-rich foods, such as kelp, may precipitate thyrotoxicosis in susceptible individuals, especially in iodine-deficient areas, and is termed Jod–Basedow disease. Amiodarone may precipitate thyrotoxicosis via iodine excess (type 1) or a drug-induced destructive thyroiditis (type 2).

Clinical Presentation

Common symptoms of thyrotoxicosis include palpitations, nervousness, shakiness, insomnia, difficulty concentrating, irritability, emotional lability, increased appetite, heat intolerance, fatigue, weakness, exertional dyspnea, hyperdefecation, decreased menses, and brittle hair. Although weight loss is more typical, approximately 10% of affected individuals gain weight likely due to a mismatch between increased metabolic demand and polyphagia. Due to changes in adrenergic tone, older individuals with thyrotoxicosis may lack many of the overt symptoms seen in younger individuals and instead present with what has been termed 'apathetic thyrotoxicosis'. Often weight loss, fatigue, and irritability are the major complaints in this age group. They may be depressed and have constipation rather than frequent stools. Atrial fibrillation, crescendo angina, and congestive heart failure are also not uncommon in this population.

Signs of thyrotoxicosis include tremors, warm moist skin, tachycardia, flow murmurs, hyperreflexia with rapid relaxation phase, and eye signs. Lid retraction or 'thyroid stare' may be seen with any cause of thyrotoxicosis and is attributed to increased adrenergic tone. True ophthalmopathy is unique to Graves' disease and may include proptosis, conjunctival injection, and periorbital edema. Patients with Graves' disease also typically have a goiter and may have a thyroid bruit from increased intrathyroidal blood flow, while patients with autonomous adenoma(s) frequently have palpable nodule(s).

Diagnosis/Investigations

Measurement of serum TSH followed by free T4 or T4 index are the initial laboratory studies when thyrotoxicosis is suspected. If free T4 (or T4 index) is normal and TSH is undetectable, a T3 level should be checked to evaluate for T3 thyrotoxicosis. Other laboratory findings that may be associated with thyrotoxicosis include mild leukopenia, normocytic anemia, transaminitis, elevated alkaline phosphatase (particularly from bone, but liver alkaline phosphatase may also be elevated), mild hypercalcemia, low albumin, and low cholesterol. Several medications including dopamine and corticosteroids may decrease TSH but should not be confused with thyrotoxicosis, as the free T4 and/or T3 are not elevated.

Once biochemical thyrotoxicosis is confirmed, the underlying etiology is usually determined by clinical findings or functional and/or structural assessment of the gland. A quantitative assessment of functional status may be obtained with radioactive iodine uptake. An inappropriately high uptake (uptake should normally be suppressed in the setting of a suppressed TSH) confirms hyperthyroidism, whereas a low uptake may be seen with the thyrotoxic phase of thyroiditis, exogenous thyroid hormone ingestion, or thyroid hormone production from an area outside of the neck. A scan with ^{123}I or ^{99m}Tc pertechnetate can be used to obtain further functional information with images depicting the distribution of trapping within the thyroid gland. Uniform distribution in a hyperthyroid patient most often suggests Graves' disease (Figure 1.4). Activity corresponding to a nodule with suppression of the rest of the thyroid suggests a toxic adenoma. A patchy distribution may be seen in toxic multinodular goiter. Structural information may be obtained with physical examination and thyroid ultrasound (Figures 1.5 and 1.6). This should be correlated with functional data to ensure that another concurrent process such as thyroid cancer is not overlooked.

Although the cause of thyrotoxicosis can usually be determined by history, physical examination, and radionuclide studies, in unclear situations the measurement of circulating thyroid autoantibodies may be helpful. A low thyroglobulin level may be useful in differentiating thyrotoxicosis factitia from other etiologies.

Management/Treatment

Complications of untreated hyperthyroidism may include atrial fibrillation, cardiomyopathy, and osteoporosis. Regardless of the etiology of the thyrotoxicosis, beta-blockers, most commonly propranolol, may be used for heart rate control and symptomatic relief. Rate control is particularly important in individuals who have developed an arrhythmia or a rate-related cardiomyopathy. Once a euthyroid state is

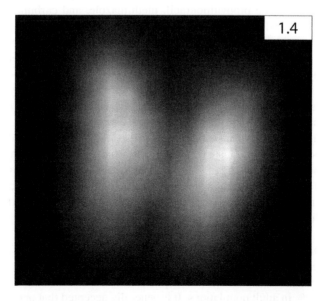

FIGURE 1.4 ^{123}I scan showing increased and homogenous uptake of radioiodine in Graves' disease.

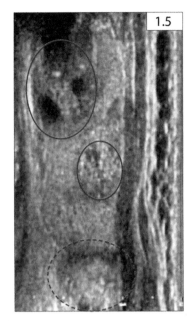

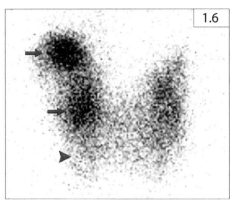

FIGURE 1.5–1.6   Right sagittal thyroid ultrasound ^{123}I scan correlation of Figure 1.5. The superior and middle nodules (circled) on ultrasound correlate with the areas of increased uptake on the scan (arrows) while the inferior nodule (dotted circle) corresponds to a relatively photopenic area and warrants further evaluation (arrowhead). (Courtesy of Dr. Susan Mandel.)

achieved, the beta-blocker is often stopped. Thyroiditis resulting in thyrotoxicosis is usually self-limiting and often requires no additional therapy, but does carry the potential for subsequent hypothyroidism. In cases of destructive thyroiditis such as amiodarone-induced thyrotoxicosis type 2, steroid therapy may be employed to decrease inflammation. Steroids can also inhibit conversion of T4 to T3.

Thionamides are the major class of drugs used in the treatment of thyrotoxicosis caused by Graves' disease or for usually brief periods in those with multinodular goiter and autonomous adenomas. Commonly utilized forms include propylthiouracil, methimazole, and carbimazole. These agents produce effective intrathyroidal iodine deficiency by inhibiting the oxidation and organic binding of thyroid iodine. Large doses of propylthiouracil may also impair the peripheral conversion of T4 to T3 by type 1 deiodinase. Since these agents inhibit the synthesis but not the release of hormones, they are not useful if there is thyroid hormone leakage from the gland without excess hormone production and also have a latent period before a clinical response is seen. Thionamides may cause hypothyroidism, particularly if given in excessive doses over longer periods of time. Potential adverse reactions include rash, arthralgia, myalgia, neuritis, agranulocytosis, hepatitis, ANCA-positive vasculitis (hepatitis and vasculitis are more common with propylthiouracil), cholestasis (which may also lead to hepatitis and is more common with methimazole), thrombocytopenia, and taste disturbance. Rash may occur in as many as 10% of patients, while agranulocytosis occurs in fewer than 1% of patients. Agranulocytosis most frequently, but not exclusively, occurs within the first few weeks or months of treatment and is often accompanied by fever and sore throat. Surgery or radioactive iodine may be considered for more definitive therapy depending upon the etiology, clinical situation, and patient preference.

Subclinical Hyperthyroidism
Subclinical hyperthyroidism is characterized by a subnormal serum TSH level and normal free T4 and T3. Subclinical hyperthyroidism is most often asymptomatic and discovered on screening. Several studies report a prevalence of <2% in adult populations. It is generally accepted that once a suppressed TSH with normal free T4 and T3 are detected, this should be reassessed, typically in 2–4 months, to determine if it

is persistent or transient, and that all patients with subclinical hyperthyroidism should undergo periodic clinical and laboratory assessment. Beyond this, there currently is no consensus as to the management of subclinical hyperthyroidism, but its treatment may be warranted in several subpopulations.

The three major concerns with subclinical hyperthyroidism are (1) progression to overt hyperthyroidism, (2) cardiac effects, and (3) skeletal effects. In individuals with subclinical hyperthyroidism attributable to nodular disease, there is a high rate of conversion to clinical hyperthyroidism and thus treatment is often considered in this population. In elderly individuals, subclinical hyperthyroidism increases the relative risk of atrial fibrillation threefold, and other adverse cardiac effects including impaired ventricular ejection fraction response to exercise have been reported. Prolonged subclinical hyperthyroidism may be associated with decreased bone mineral density, particularly in postmenopausal women. These risks are considered in developing an individualized treatment plan. In most other individuals, treatment may be unnecessary, and for individuals in which treatment is deferred, thyroid tests are typically performed every 6 months.

Graves' Disease

Definition/Overview

Graves' disease, or as it is known in parts of Europe, von Basedow's disease, is an autoimmune disorder in which stimulatory autoantibodies directed against the TSH receptor (TSHRAbs) result in TSH-independent stimulation of the thyroid gland causing production and secretion of thyroid hormone. Histologically, hyperplastic columnar epithelium is evident (Figure 1.7). Extrathyroidal manifestations may include ophthalmopathy, pretibial myxedema, and, rarely, thyroid acropathy. Thyroid enlargement with hormone excess is typical, but any of the components, thyroid disease, infiltrative orbitopathy and ophthalmopathy, or infiltrative dermopathy may occur and often run largely independent courses.

Epidemiology/Etiology

Graves' disease has an incidence of between 0.3 and 1.5 cases per 1,000 population per year with a female-to-male ratio of between 5 and 10 to 1. The typical age of presentation is between 30 and 60 years. Although it is by far the most common cause of hyperthyroidism in individuals younger than age 40, it is very uncommon in children under 10 years old. Smoking has been associated with a greater propensity to develop ophthalmopathy and the worsening of ophthalmopathy with antigen release after radioactive iodine therapy.

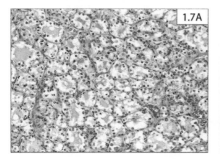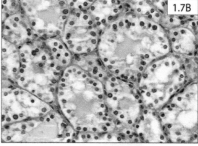

FIGURE 1.7 Graves' disease. (A) At lower power, hyperplastic columnar epithelium with increased infolding is noted. (B) At higher power, clear vacuoles in the colloid are evident with the increased activity of the epithelium from increased thyroid hormone production leading to scalloping of the colloid. (Courtesy of Dr. James Connolly.)

The thyroid component of Graves' disease is genetically related to autoimmune thyroiditis, particularly Hashimoto's disease, with both often occurring within the same families. The frequency of other autoimmune disorders including type 1 diabetes, pernicious anemia, myasthenia gravis, Addison's disease, Sjögren's syndrome, lupus erythematosus, rheumatoid arthritis, and idiopathic thrombocytopenic purpura is also increased in Graves' disease patients and their families. There have been reports that in susceptible individuals SARS-CoV-2 infection or vaccination may worsen or precipitate autoimmune thyroid disease.

Although the TSH receptor is the primary autoantigen of Graves' disease, autoantibodies against TPO and thyroglobulin are also common. Thyroid-directed T-cell-mediated autoimmunity can also be shown. Extrathyroidal TSH receptor messenger ribonucleic acid (mRNA) and receptor protein have been reported in many other tissues including retro-orbital adipocytes, muscle cells, and fibroblasts, and may play a role in the extrathyroidal manifestations not seen in other forms of thyrotoxicosis. The expression may trigger lymphocyte migration into affected tissues. TSHRAbs may be stimulating, blocking, or neutral. Stimulating TSHRAbs bind to the TSH receptor activating adenylate cyclase, inducing thyroid growth, increasing vascularity, and increasing thyroid hormone production and secretion. Changes in the balance between blocking and stimulating antibodies may lead to fluctuations in thyroid hormone levels.

Clinical Presentation

Most patients with Graves' disease have a diffuse goiter. The gland is frequently enlarged two to three times more than normal but may be much larger. This enlargement is usually symmetric and there is a smooth or lobular surface to the gland. The consistency of the gland may vary from soft to firm and rubbery, but is often more spongy than that seen in Hashimoto's disease. In more 'severe' cases, a bruit or thrill may be present with increased intrathyroidal blood flow, which is more common with a larger goiter.

Although thyroid-associated ophthalmopathy is closely associated with Graves' hyperthyroidism, either condition may exist without the other; it may predate (20%), coincide with (40%), or follow successful treatment of hyperthyroidism (40%). Thyroid-associated ophthalmopathy results from enlargement of the extraocular muscles and intraorbital fat with an increase in retro-ocular pressure, caused by lymphocytic infiltration, edema, and later fibrosis. This results in proptosis and impairment of extraocular muscle function. As a result, ophthalmoplegia, diplopia, chemosis, papilledema, or corneal ulceration may occur (Figures 1.8–1.12).

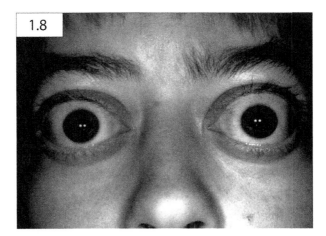

FIGURE 1.8 Normally, the upper lid is located 1–1.5 mm below the superior limbus, and the lower lid is located at the inferior limbus. This figure demonstrates upper lid retraction (Dalrymple sign) with temporal flare and scleral show in Graves' ophthalmopathy. (Courtesy of Dr. Richard Dallow.)

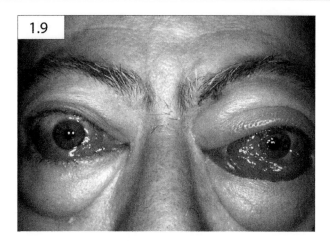

FIGURE 1.9   Marked periorbital edema and chemosis are demonstrated. (Courtesy of Dr. Richard Dallow.)

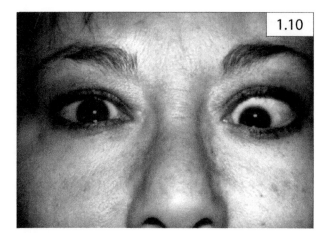

FIGURE 1.10   Ophthalmoplegia with downward gaze is shown. (Courtesy of Dr. Richard Dallow.)

Thyroid-associated dermopathy is seen in 5%–10% of patients with Graves' disease and is closely associated with ophthalmopathy. It is generally over the shin (pretibial myxedema) but can be seen over the toes, forehead, neck, or in areas of trauma (Figures 1.13 and 1.14). It presents as painless thickening of the skin in hyperpigmented nodules or plaques. Thyroid acropachy, (clubbing of the digits and periosteal bone formation) is seen in less than 1% of patients and is usually associated with longstanding disease (Figures 1.15–1.17). Almost all patients with acropachy also have thyroid-associated ophthalmopathy and dermopathy. Generalized lymphadenopathy, occasionally with splenic and thymic enlargement, may also be seen.

Differential Diagnosis

The diffuse goiter of Graves' disease may be confused with the goiter of other thyroid diseases but can often be differentiated based on laboratory studies or radioactive iodine uptake. Mild bilateral exophthalmos may be familial and also sometimes occurs in patients with Cushing's syndrome, cirrhosis, uremia, chronic obstructive pulmonary disease, or superior vena cava syndrome. Unilateral exophthalmos, even when associated with thyrotoxicosis, should raise consideration of another local cause, including orbital

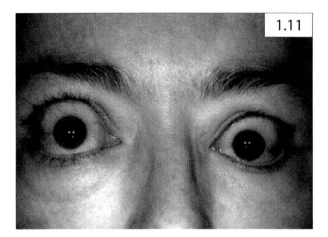

FIGURE 1.11   Lid retraction with proptosis and conjunctival injection is shown. (Courtesy of Dr. Richard Dallow.)

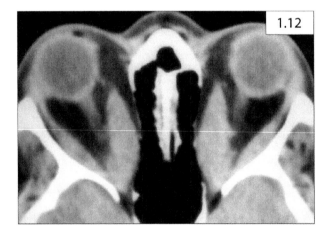

FIGURE 1.12   Orbital CT demonstrating the classic findings in Graves' ophthalmopathy with thickened recti muscles but sparing of the tendons. Exophthalmos with bilateral anterior displacement of the globes is also shown.

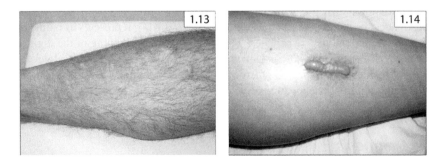

FIGURE 1.13–1.14   Skin changes. Subtle findings of pretibial myxedema with painless thickening of the skin over the shin are shown. (Courtesy of Dr. Pamela Hartzband.) Thyroid-associated dermopathy is evident as skin thickening after a skin biopsy. (Courtesy of Dr. Arturo Rolla.)

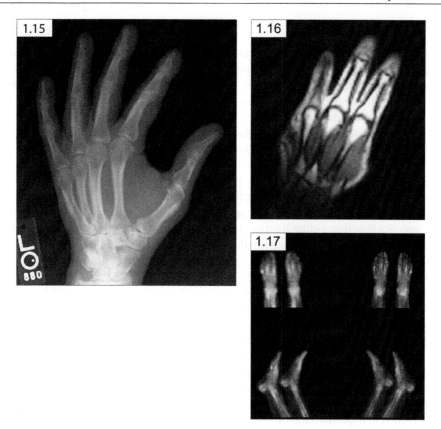

FIGURE 1.15–1.17   Thyroid acropachy. Thyroid acropachy is characterized by clubbing of the fingers and toes often with soft tissue swelling over the distal small joints. Soft tissue swelling with periosteal or endocortical thickening or subperiosteal reaction may be seen on radiographs. (Courtesy of Drs. A. Rolla and P. Hartzband.) Soft tissue swelling with periosteal or endocortical thickening or subperiosteal reaction seen on MRI. (Courtesy of Drs. A. Rolla and P. Hartzband.)   Soft tissue swelling with periosteal or endocortical thickening or subperiosteal reaction seen on bone scan. (Courtesy of Drs. A. Rolla and P. Hartzband.)

neoplasm, carotid–cavernous sinus fistulae, cavernous sinus thrombosis, orbital pseudotumor, or other infiltrative disorders.

Diagnosis/Investigations

Thyroid tests in Graves' disease are consistent with thyrotoxicosis, usually with a suppressed TSH and elevated free T4. Often there is a proportionally greater increase in T3 than T4 concentrations in Graves' disease (this can also be seen with autonomous nodules). If free T4 levels are unexpectedly normal, T3 should be measured to evaluate for T3 thyrotoxicosis.

Measurement of radioactive iodine uptake may be useful in differentiating Graves' disease, where uptake is inappropriately normal or high, from painless thyroiditis, where uptake is low during the thyrotoxic phase.

Measurement of TSHRAbs is usually not necessary in hyperthyroid patients with Graves' disease with an intact thyroid gland as thyrotoxicosis already serves as an internal bioassay of autoantibody activity. In individuals with possible euthyroid Graves' ophthalmopathy, measurement of TSHRAbs may aid in diagnosis, especially if eye findings are unilateral. Similarly, in pregnant women with a prior history of Graves' disease and thyroid ablation, who therefore do not have an internal bioassay of activity, maternal TSHRAbs may be useful in predicting neonatal thyrotoxicosis.

Management/Treatment

The mainstay of pharmacologic therapy for Graves' disease is the thionamides. As described in the thyrotoxicosis section, these drugs inhibit thyroid hormone production. Thionamide drugs may also directly decrease the autoimmunity in Graves' disease by both decreasing antigen expression and cytokine release from the thyroid as well as potential nonspecific immunosuppression leading to decreased lymphocytic infiltration and antigen presentation. Up to 40% of patients previously treated with thionamides remain euthyroid 10 years after discontinuation of antithyroid therapy. Individuals with persistently high levels of TSHRAbs or a T3 to T4 ratio of greater than 20 are more likely to relapse after cessation of antithyroidal drugs.

Radioactive iodine is often considered the preferred treatment for patients with Graves' disease in North America and is particularly attractive for those who have relapsed after discontinuation of antithyroid drugs, who would not tolerate a relapse, or are at increased risk of atrial fibrillation due to comorbid conditions or age. Radioactive iodine treatment is contraindicated in pregnant women and those who are breastfeeding. It can induce worsening ophthalmopathy, particularly in smokers, but this risk can be reduced with high-dose glucocorticoid therapy (for example, 30–40 mg of prednisone daily, with a taper over weeks to months).

Treatment regimens may vary from center to center and include administering either an ablative dose or a calculated smaller dose of radioiodine. If used, antithyroid drugs are stopped 3–4 days before radioiodine to allow for its effective uptake and may be resumed 3–4 days after in individuals at high risk for radiation thyroiditis. Since it is radioprotective, pretreatment with propylthiouracil is generally avoided or a higher dose of radioactive iodine is used at the time of treatment. Typically, a response is seen within 3 months, but since radioiodine may work slowly, it is usual to wait 6 months before giving another dose for persistent hyperthyroidism. By 1 year, permanent hypothyroidism occurs in the vast majority of those given high-dose radioiodine, while those given a lower dose may develop hypothyroidism later and are at higher risk for recurrent hyperthyroidism.

Subtotal thyroidectomy may be preferred in patients with a large goiter, a coexistent thyroid nodule not proven to be benign, or when rapid control is required such as therapy-resistant Graves' disease during pregnancy. Preferably, the patient is treated with antithyroidal agents until euthyroid and an appropriate beta-blockade are instituted. Inorganic iodide may be administered for 7–10 days prior to surgery to decrease the vascularity of the gland.

During pregnancy, TSHRAbs, blocking or stimulating, may cross the placenta and affect fetal thyroid function. Regular fetal monitoring for evidence of fetal thyrotoxicosis or goiter is therefore important in cases where the mother has a history of Graves' disease, whether or not there has been prior maternal thyroidectomy or ablation.

Treatment of Graves' ophthalmopathy, thyroid eye disease, may include applying cool compresses to the eyes or using lubricating eye drops or gel to help maintain moisture. Sunglasses may help protect the eyes from the sun and wind. Elevating the head of the bed may help reduce swelling and pressure on the eyes. The use of prisms may aid with double vision. Medical treatments include steroids or teprotumumab, an insulin-like growth factor-1 receptor antagonist antibody. Surgical treatments include surgical repositioning of the eyelid(s) to help reduce irritation, eye muscle surgery, and orbital decompression surgery.

Hypothyroidism

Definition

Hypothyroidism results from thyroid hormone deficiency in target tissues. Primary hypothyroidism is defined as decreased secretion of thyroid hormone by factors affecting the thyroid gland itself. Central hypothyroidism is due to factors interfering with TSH release from the pituitary (secondary hypothyroidism) or TRH release from the hypothalamus (tertiary hypothyroidism). In rare instances, thyroid hormone resistance may lead to hypothyroidism despite normal or elevated thyroid hormone levels. Hypothyroidism is a graded phenomenon, which in its most severe form can result in myxedema.

Epidemiology/Etiology

The most common causes of hypothyroidism are autoimmune thyroid disease, hypothyroidism after surgery, or radioactive iodine. Primary hypothyroidism is relatively common and affects 4%–8% of the general population. Hypothyroidism is much more common in women than men with a female-to-male ratio of up to 8–10 to 1. The mean age of diagnosis is mid-50s.

Central hypothyroidism is causal 1 in 20 to 1 in 200 individuals with hypothyroidism, frequently after damage to the hypothalamus or pituitary by tumor, trauma, or an infiltrative disease. Thyroid hormone resistance syndromes are seldom the cause of hypothyroidism with only approximately 1,000 registered patients worldwide. Hypothyroidism may also be caused by iodine deficiency (decreased substrate for synthesis) or transiently by iodine excess via the Wolff–Chaikoff effect (inhibition of iodide organification by inorganic iodide excess). Many drugs, including lithium, interferon, amiodarone, and antithyroid agents, may cause hypothyroidism. Rare causes of hypothyroidism include infiltrative diseases such as sarcoidosis, cystinosis, hemochromatosis, progressive systemic sclerosis, amyloidosis, Riedel's thyroiditis with fibrosis, infectious diseases, thyroid dysgenesis, and consumptive hypothyroidism (excessive type 3 iodothyronine deiodinase activity).

Clinical Presentation

The symptoms of hypothyroidism are often nonspecific and include fatigue, cold intolerance, depression, mild weight gain, weakness, joint aches, constipation, dry skin, hair loss, and menstrual irregularities. Common signs of moderate to severe hypothyroidism include diastolic hypertension, bradycardia, coarse hair, diffuse hair loss (especially the outer third of the eyebrows), dry brittle nails, periorbital swelling, carpal tunnel syndrome, and a delayed relaxation phase of deep tendon reflexes. Other less common presentations may include yellowing of the skin (carotenoderma), myxedema (pale, waxy, edematous skin without pitting), acropachy, ventricular arrhythmias, and congestive heart failure (particularly in association with underlying cardiac disease). Retarded growth and delayed bone age may be seen in hypothyroid children. In primary hypothyroidism, the thyroid usually has a firm consistency. Its size can be quite variable.

When myxedema coma occurs, it is usually in elderly patients with hypothyroidism and a superimposed precipitating event. Hypothermia, bradycardia, and hypoventilation are common. Ileus is usually present, and pericardial, pleural, and peritoneal effusions may be seen. Central nervous system (CNS) manifestations may include confusion, seizures, or coma.

Diagnosis/Investigations

TSH is elevated in individuals with primary gland failure but may be normal or low in individuals with central hypothyroidism. Although central hypothyroidism is relatively uncommon, the free T4 or T4 index should also be checked if this is suspected. Other laboratory findings associated with hypothyroidism may include normochromic, normocytic anemia or iron deficiency anemia in the setting of excessive menstrual bleeding, hyponatremia, hypercholesterolemia, and elevated creatine phosphokinase.

Management/Treatment

The standard treatment for hypothyroidism is thyroid hormone replacement, usually with oral levothyroxine (LT4). In primary hypothyroidism, therapy is titrated to a normal TSH (typical goals are 0.3–3.0 µIU/mL) unless otherwise indicated (for example, those with a history of thyroid cancer may have a lower

TSH goal). In an adult, the full replacement dose is often around 1.6 µg/kg/day. Elderly patients or those with known or suspected cardiac disease are often started on lower doses of LT4 (typically 25 µg/day) and increased slowly until TSH is normal. In central hypothyroidism, trough free T4 or T4 index levels should be followed instead and therapy adjusted as needed to keep troughs in the middle of the normal range. Since the bioavailability of different thyroid hormone brand name preparations are often not equivalent, brand changes should not be made without retitrating the dose. Even if a bioequivalent substitution is made, consider rechecking the TSH in 8 weeks. In general, it takes 6–8 weeks for TSH levels to reach equilibrium after a dose adjustment.

If myxedema coma is diagnosed or suspected, the treatment includes rapid repletion of thyroid hormone deficit, stress doses of glucocorticoids (at least until adrenal function can be evaluated), and treatment of any precipitants. Initially, treatment with intravenous levothyroxine is usually employed, as absorption may be variable in the setting of associated gut edema. An intravenous loading dose of 200–500 µg of levothyroxine is commonly recommended, followed by daily intravenous administration of 50–100 µg. Lower daily doses are used in elderly patients and for those in whom myocardial ischemia is likely. The role of intravenous T3 remains controversial and is usually reserved for individuals with low cardiovascular risk with some practitioners advocating additional intravenous T3 at 10 µg every 8 hours for such patients.

Untreated or inadequately treated hypothyroidism during pregnancy may increase maternal and fetal complications including fetal death. Even mild, asymptomatic maternal hypothyroidism may affect the cognitive function of the offspring. TSH measurement should be performed before pregnancy or as early as possible during the first trimester for those with known thyroid disease. Since thyroid hormone requirements often increase during the first and second trimesters of pregnancy, in women with known hypothyroidism one strategy has been to increase thyroid hormone dose by about 30% when pregnancy is confirmed and then to follow the serum TSH level every 6 weeks during pregnancy to ensure that the requirement for levothyroxine has not changed.

Subclinical Hypothyroidism
Subclinical hypothyroidism is characterized by a mildly increased TSH in the setting of normal free T4 and T3. Subclinical hypothyroidism is most often asymptomatic and discovered on screening. The prevalence has been estimated at between 1% and 10% of the adult population.

The major concerns with subclinical hypothyroidism are (1) progression to overt hypothyroidism, (2) cardiovascular effects, (3) hyperlipidemia, and (4) neuropsychiatric effects. Individuals with TSH levels >10 µIU/mL or with TSH levels between 5 and 10 µIU/mL and goiter and/or positive antithyroid peroxidase antibodies have the highest rates of progression to overt hypothyroidism and are therefore often treated with levothyroxine. Beyond this, treatment of subclinical hypothyroidism remains controversial.

Thyroiditis

Thyroiditis rather broadly refers to inflammation of the thyroid gland and comprises a large group of diverse conditions. Since these disorders may be grouped in various ways and there may be multiple names for the same conditions, these conditions may at first seem confusing. Many of the commonly used names are listed in Table 1.2; the major syndromes are described in the following and summarized in Table 1.3.

In postpartum thyroiditis, painless thyroiditis, and subacute thyroiditis, inflammatory destruction of the thyroid may lead to transient thyrotoxicosis, as preformed thyroid hormone is released from the damaged gland. Due to the destructive nature of these processes, thyrotoxicosis may be preceded by a significant increase in serum thyroglobulin. Reflecting the ratio of stored hormone in the gland, serum T4 concentrations are often elevated proportionally higher than T3 concentrations in contrast to Graves' disease or autonomous adenomas in which T3 may be preferentially elevated. As thyroid hormone stores

TABLE 1.2 Forms of Thyroiditis

TYPE	OTHER NAMES OR SUBTYPES
Hashimoto's thyroiditis	Chronic lymphocytic thyroiditis, chronic autoimmune thyroiditis, lymphadenoid goiter, struma lymphomatosa
Postpartum thyroiditis	Painless postpartum thyroiditis, subacute lymphocytic thyroiditis
Silent thyroiditis	Painless (sporadic) thyroiditis, subacute lymphocytic thyroiditis
Subacute thyroiditis	Painful subacute thyroiditis, de Quervain's thyroiditis (subacute) granulomatous thyroiditis, giant cell thyroiditis
Suppurative thyroiditis	Infectious thyroiditis, pyogenic thyroiditis, bacterial thyroiditis, acute (suppurative) thyroiditis
Riedel's thyroiditis	Reidel's struma
Thyroiditis	Fibrous thyroiditis
Drug-induced	Amiodarone, lithium, interferon-alpha, interleukin 2, sunitinib, checkpoint inhibitors
Other	Radiation-induced, traumatic

are depleted and destruction continues, there may be progression to overt hypothyroidism. Hashimoto's thyroiditis, painless thyroiditis, and postpartum thyroiditis all have an autoimmune basis.

Hashimoto's Thyroiditis

Hashimoto's thyroiditis often begins clinically with gradual enlargement of the thyroid gland and eventual development of hypothyroidism. If untreated, the goiter may slowly increase in size. The goiter is diffuse and firm with the gland variably being normal to four times the normal size at diagnosis. Associated pain and tenderness are unusual but may be present. In addition to the symptoms of hypothyroidism, about one-quarter of patients with Hashimoto's thyroiditis develop other musculoskeletal complaints including chest pain, fibrositis, or arthritis.

Antithyroid autoantibodies are detectable in more than 95% of patients with Hashimoto's thyroiditis, with high serum TPO antibodies present in 90% of patients and high serum thyroglobulin antibodies detectable in 50%–80% of patients. Elevated antibodies may also be detected in 5%–15% of the general population, the majority of whom have normal thyroid function. The ultrasound appearance of the gland is remarkable for a heterogeneous echotexture often with multiple ill-defined hypoechoic patches or pseudonodules. Histology often reveals lymphocytic infiltration with germinal center formation and fibrosis (Figure 1.18). A radioactive iodine (RAI) scan contributes little to the diagnosis. Uptake may be low, normal, or elevated with an irregular pattern.

With the institution of LT4 treatment, goiter size often decreases within months, whether the patient is euthyroid or hypothyroid. This is especially true in younger individuals, as there is likely less fibrosis present. If the goiter is small and the patient is euthyroid and asymptomatic, no treatment is required. Although controversial, some physicians consider therapy if the TSH is elevated and free T4 is normal since the eventual onset of hypothyroidism is likely in such patients (estimated at 2%–5% per year). Antibody levels may spontaneously dissipate and up to 20% of initially hypothyroid patients will later recover and have normal thyroid function if thyroid hormone withdrawal is attempted.

Postpartum and Painless Thyroiditis

Postpartum thyroiditis is most common in women with a high serum TPO antibody concentration in the first trimester of pregnancy or immediately after delivery. Women with type 1 diabetes are at particular risk with up to 25% developing postpartum thyroiditis. Thyrotoxicosis typically is noted by 3–4 months after delivery and lasts 1–2 months. This may be followed by a hypothyroid phase lasting 4–6 months.

TABLE 1.3 Overview of Thyroiditis Syndromes

CHARACTERISTIC	HASHIMOTO'S THYROIDITIS	POSTPARTUM THYROIDITIS	SILENT THYROIDITIS	SUBACUTE THYROIDITIS	SUPPURATIVE THYROIDITIS	RIEDEL'S THYROIDITIS
Thyroid pain	No	No	No	Yes	Yes	No
Typical neck exam	Firm symmetric goiter	Small, nontender gland	Small, nontender gland	Tender and swollen gland	Tender thyroid mass	Rock-hard, fixed, painless gland
Sex ratio (F:M)	8–15:1	—	2:1	5:1	1:1	3–4:1
Cause	Autoimmune	Autoimmune	Autoimmune	? Viral	Infectious	Unknown
Associations	HLA DR3, DR4, DR5	HLA DR3, DR5	HLA DR3	HLA Bw-35	Pre-existing thyroid disease immune-compromised; structural abnormalities	Systemic fibrosis; hypoparathyroidism from fibrosis
Temporal course	Chronic	Episodic: 70% recurrence with pregnancy	Episodic: recurrence rate unknown	Episodic: <2%–4% recurrence rate	May be fatal if untreated	Progressive
ESR	Normal	Normal	Normal	Elevated	Elevated	Normal
TPO antibodies	Elevated	Elevated	Elevated	Transient mild increase	Absent	Elevated in 2/3 of patients
Thyroid hormonal status	Hypothyroid or euthyroid	Thyrotoxic, hypothyroid, or both	Thyrotoxic, hypothyroid, or both	Thyrotoxic, hypothyroid, or both	Usually euthyroid	Euthyroid but may progress to hypothyroid
Histology	Lymphocytic infiltrate, germinal centers, fibrosis	Lymphocytic infiltrate	Lymphocytic infiltrate	Giant cells, granulomas	Abscess	Dense fibrosis
Typical treatments	Levothyroxine or observation	Observation/ variable	Observation/ variable	NSAIDs or glucocorticoids	Surgical abscess drainage and antibiotics	Surgery, glucocorticoids, tamoxifen, methotrexate

NSAID, nonsteroidal anti-inflammatory drug.

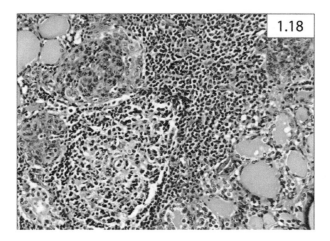

FIGURE 1.18 Hashimoto's thyroiditis. There is a profuse mononuclear infiltrate with germinal center formation. Thyroid follicles are small and reduced in number. (Courtesy of Dr. Tad Wieczorek.)

There is recovery of normal thyroid function within a year in 80% of women; however, 50% of affected women develop chronic hypothyroidism within 7 years. There is about a 70% chance of recurrence with subsequent pregnancies.

Other than the lack of a temporal relationship with pregnancy, the presentation and clinical course of painless thyroiditis are similar to that of postpartum thyroiditis. About 50% of individuals with painless thyroiditis will have a small, firm, nontender gland, and about 20% of affected individuals will develop chronic hypothyroidism. An elevated serum TPO antibody titer is detectable in about 50% of individuals with painless thyroiditis at the time of presentation. The titers are on average lower than those seen in Hashimoto's thyroiditis but cannot be used to distinguish the two on an individual basis. A low or undetectable radioactive iodine uptake (RAIU) can usually differentiate thyroiditis from other forms of thyrotoxicosis with suppressed TSH; however, during the recovery phase of thyroiditis, RAIU may be normal or elevated and can be potentially misleading if not correlated with TSH and thyroid hormone levels. On ultrasound, the gland is usually hypoechogenic with normal to low vascularity. Histology is remarkable for a lymphocytic infiltrate.

If thyrotoxicosis is present, beta-blockers may be used for symptomatic relief. Since there is not an actual increase in thyroid hormone production but instead a release of thyroid hormone with damage to the gland, thionamides should not be used. If chronic hypothyroidism develops, LT4 therapy may be required. Transient hypothyroidism usually does not require additional therapy.

Painful Subacute Thyroiditis

Subacute thyroiditis frequently follows a viral upper respiratory tract infection or sore throat and begins with a prodrome of generalized myalgia, pharyngitis, low-grade fever, and fatigue. Mumps, influenza, COVID-19 (SARS-CoV-2), and other viral infections have been implicated. Interestingly, subacute thyroiditis has also been reported after vaccination for SARS-CoV-2 or influenza. With the development of subacute thyroiditis, fever and severe neck pain often with swelling are noted. Approximately half of affected individuals develop symptomatic thyrotoxicosis, which may last several weeks, and hypothyroidism may subsequently develop. Five percent of patients develop chronic hypothyroidism, usually mild, while the rest have normalization over 6–12 months. The recurrence rate is estimated to be between 2% and 4%. On histology and cytology, giant cells and granulomas may be seen (Figure 1.19). As SARS-CoV-2 has been identified as a potential viral trigger, checking for SARS-CoV-2 infection should be considered in patients with subacute thyroiditis.

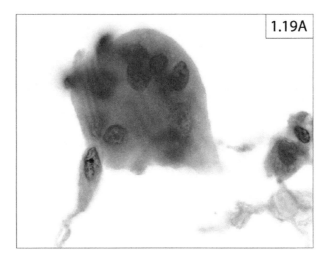

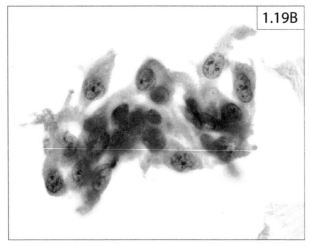

FIGURE 1.19   Subacute thyroiditis cytology. (A) Giant cell; (B) granuloma. (Courtesy of Dr. Tad Wieczorek.)

The treatment for painful subacute thyroiditis is designed to provide symptomatic relief. Nonsteroidal anti-inflammatory agents can frequently be used to control mild thyroid pain. For more severe pain or significant thyrotoxicosis, high-dose glucocorticoids (prednisone 40 mg/day) can provide relief and are usually tapered over 4–6 weeks.

Suppurative Thyroiditis

The thyroid gland is normally highly resistant to infection. This has been attributed to its location and encapsulation, high vascularity, high iodide content, the generation of hydrogen peroxide during synthesis of thyroid hormone, and extensive lymphatic drainage. Suppurative thyroiditis is most likely to occur in individuals with congenital anomalies such as a pyriform sinus fistula or persistent thyroglossal duct, those with preexisting thyroid disease such as a degenerating thyroid nodule, or those who are otherwise immunocompromised or debilitated including individuals with acquired immunodeficiency syndrome (AIDS) or cancer.

Patients with suppurative bacterial thyroiditis usually present with fever, dysphagia, dysphonia, anterior neck pain, and local lymphadenopathy, and have a tender erythematous thyroid mass. The patient is very uncomfortable and may sit with a flexed neck to avoid pressure on the thyroid. In children, suppurative thyroiditis affecting the left lobe of the thyroid is most commonly a result of direct extension from a pyriform sinus fistula (this tract rarely develops on the right), while a midline infection raises the possibility of a persistent thyroglossal duct. In adults, symptoms may not be as obvious as in children and they may instead present with a vague, slightly painful mass in the thyroid region, often without fever. This presentation is more common with fungal infections, parasitic infections, and mycobacterial thyroiditis. Fine needle aspiration (FNA) under ultrasound guidance with gram's stain and culture is the diagnostic test of choice when suppurative thyroiditis is suspected and may also provide therapeutic drainage. Treatment includes surgical drainage and appropriate antibiotics.

Reidel's Thyroiditis

Patients with Reidel's thyroiditis often present with a painless, extremely hard, fixed goiter that is often described as 'rock-hard' or 'wood-like'; malignancy is often initially suspected. They may have dyspnea, hoarseness, aphonia, or dysphagia from tracheal or esophageal compression. Most patients are initially euthyroid at presentation, and the disease may remain stable over many years or progress slowly to hypothyroidism. Hypoparathyroidism from fibrosis of adjacent parathyroid glands may also be present.

An open biopsy is usually required to diagnose Reidel's thyroiditis. The firmness of the gland and paucity of thyroid follicular cells often leads to an inadequate FNA biopsy. For this reason and to differentiate from the fibrotic changes associated with anaplastic thyroid carcinoma, a surgical biopsy is preferred for diagnosis.

The management of Reidel's thyroiditis depends upon the clinical features of the disease and has been largely empiric. In more advanced cases, surgical intervention may be required to relieve compression. With less advanced disease, corticosteroids and tamoxifen have both been used successfully, either alone or in combination. Steroids may reduce inflammation and decrease the actions of fibrinogenic cytokines, while it is believed that the response to tamoxifen is due to the inhibition of fibroblast proliferation by transforming growth factor (TGF)-beta as opposed to antiestrogen effects. Methotrexate is usually reserved for those with progressive Reidel's thyroiditis not responsive to other therapies. Since one-third of patients with Reidel's thyroiditis will develop an extracervical manifestation of multifocal fibrosclerosis such as retroperitoneal fibrosis, mediastinal fibrosis, or sclerosing cholangitis, screening for these other conditions should also be considered.

Drug-Induced Thyroiditis

A number of drugs, including amiodarone, interferon-alpha, lithium, and interleukin-2 (IL-2), can cause thyroiditis, which may present with hypothyroidism or thyrotoxicosis. Interferon-alpha and IL-2 have both been associated with painless lymphocytic thyroiditis. This is likely through an enhancement of underlying autoimmune processes, as induction of and increased anti-TPO antibody titers have been detected with exposure.

Tyrosine kinase inhibitors, especially sunitinib, may cause a destructive thyroiditis. Immune checkpoint inhibitors are also associated with thyroiditis. PD-1 inhibitors are associated with greater risk of thyroid dysfunction relative to CTLA-4 inhibitors, although the highest risk occurs with combined anti-CTLA-4 and anti-PD-1 treatment.

Lithium and amiodarone cause thyroid dysfunction via multiple different mechanisms. For example, amiodarone can cause iodine-induced disease or a destructive thyroiditis (Table 1.4). For differentiating between types 1 and 2 amiodarone-induced thyrotoxicosis, RAIU, IL-6 levels, and Doppler ultrasound for vascularity have all been proposed, but in clinical practice, it often remains difficult to distinguish between the two. As such, some clinicians treat both concurrently using a combination of thionamide and steroids. Those with type 2 disease typically have a more rapid response to this strategy than those with type 1 disease, allowing tailoring of therapy to the underlying etiology based upon response. Thyroidectomy may be advisable for some patients.

TABLE 1.4 Amiodarone-Induced Thyroid Dysfunction

	TYPE 1	TYPE 2	HYPOTHYROID
Mechanism	Iodine excess	Destructive thyroiditis	Iodine excess
Presentation	Thyrotoxicosis	Thyrotoxicosis	Hypothyroidism
Thyroid antibodies	Absent or present	Usually initially absent	Often present
RAI uptake	Low in iodine-sufficient areas Variable in iodine-deficient areas	<5%	Low in iodine-sufficient areas
Doppler ultrasound	Hypervascular	Reduced blood flow	Variable
IL-6	Normal to mild elevation	Markedly elevated	Normal
Preferred treatment	Thionamides (possible potassium perchlorate and/or surgery)	Glucocorticoids	Levothyroxine

Thyroid Nodules

Definition/Overview

Although the normal thyroid gland is fairly homogeneous, nodules are not infrequent with about 5% of women and 1% of men in iodine-sufficient areas having palpable thyroid nodules. In autopsy series, thyroid nodules are detected in 19%–67% of the population, with higher frequencies noted in women and the elderly. The main clinical concern with thyroid nodules is that of thyroid cancer, which occurs in 5%–10% of nodules, although it is estimated that only 1 in 15 cases of thyroid cancer are diagnosed premortem.

Approximately 1 in 10 to 1 in 20 solitary nodules are autonomous, with this being more common in Europe than in the USA. Thyrotoxicity is related to the amount of autonomous tissue and is more common in nodules over 3 cm in diameter. In some individuals, multiple autonomous nodules may be present, and such a toxic adenomatous goiter is sometimes referred to as Plummer's disease.

Clinical Presentation

Thyroid nodules are often asymptomatic, and it is not unusual for them to go unrecognized by the patient, instead being noted by an acquaintance or family member, on routine examination, or incidentally on an unrelated radiologic study. When patients identify nodules themselves, it is often in the setting of increased awareness of the neck such as after a sore throat or cough. Occasionally, a painful, rapid expansion may be seen, which may be due to acute hemorrhage.

Large goiters, particularly those with substernal components, may cause venous congestion or tracheal compression (Figures 1.20–1.22). Patients may present with difficulty breathing, particularly when lying flat, or experience a feeling of worsening asthma symptoms. Patients with venous congestion may note facial fullness when they extend their arms above their head, referred to as Pemberton's sign (Figures 1.23 and 1.24). Pemberton's sign is caused by clavicular motion during arm elevation that compresses major venous structures within a narrowed thoracic inlet against a relatively fixed and enlarged thyroid, much like the movement of a nutcracker (Figure 1.25).

Patients with toxic adenomas may not have thyrotoxic symptoms at presentation. Those with symptomatic toxic adenomas tend to be older than individuals with Graves' disease, and the onset of thyrotoxicosis is generally slower than in Graves' patients. When autonomy is longstanding, the normal thyroid tissue that surrounds the nodule is often atrophic.

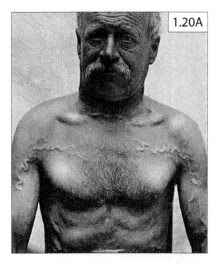
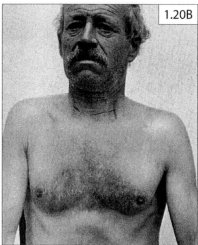

FIGURE 1.20   (A) A man with retrosternal goiter causing venous congestion. (B) Six months after resection, venous congestion has resolved. (From *Le Goitre* by F. de Quervain, 1923.)

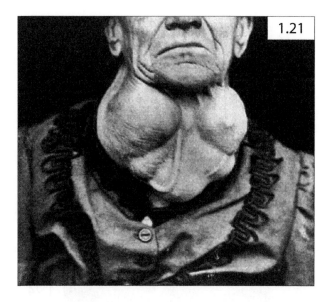

FIGURE 1.21   Goiter with multiple visible thyroid nodules. (From *Le Goitre* by F. de Quervain, 1923.)

Differential Diagnosis

The differential of thyroid mass is quite broad, as adenomas, carcinomas, thyroid cysts, hemiagenesis, thyroiditis, parathyroid lesions (including cysts, adenomas, and carcinomas), thyroid sarcoma, thyroid lymphoma, and metastatic cancer may also present as a thyroid mass on exam or ultrasound.

Diagnosis/Investigations

Current diagnostic algorithms in the evaluation of thyroid nodules focus on the risk of malignancy, evidence of autonomy, and symptoms of compression or obstruction. Factors that increase the likelihood of thyroid malignancy include age younger than 20 or older than 60 years, prior exposure to ionizing

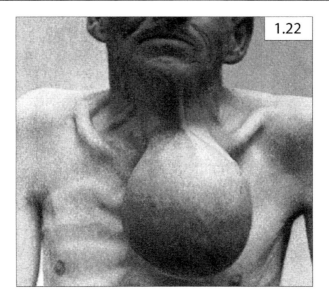

FIGURE 1.22 Large pendulous cystic nodule. (From *Le Goitre* by F. de Quervain, 1923.)

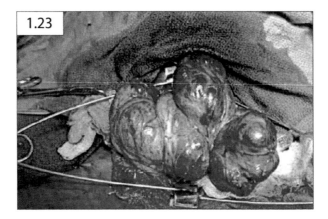

FIGURE 1.23 The goiter is shown exposed during resection. (Courtesy of Dr. Sareh Parangi.)

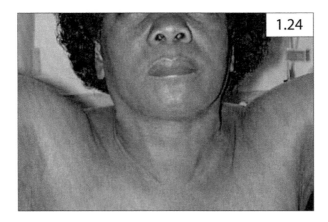

FIGURE 1.24 Goiter. On physical exam there is venous engorgement with arms raised above the head (Pemberton's sign). (Courtesy of Dr. Sareh Parangi.)

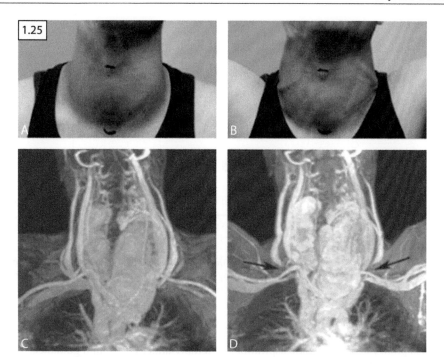

FIGURE 1.25 Pemberton's sign: Caused by clavicular motion during arm elevation that compresses major venous structures within a narrowed thoracic inlet against a relatively fixed and enlarged thyroid. (From Werner & Ingbar's *The Thyroid: A Fundamental and Clinical Text*, 11th Edition, 2021 (Wolters Kluwer), Page 261, Figure 16-2.)

radiation to the head or neck, family history of medullary or papillary thyroid cancer, and stigmata or family history of familial predisposing syndromes such as Gardner's syndrome (colonic polyps, osteomas, and soft tissue tumors), Carney complex (cardiac myxomas and spotty pigmentation), and Cowden's syndrome (hamartomas and neoplasia). Physical findings suggestive of malignancy include a hard, nontender nodule, fixed to adjacent tissue, and local lymphadenopathy.

Serum TSH should be measured in all patients with nodular disease. In most instances, serum TSH is normal and then further diagnostic evaluation is performed with ultrasound and FNA biopsy. If the TSH is low, isotopic scanning with ^{131}I or ^{123}I is often performed to determine if there is evidence of autonomy. Although not commonly performed, if the TSH is not suppressed but there is a high index of suspicion for autonomy, exogenous thyroid hormone can be administered prior to imaging to demonstrate nonsuppressibility (Figure 1.26). Nodules that exhibit evidence of autonomous function have a low risk of malignancy, although there have been reports of malignancy in autonomous nodules, particularly in those found to be a follicular variant of papillary cancer.

Thyroid ultrasound can be used as an adjunct to physical examination for screening high-risk individuals (for example, those with hereditary syndromes or prior radiation exposure), or for guidance of FNA. Ultrasonography more accurately detects the presence, location, and size of nodules within the thyroid gland than examination alone, as 40%–60% of thyroid nodules between 1 and 2 cm in diameter are not palpable on examination. Thyroid ultrasound can provide information including consistency, echogenicity, patterns of calcification, and Doppler blood flow. Nodules that are principally solid, hypoechoic, have irregular margins, contain microcalcifications, lack a halo, are taller than wide, or have increased vascular flow are of more concern for malignancy, but ultrasound characteristics alone are usually not sensitive or specific enough for diagnostic purposes.

FNA biopsy is considered the most accurate test (diagnostic accuracy exceeding 90%) for the diagnosis of thyroid nodules. Biopsy is usually performed with a 27- or 25-gauge needle with sampling

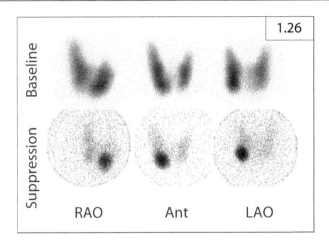

FIGURE 1.26 Thyroid scintigraphy (suppression scan). RAO, anterior, and LAO views are shown. In the top panel, ^{123}I thyroid scintigraphy shows iodine uptake by the thyroid. In the lower panel, after treatment with exogenous thyroid hormone, an autonomous area becomes apparent in the right inferior portion of the gland as the normal surrounding tissue is suppressed.

performed via capillary action or gentle aspiration, preferably under ultrasound guidance. Typical thyroid cytology findings include thyroid epithelial cells arranged in macrofollicles (Figure 1.27A) and microfollicles (Figure 1.27B). FNA results are usually categorized into one of the following diagnostic categories: benign (negative), suspicious (indeterminate), malignant (positive), or unsatisfactory (nondiagnostic or insufficient). Although follicular neoplasm (microfollicular lesion) can be diagnosed by cytology, the distinction between follicular adenoma and carcinoma requires pathologic evaluation of a surgical specimen.

Since it is difficult to differentiate between thyroid and parathyroid tissue on FNA, if it is unclear on ultrasound if the area is a thyroid nodule or parathyroid adenoma, then the serum calcium should be checked and the aspirate evaluated for parathyroid hormone on washout. Parathyroid adenomas are typically extrathyroidal and hypoechoic on ultrasound. If the fluid removed from a cyst is clear and waterlike, then it may be a parathyroid cyst. The diagnosis can be confirmed by analyzing the fluid for parathyroid hormone level; although it is infrequent for parathyroid cysts to cause hyperparathyroidism, serum calcium should still be checked in this setting.

Although more expensive than ultrasound, computed tomography (CT) or magnetic resonance imaging (MRI) can help evaluate substernal goiters and define the relationship of nodules to surrounding structures. This is most helpful if there is evidence of venous obstruction or difficulty breathing. Chest X-ray, barium swallow, and pulmonary function tests with flow volume loop may also be used to determine the extent of obstruction.

Management/Treatment

Nodules with malignant or indeterminate aspirates are usually treated surgically with the extent of surgery and follow-up therapy, if any, based on the clinical situation. Various surgical specimens are shown in Figures 1.28–1.31. Obstructive goiters are generally treated surgically, although radioactive iodine treatment has been used in a limited fashion. Autonomous nodules without TSH suppression are often observed and may involute, stay the same, or grow. Once there is evidence of thyrotoxicosis, autonomous nodules are generally treated with radioiodine or surgery.

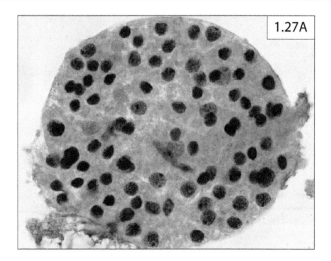

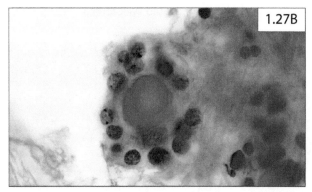

FIGURE 1.27   (A) Macrofollicle. (B) Microfollicle. (Courtesy of Dr. Tad Wieczorek.)

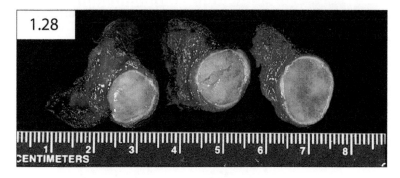

FIGURE 1.28   Papillary carcinoma. (Courtesy of Dr. Tad Wieczorek.)

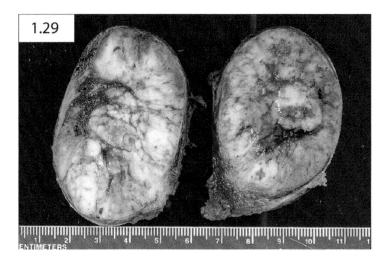

FIGURE 1.29 Follicular carcinoma. (Courtesy of Dr. Tad Wieczorek.)

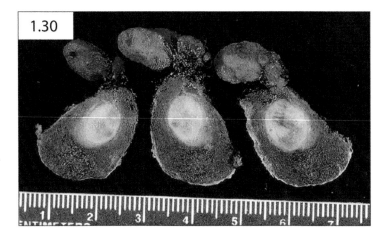

FIGURE 1.30 Follicular adenoma. (Courtesy of Dr. Tad Wieczorek.)

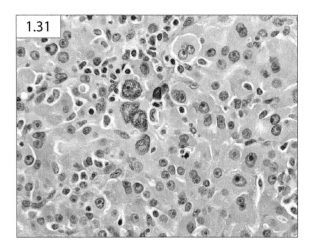

FIGURE 1.31 Anaplastic carcinoma histology. (Courtesy of Dr. Tad Wieczorek.)

THYROID CANCER

Louis G. Portugal and Alexander J. Langerman

Definition/Overview

In the USA, there are approximately 40,000 new cases of thyroid cancer diagnosed yearly, about 2% of all malignancies, although this rate has been increasing due in part to more sensitive diagnostic methods resulting in earlier diagnosis. Fortunately, thyroid cancer is a very treatable disease, with only 1,500 disease-specific deaths occurring per year. Females are three times more likely to present with a thyroid nodule to be evaluated for cancer, but a thyroid nodule in a male is more suspicious for malignancy. A history of radiation exposure or positive family history, as well as physical examination findings, such as associated lymphadenopathy, also increase the likelihood of cancer. Even though most thyroid nodules encountered by clinicians will be benign, a prompt workup is necessary to ensure early and appropriate treatment can be instituted for those with malignancy.

Etiology

The primary risk factors for thyroid carcinoma are a family history of thyroid cancer or related genetic syndromes and a personal history of radiation exposure. In the 1940s and 1950s, low-dose irradiation was commonly used to treat acne, adenotonsillar hypertrophy, thymus enlargement, and other conditions. As reports of childhood thyroid cancer emerged, the practice was largely abandoned. Any patient with a history of radiation to the face, neck, or chest is at increased risk of developing thyroid neoplasms. Patients with this type of radiation exposure have up to a 50% chance of harboring cancer in a thyroid nodule and have a higher chance of cervical metastasis. The most common histology of postradiation thyroid cancer is papillary.

In 1986, a reactor at the nuclear power plant in Chernobyl suffered a meltdown and explosion resulting in extensive radiation exposure to the surrounding area. Located in the northern part of what is now Ukraine, Chernobyl is close to the Ukraine–Belarus border and Belarus actually received the majority of the fallout. In the months following the explosion, radioactivity was detected as far away as the United Kingdom. Local children exposed to the fallout had a 60-fold increase in thyroid carcinoma. A connection has been made between exposure to this disaster and a particular gene rearrangement (RET/PTC) in papillary thyroid cancers.

The full spectrum of genetic abnormalities resulting in thyroid cancer is actively being investigated. Certain familial syndromes such as Gardner's (autosomal dominant syndrome of colonic polyps, osteomas, and soft tissue tumors) and Cowden's (autosomal dominant syndrome of multiple hamartomas) are associated with well-differentiated thyroid cancer. The multiple endocrine neoplasia syndromes IIA and IIB are associated with medullary thyroid cancer.

Pathophysiology

The pathophysiology of thyroid cancer is influenced by the specific histologic diagnosis.

Well-Differentiated Thyroid Cancer

Papillary Thyroid Cancer

Papillary thyroid cancer (PTC) is the most common histology, accounting for 80% of all thyroid cancers. It has a bimodal distribution with peaks in the 20s–30s and 50–60s. PTC has a propensity for lymphatic spread, and up to 80% of patients can present with microscopic disease in the lymph nodes. Indeed, the finding of cystic or calcified cervical lymph nodes should raise immediate suspicion for PTC. There is also a high incidence of multicentricity within the thyroid with up to 80% of thyroidectomy specimens demonstrating additional foci of PTC in the contralateral lobe.

Histologically, PTC is made of malignant epithelium usually forming papillae with characteristic nuclear clearing ('Orphan Annie eyes') and intranuclear inclusions and grooves (Figure 1.32). Concentric calcifications called psammoma bodies are seen in roughly half of specimens. Other histologic variations include the follicular type, whose behavior is more similar to follicular cell carcinoma, a diffuse sclerosing type with a lack of papillae but many psammoma bodies, and the more clinically aggressive tall and columnar cell types.

Although there are no pathognomonic ultrasound findings, PTC is usually hypodense to surrounding thyroid tissue and can be partially or entirely cystic (Figure 1.33). Microcalcifications, or eggshell-like peripheral calcifications, while present in some benign processes, increase with the likelihood of PTC. FNA is highly sensitive and specific for PTC (Figure 1.33), and most patients will proceed to surgery knowing their diagnosis ahead of time (Figures 1.34–1.40).

Noninvasive follicular thyroid neoplasm with papillary-like nuclear features (NIFTP) is the term now used for noninvasive encapsulated follicular variant of papillary thyroid carcinoma (EFVPTC). It is now considered indolent or premalignant. Surgical excision is required for diagnosis and therapy, but total thyroidectomy and radioactive iodine therapy are not.

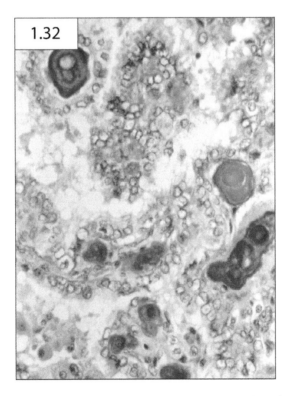

FIGURE 1.32 Histology of papillary thyroid cancer demonstrating central nuclear clearing (Orphan Annie eyes) and psammoma bodies.

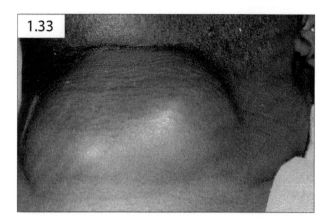

FIGURE 1.33 Patient with papillary thyroid cancer of the thyroid isthmus presenting as an invasive anterior neck mass that is firm and minimally mobile on physical exam.

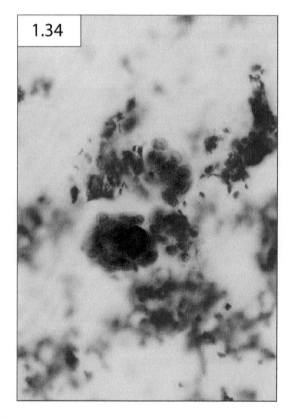

FIGURE 1.34 Cytology from fine needle aspiration biopsy of a thyroid mass demonstrating papillary fronds consistent with papillary thyroid cancer.

Follicular Cell Cancer

In most regions, follicular cell carcinoma represents 5%–15% of all thyroid cancers. This increases to 40% in areas that are endemic for goiter from iodine deficiency. The median age at diagnosis is 50. Follicular cancer tends to spread hematogenously, with 10%–15% of patients presenting with systemic metastasis, with lung being the most common site, followed by bone, liver, brain, and other sites. These are iodine-avid tumors, with three-quarters able to concentrate iodine.

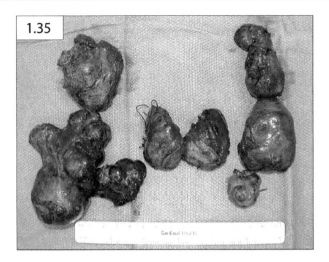

FIGURE 1.35 Surgical specimen of a total thyroidectomy (specimen in center) surrounded by bilateral neck dissections demonstrating a metastatic papillary thyroid cancer that extensively involved both jugular lymph node chains. This demonstrates the potential for thyroid cancer to present primarily with cervical metastasis with minimal clinical changes in the thyroid gland.

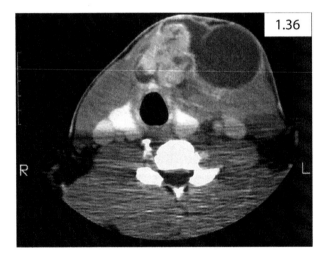

FIGURE 1.36 Axial CT scan of a patient demonstrating the growth pattern of papillary thyroid cancer arising from the isthmus and invading the strap muscles anteriorly.

For most follicular cancers, FNA can only make the diagnosis of a follicular lesion. The diagnosis of cancer relies on features detected during permanent sectioning, namely, extracapsular spread or vascular invasion (Figure 1.41). If a follicular lesion presents with local extrathyroid spread or regional or distant metastasis, a preoperative diagnosis of follicular cancer can more assuredly be made. Minimally invasive follicular cancer is defined as those nodules with only capsular invasion, and is believed to be similar in prognosis and behavior to benign follicular adenomas. Moderately invasive follicular cancers are those demonstrating vascular invasion, and widely invasive are those with spread beyond their capsules.

Hurthle Cell Cancer
Hurthle cell thyroid cancer is very similar to follicular cancer and indeed may be a variant thereof. The hallmark is large, mitochondria-rich cells with eosinophilic cytoplasm. The presentation, reliance on

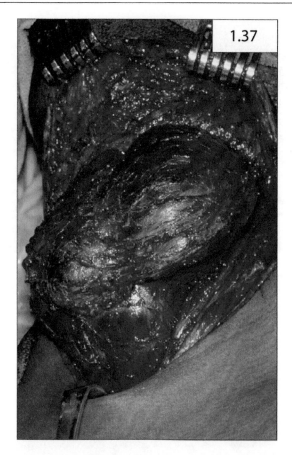

FIGURE 1.37 Surgical findings of the patient in Figure 1.36 demonstrating the growth pattern of papillary thyroid cancer arising from the isthmus and invading the strap muscles anteriorly. The picture is oriented with the superior part of the neck at the top.

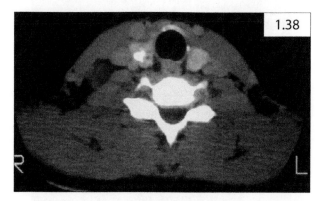

FIGURE 1.38 Axial CT scan of a patient with calcifications within the right thyroid lobe harboring papillary thyroid cancer. Papillary thyroid cancer should always be considered in patients demonstrating calcifications within the thyroid gland on radiographic imaging.

permanent sectioning for diagnosis, and penchant for hematogenous spread are the same as follicular cancer. However, some authors believe Hurthle cell cancer to be a more aggressive entity, demonstrating up to one-third as multicentric and one-quarter with lymph node spread at diagnosis. Hurthle cell cancers are less iodine avid than follicular cancers, but they do tend to produce thyroglobulin.

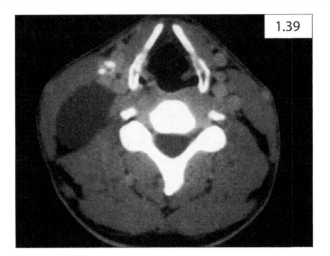

FIGURE 1.39   CT scan of the patient in Figure 1.41 at a higher axial plane in the neck. Findings include metastatic thyroid cancer to the right cervical region manifesting as a cystic neck mass as well as neck mass with calcifications. The differential diagnosis of any patient presenting with a cystic neck mass or lymph node with calcification should always include metastatic papillary thyroid cancer.

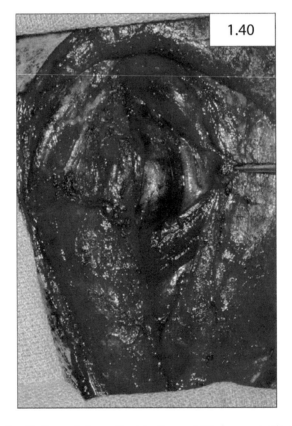

FIGURE 1.40   Intraoperative findings of the patient in Figure 1.38 demonstrating the cystic neck mass just medial to the right sternocleidomastoid. The picture is oriented with the superior part of the neck at the top.

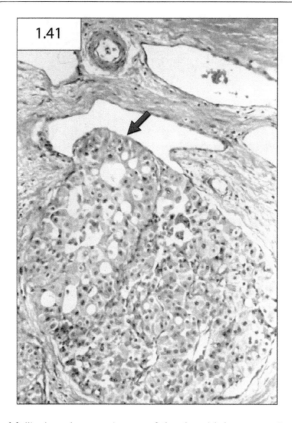

FIGURE 1.41 Histology of follicular adenocarcinoma of the thyroid demonstrating angioinvasion (arrow).

Insular Thyroid Cancer

Insular thyroid cancer is a rare disease entity distinguished by the identification of small clusters of malignant cells similar in appearance to pancreatic islet cells. Insular thyroid cancer can occur in association with papillary or follicular cancer or as an independent process. Insular carcinoma arising independently is associated with a more aggressive clinical course. These lesions are typically iodine avid.

Medullary Thyroid Cancer

Medullary thyroid cancer (MTC) arises from the parafollicular C-cells of neural crest origin. Approximately two-thirds arise spontaneously, usually as a solitary nodule in patients in their sixth or seventh decade, with equal distribution between females and males. The remaining third are associated with familial autosomal dominant mutations of the RET protooncogene, either in isolation or as part of the syndromes of multiple endocrine neoplasia (MEN) 2A and 2B. Familial MTC is associated with multicentricity.

Measurement of serum calcitonin can be useful in the diagnosis of MTC and can be used for postoperative monitoring for recurrence. Up to half of patients will present with local or distant disease; the favored sites of spread are cervical lymph nodes, then mediastinum, lung, liver, and bone. Some patients may present with pain from local invasion. The overall clinical behavior is more aggressive than the aforementioned differentiated thyroid cancers but less aggressive than anaplastic cancer.

Anaplastic Thyroid Cancer

Anaplastic thyroid cancer is an uncommon entity, accounting for less than 2% of thyroid cancers but causing the most deaths. The prognosis is grim, with fewer than 10% of patients surviving beyond 5 years, and most patients only surviving 3–6 months after diagnosis. The typical presentation is a female in her 50s

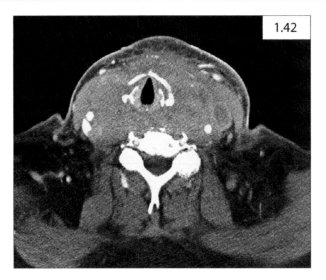

FIGURE 1.42   Axial CT scan demonstrating invasive anaplastic thyroid cancer invading the larynx and encasing the great vessels.

or 60s with a rapidly enlarging thyroid mass. Half of patients present with metastatic disease, primarily mediastinum and lung, followed by bone and brain (Figures 1.42 and 1.43).

Respiratory symptoms are common, and airway management with a tracheotomy is often necessary. In some patients, extensive tracheal invasion requires endoluminal stenting to alleviate asphyxiation. Anaplastic cancer is believed to be on the far end of a spectrum of dedifferentiation of thyroid cells, as evidenced by common genetic alterations, especially with papillary cancer. Most anaplastic cancers have lost their ability to concentrate iodine or elaborate thyroglobulin.

Thyroid Lymphoma
Primary thyroid lymphoma is uncommon, accounting for approximately 2% of thyroid malignancies. Many patients have a history of autoimmune thyroiditis, particularly Hashimoto's, and 85% of thyroid

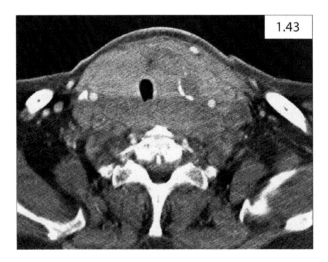

FIGURE 1.43   Axial CT scan demonstrating invasive anaplastic thyroid cancer encasing the tracheal airway.

lymphoma specimens have thyroiditis features present histologically. A typical presentation is enlargement of a previously existing goiter, or as a rapidly enlarging thyroid or cervical mass. 'B' symptoms such as fever, weight loss, and night sweats can also be present.

Thyroid lymphomas are typically non-Hodgkin's lymphomas of the B-cell type, though T-cell lymphomas can occur, particularly in human T-lymphotropic virus (HTLV)-endemic areas. Many patients have laboratory evidence of longstanding hypothyroidism, with elevated TSH and antithyroid peroxidase or thyroglobulin antibodies. Elevated immunoglobulins or lactate dehydrogenase can also be seen. Traditionally, an incisional or excisional biopsy was needed to establish the diagnosis accurately, sent fresh for lymphoma workup. However, advances in flow cytometry have made diagnosis by FNA more reliable when performed by experienced clinicians.

Clinical Presentation

The first discovery of a thyroid nodule is often made on physical examination or is an incidental finding on imaging workup for another reason. Thyroid nodules are not uncommon, with studies reporting 30%–50% of individuals harboring incidental nodules. The vast majority of nodules will be benign, with less than 10% representing malignancy. Certain features of the history and physical exam may suggest a malignancy. As mentioned earlier, patients with a history of radiation exposure or family history are at increased risk. In addition, a history of a rapidly enlarging mass is more suspicious for malignancy (Figure 1.33); however, a rapidly enlarging, painful thyroid mass may represent hemorrhage into a benign cyst. More aggressive thyroid cancers can manifest early with respiratory symptoms, due either to airway compression, invasion of the trachea, or compression or invasion of the recurrent laryngeal nerves leading to vocal cord dysfunction.

Most patients presenting with thyroid cancer are euthyroid. Symptoms of hyper- or hypothyroidism do not rule out cancer but may prompt further workup for a benign cause.

Nodules that are greater than 1 cm can usually be palpated. Fixation to surrounding structures and palpable cervical lymphadenopathy increase the suspicion of malignancy, though in particular, lymphadenopathy can occur in benign processes such as Graves' and Hashimoto's. History and physical examination findings that are more indicative of a malignant process are summarized in Table 1.5. Well-differentiated thyroid cancers (papillary, follicular, and Hurthle cell) can be staged using one of four grading systems: AJCC, AGES, AMES, or MACIS. Again, depending on the histology, cancer of the thyroid has many different presentations and behaviors.

TABLE 1.5 History and Physical Examination Findings Suggestive of Thyroid Cancer

History
Family history of multiple endocrine neoplasia, or medullary thyroid cancer
Personal history of head and neck irradiation or radiation exposure
Symptoms of airway compression or voice changes
Symptoms of hemoptysis
Rapid tumor growth
Physical Examination
Very firm or hard nodule
Fixation of nodule to surrounding structures
Regional lymphadenopathy including cystic neck mass
Distant metastases
Large nodule (>4 cm)

Differential Diagnosis

The primary differential diagnosis is between benign and malignant processes. Thyroid cancer typically presents as a nodule and may not be able to be distinguished from a benign adenoma without surgical excision. Metastases from renal cell, melanoma, breast, and lung cancer can also present as thyroid nodules. Multinodular goiters usually represent benign processes, but large or suspicious nodules must be investigated independently, as they carry the same risk for carcinoma. Diffuse thyroid enlargement may be benign goiter, an inflammatory or infectious process, or neoplastic infiltration.

Diagnosis

Palpation of the thyroid, and appreciating the overall size and consistency of the thyroid as well as the character of any nodules is the first step in diagnosis. Tenderness, fixation to surrounding structures, and associated cervical lymphadenopathy should be appreciated (Table 1.5). A screening TSH can be ordered to evaluate for functional nodules. FNA is the mainstay of the workup for a thyroid nodule. A 27-gauge needle loaded on a syringe is inserted into a palpable nodule, while gentle suction is maintained with backpressure on the syringe plunger. Several passes are made in different directions taking care to stay within the nodule. The hub of the needle is watched for the return of serous material. Aspiration of blood decreases the interpretability of the FNA, and if this occurs, the needle should be taken out, pressure should be held, and the FNA should be reattempted with a fresh needle. Multiple samples should be taken and spread among slides for both air-dry and cytologic fixation. Involvement of experienced clinicians in the process of FNA increases the diagnostic yield. If the nodule is found to be cystic and fluid-filled, the fluid should be sent for cytology. Bloody fluid may represent hemorrhage into a cyst or carcinoma. If a lesion is found on imaging to have both solid and cystic components, an attempt should be made to sample the solid component.

As mentioned earlier, FNA is highly sensitive and specific when diagnosing PTC. Follicular and Hurthle cell nodules cannot be distinguished between benign and malignant on FNA alone. Anaplastic cancer and thyroid lymphoma may require additional tissue from an incisional biopsy to make the diagnosis accurately. Nondiagnostic FNA should never be interpreted as negative for cancer.

Ultrasonography is very useful for evaluating the thyroid. It can detect additional nonpalpable nodes or differentiate between nodules and lobar hypertrophy. Certain characteristics of nodules, such as calcifications or cystic components, can increase the suspicion of cancer. Ultrasound can also be used to evaluate regional lymphatics and can be used to guide FNA for nonpalpable nodules or for sampling the solid component of a cystic nodule.

CT and MRI scans of the thyroid usually do not add much to the workup of thyroid cancer. For patients with well-differentiated thyroid cancers who are being considered for postoperative radioactive iodine therapy (see later), use of CT with iodinated contrast media is contraindicated because it delays treatment for up to 3 months. If imaging must be obtained in these patients, such as for suspicion of tracheal invasion or to evaluate substernal extension, MRI is preferred. Postoperatively, MRI is also better at distinguishing recurrent disease from postoperative fibrosis. In patients who present with massive, rapidly enlarging goiters suspicious for anaplastic carcinoma or lymphoma where tissue diagnosis or airway management is needed, a CT with contrast is appropriate for surgical planning.

Radionucleotide scanning with radioactive iodine is useful for assessing the functionality of a nodule but is not useful in determining the risk for cancer. Nodules that fail to take up iodine on scan are referred to as cold nodules. Traditionally, cold nodules have been considered higher risk for cancer. However, the majority of patients with thyroid nodules are cold on scan, making radionucleotide ineffective in screening for cancer risk. Additionally, hyperfunctional or hot nodules have been traditionally considered to be benign but numerous cases have been reported of hot nodules harboring thyroid cancer. The primary role of radionucleotide scanning is for ablation and posttreatment surveillance.

Management/Treatment

Surgery is the primary treatment for most thyroid cancers. For some well-differentiated thyroid nodules, there is controversy regarding the extent of surgical resection (lobectomy versus subtotal or total thyroidectomy). However, the basic guiding principles are as follows:

- If a patient has no worrisome risk factors and a favorable histology (e.g., a young woman with an isolated <4 cm papillary cancer without worrisome features with no extracapsular spread or nodal involvement), a lobectomy may be appropriate and spares the patient a lifetime of thyroid hormone replacement.
- If unfavorable features are seen in permanent histology after a lobectomy, such as vascular invasion or diffuse infiltration of the thyroid, removal of the contralateral lobe is indicated.
- If there is high suspicion for multicentricity (e.g., large papillary thyroid cancers and familial medullary thyroid cancer), or at least some disease in the contralateral lobe, an upfront total thyroidectomy is indicated or removal of the contralateral lobe after unilateral lobectomy.
- If postoperative radioactive iodine is planned for aggressive histology or known extrathyroid disease, a total thyroidectomy permits more effective detection and treatment of residual local and distant microscopic disease (see later).

The standard surgical approach is through a small horizontal incision just above the clavicle. The strap muscles are divided in the midline down to the gland. One lobe is removed at a time if both are being taken, with care to preserve the parathyroid glands and recurrent laryngeal nerves.

In patients with clinically apparent nodal disease in the central compartment or lateral cervical lymph node chains, a neck dissection is warranted to remove gross disease. En bloc lymphadenectomy is preferred in these situations over removal of individual nodes given the high incidence of microscopic disease. The role of neck dissection in the clinically negative neck is more controversial.

Radioactive iodine (^{131}I) has proven a very effective treatment for microscopic and distant disease in well-differentiated thyroid cancer (i.e., cancers able to uptake and concentrate the radioiodine). The typical sequence of treatment is total thyroidectomy, followed by a 4–6-week period of thyroid withdrawal during which time the TSH level is allowed to rise to greater than 30 µIU/mL. Then, while maximal stimulation of any remaining thyroid tissue is occurring, whole-body radioiodine scanning is performed, followed the next day by ^{131}I ablation (Figure 1.44). As an alternative to thyroid hormone withdrawal, recombinant thyrotropin alfa may be used as an adjunctive treatment for radioiodine ablation of thyroid tissue remnants in patients who have undergone a near-total or total thyroidectomy for well-differentiated thyroid cancer and who do not have evidence of distant metastatic thyroid cancer.

After ablation, the patient is started on thyroid suppression therapy with levothyroxine to maintain a low level of TSH through feedback mechanisms on the hypothalamus. The target level of TSH is determined by the aggressiveness of the cancer, with lower or undetectable levels desired for higher-risk patients. Serum thyroglobulin (Tg) is followed for recurrence. Recombinant thyrotropin alfa may be used as an adjunctive diagnostic tool to improve the sensitivity of Tg testing. In patients with antithyroglobulin (anti-Tg) antibodies, Tg levels cannot be accurately followed with the standard assays, but Tg mass spectrometry can be used. In these patients, the level of anti-Tg has been shown somewhat to correlate with recurrence.

In contrast to patients with well-differentiated thyroid cancer, chemotherapy and radiation are the primary treatment modalities for patients with anaplastic cancer or thyroid lymphoma, and there is no role for radioactive iodine. For lymphoma, the treatment regimen is driven by the specific types of cells involved, but the most common for non-Hodgkin's lymphoma is a combination of cyclophosphamide, doxorubicin, and vincristine in combination with radiotherapy. Treatment for anaplastic cancer is largely experimental, with some combination of chemotherapy, external beam radiation, and surgical debulking performed as much for palliation as curative intent. The main role of surgery in both anaplastic cancer and thyroid lymphoma is obtaining tissue for diagnosis and airway management with a tracheotomy.

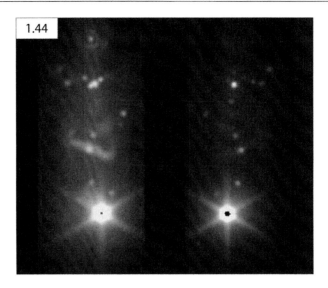

FIGURE 1.44   Radioactive iodine uptake scan with ^{131}I demonstrating metastatic papillary thyroid cancer. The large starburst pattern in the lower part of the image is consistent with metastasis to the pelvic bone.

Patients with a family history of medullary thyroid cancer who are positive for the RET mutation often undergo prophylactic thyroidectomy at a young age. Total thyroidectomy with central compartment neck dissection is the minimum treatment for any patient presenting with clinically evident MTC. Further neck dissection is based on clinical findings.

BIBLIOGRAPHY

Burch HB, Perros P, Bednarczuk T, Cooper DS, Dolman PJ, Leung AM, Mombaerts I, Salvi M, Stan MN. Management of Thyroid Eye Disease: A Consensus Statement by the American Thyroid Association and the European Thyroid Association. *Thyroid* 2022 December;32(12):1439–1470. doi: 10.1089/thy.2022.0251. Epub 2022 December 8. PMID: 36480280. PMCID: PMC9807259.

De Filippis EA, Sabet A, Sun MR, Garber JR. Pemberton's Sign: Explained Nearly 70 Years Later. *J Clin Endocrinol Metab* 2014 June;99(6):1949–1954. doi: 10.1210/jc.2013-4240. Epub 2014 Mar 19. PMID: 24646105.

Duntas LH, Jonklaas J. COVID-19 and Thyroid Diseases: A Bidirectional Impact. *J Endocr Soc* 2021 April 27;5(8):bvab076. doi: 10.1210/jendso/bvab076. PMID: 34189381. PMCID: PMC8135350.

Ferrari SM, Fallahi P, Galetta F, Citi E, Benvenga S, Antonelli A. Thyroid Disorders Induced by Checkpoint Inhibitors. *Rev Endocr Metab Disord* 2018 December;19(4):325–333. doi: 10.1007/s11154-018-9463-2. PMID: 30242549.

Haugen BR, Alexander EK, Bible KC, Doherty GM, Mandel SJ, Nikiforov YE, Pacini F, Randolph GW, Sawka AM, Schlumberger M, Schuff KG, Sherman SI, Sosa JA, Steward DL, Tuttle RM, Wartofsky L. 2015 American Thyroid Association Management Guidelines for Adult Patients with Thyroid Nodules and Differentiated Thyroid Cancer: The American Thyroid Association Guidelines Task Force on Thyroid Nodules and Differentiated Thyroid Cancer. *Thyroid* 2016 January;26(1):1–133. doi: 10.1089/thy.2015.0020. PMID: 26462967. PMCID: PMC4739132.

Nikiforov YE, Seethala RR, Tallini G, Baloch ZW, Basolo F, Thompson LD, Barletta JA, Wenig BM, Al Ghuzlan A, Kakudo K, Giordano TJ, Alves VA, Khanafshar E, Asa SL, El-Naggar AK, Gooding WE, Hodak SP, Lloyd RV, Maytal G, Mete O, Nikiforova MN, Nosé V, Papotti M, Poller DN, Sadow PM, Tischler AS, Tuttle RM, Wall KB, LiVolsi VA, Randolph GW, Ghossein RA. Nomenclature Revision for Encapsulated Follicular

Variant of Papillary Thyroid Carcinoma: A Paradigm Shift to Reduce Overtreatment of Indolent Tumors. *JAMA Oncol* 2016 August 1;2(8):1023–1029. doi: 10.1001/jamaoncol.2016.0386. PMID: 27078145. PMCID: PMC5539411.

Werner and Ingbar's the Thyroid. In: Braverman LE, Cooper DS, Kopp P, ed. *A Fundamental and Clinical Text*, 11th edition, Philadelphia, PA: Wolters Kluwer, 2021.

Diabetes Mellitus

2

Alalah Mazhari, Mary Ann Emanuele, and Gerald Charnogursky

INTRODUCTION

Diabetes mellitus is a disease that afflicts more than 400 million people worldwide. The areas most affected are Africa, the eastern Mediterranean region, and Southeast Asia. Data from the National Health Interview Survey (2016 and 2017) estimated the prevalence of diagnosed type 2 diabetes (T2DM) among adults in the United States was 8.5%, and other national databases, such as the Centers for Disease Control and Prevention Diabetes Surveillance System, reported a prevalence of diagnosed diabetes of approximately 7%. In the United States, the lifetime risk for developing diabetes in an individual born after 2000 is 33% for Caucasians and 50% for Hispanics. These numbers reflect the explosion of obesity in the US and worldwide. Type 1 diabetes (T1DM), accounting for about 10% of people with diabetes mellitus, is an autoimmune disease in which the insulin-producing β-cells of the pancreas are destroyed. Treatment relies solely on the use of insulin.

T2DM, seen in almost 90% of the diabetic population, has several pathophysiologic loci. These include insulin resistance at hepatic, skeletal muscle and adipocyte level, relative or absolute hypoinsulinemia, decreased GLP-1 secretion and increased resistance to GLP-1, and enhanced glucose absorption from the proximal convoluted tubule in the kidney. Insulin resistance, in addition to participating in the development of hyperglycemia, can also lead to hypertriglyceridemia, low HDL cholesterol, hypertension, and truncal obesity, and this constellation of features is commonly referred to as metabolic syndrome. The treatment of T2DM initially relies on the use of oral agents and subcutaneously injected medications that augment insulin secretion, reduce excessively high glucagon levels, decrease insulin resistance, or interrupt intestinal carbohydrate absorption. These agents may be used in combination with a variety of insulins as pancreatic function wanes.

RETINOPATHY

Definition/Overview

Retinopathy is the most common microvascular complication of diabetes and accounts for 10,000 cases of new blindness per year. This complication is seen in both T1DM and T2DM, but since the onset of

DOI: 10.1201/9781003100669-2

T2DM can be insidious, it may develop many years before diagnosis. There is evidence that retinopathy may begin to develop 7–10 years before the clinical diagnosis of T2DM. Retinopathy is known to initially worsen, and then improve as better glycemic control is instituted. It may also progress with pregnancy, with improvement after delivery. Treatment protocols utilizing intravitreal anti–vascular endothelial growth factor (anti-VEGF) therapies in retinal diseases continue to evolve. In the management of neovascular age-related macular degeneration (nAMD), extending the treatment interval can maintain significant visual acuity while reducing the treatment burden. For patients with diabetic retinopathy (DR), early intervention with anti-VEGF therapies has reduced vision-threatening complications as well as slowed disease progression. The role of persistent subretinal and intraretinal fluid in determining response to treatment in patients with nAMD must also be addressed and follow-up with a retinal specialist is crucial.

Etiology

The major mechanism for the development of retinopathy is chronic hyperglycemia. Accumulation of polyols and advanced glycosylation end products, oxidative stress, and protein kinase C activation may mediate the effects of hyperglycemia. Excessive levels of intraocular vascular endothelial growth factor, a deficiency of pigment epithelium-derived factor (a protein that inhibits neovascularization), and reduced concentrations of transforming growth factor-β (a protein that may inhibit endothelial proliferation) may play a role. Insulin-like growth factor 1 seems to be permissive in the development of retinopathy. In addition to these chemical factors, genetic factors seem to play a role, as genetic clustering of retinopathy has been reported.

Pathophysiology

Diabetic retinopathy may be divided into pre-proliferative (or background) retinopathy and the more serious proliferative retinopathy. First, there is the pre-proliferative phase. Because of the alterations described in the preceding 'Etiology' section, there is loss of the vascular supporting cells, the pericytes, which allow for the development of microaneurysms, small outpouching from the capillaries of the retina, as well as dot intraretinal hemorrhages (Figure 2.2, compared to Figure 2.1, the normal fundus). There may be a progressive increase in the number of hemorrhages as well as the development of cotton wool spots, both manifestations of regional ischemia due to microvascular disease.

Proliferative retinopathy develops because of the formation of new blood vessels, the process of neovascularization (Figure 2.2). This is likely due, at least in part, to the growth factor imbalance described earlier, as well as to loss of pericytes, which may have a contractile function regulating retinal blood flow. This dysregulation may lead to ischemia, an additional stimulus to neovascularization. The new and fragile blood vessels grow into the vitreous where they may burst, with the vitreous hemorrhage causing visual loss (Figure 2.4). Scarring in the hemorrhage attaching to the retina can then retract causing retinal detachment and more visual problems.

Excess VEGF may cause disruption of the blood–retinal barrier. This can lead to macular edema, which may result in substantial central visual loss. When the fluid elements of this macular edema reabsorb, the lipid and lipoprotein elements remaining cause hard exudates (Figure 2.3).

Clinical Presentation

There is a progression from microaneurysms and dot hemorrhages to neovascularization (Figures 2.1–2.3). After neovascularization, its attendant problems, vitreous hemorrhage, retinal detachment, and glaucoma may follow (Figure 2.4). Macular edema can occur anywhere during the course of this progression.

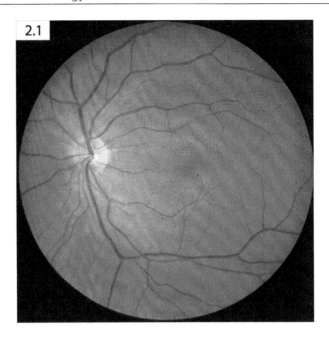

FIGURE 2.1 Normal fundus. (Courtesy of Dr. Mark Dailey.)

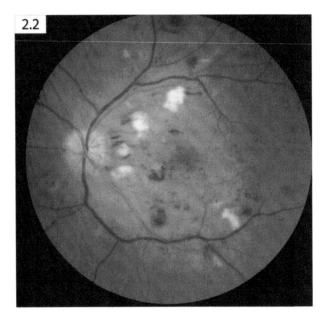

FIGURE 2.2 Microaneurysms, flame hemorrhages, cotton wool spots, and neovascularization of the disc. (Courtesy of Dr. Mark Dailey.)

Diagnosis

The traditional method of detection of diabetic retinopathy is by ophthalmoscopic physical examination, preferably through dilated pupils. However, a variety of photographic techniques may complement

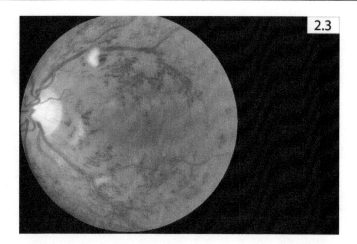

FIGURE 2.3   Hard exudates. (Courtesy of Dr. Mark Dailey.)

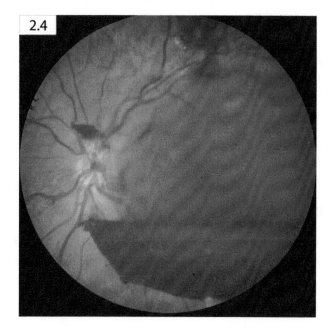

FIGURE 2.4   Large preretinal hemorrhage. (Courtesy of Dr. Mark Dailey.)

physical examination or even replace it. Fluorescein angiography is a useful method for characterization of the retinal vasculature (Figure 2.5).

Management/Treatment

Observational as well as interventional studies have shown that maintenance of good glycemic control is of ocular benefit. Several prospective trials have documented the importance of good blood pressure control in ocular protection and, in fact, there was a 47% reduced risk of deterioration in visual acuity in the United Kingdom Prospective Diabetes Study.

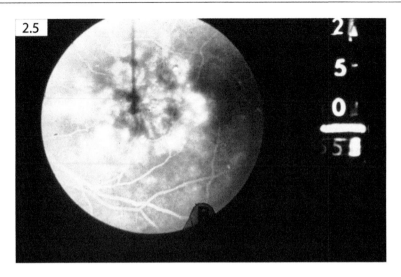

FIGURE 2.5   Fluorescein angiogram showing vascular leakage. (Courtesy of Dr. Mark Dailey.)

In addition, several eye-specific treatments are effective. Panretinal scatter photocoagulation benefits people with proliferative retinopathy or neovascular glaucoma. Focal photocoagulation may be used for macular edema. Vitrectomy can be used for nonclearing vitreous hemorrhage or traction detachment of the retina. Newer approaches, such as blockade of VEGF, are also very effective.

NEPHROPATHY

Definition/Overview

Diabetic nephropathy is the leading cause of renal failure in individuals on dialysis. It has been generally defined as the presence of more than 500 mg albumin in a 24-hour urine collection. This is overt nephropathy. However, patients first go through stages of lesser protein spillage, termed microalbuminuria. Proteinuria occurs in 15%–40% of individuals with T1DM, the prevalence peaking at 15–20 years of diabetes duration. The prevalence varies from 5% to 20% in patients with T2DM.

Etiology

At most, probably no more than 40% of diabetic people develop nephropathy. It is clear that there is familial clustering of this complication, and, thus, genetic susceptibility plays a role in the development of nephropathy in both T1DM and T2DM. On this background, several modifiable factors lead to the clinical initiation and progression of nephropathy including hyperglycemia and hypertension. Other etiological factors include glomerular hyperfiltration, proteinuria itself, smoking, dyslipidemia, and dietary factors including protein and fat.

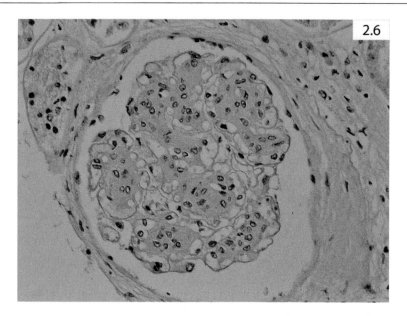

FIGURE 2.6 Glomerulus from a patient with advanced diabetic nephropathy stained with PAS. Nodular mesangial expansion is seen (Kimmelstiel–Wilson nodules). (Courtesy of Dr. Maria Picken.)

Pathophysiology

The classic histological changes of diabetic nephropathy are increased glomerular basement membrane (GBM) width and mesangial expansion (Figures 2.6 and 2.7). Not only is the GBM thickened, but it is biochemically and functionally defective, allowing for albumin leakage into the urine. The defective

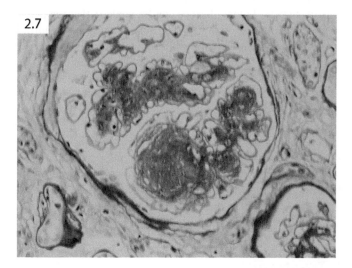

FIGURE 2.7 Glomerulus from a patient with advanced diabetic nephropathy stained with H&E. Nodular mesangial expansion is seen (Kimmelstiel–Wilson nodules). (Courtesy of Dr. Maria Picken.)

function of the GBM coupled with increased transglomerular pressure (caused by excessive constriction of the efferent glomerular arteriole compared to the afferent arteriole) leads to proteinuria. The expansion of the mesangium decreases glomerular capillary luminal space and, thus, reduces glomerular filtration.

The mechanistic role of hyperglycemia in the pathophysiology is complex and mediated through an increase in growth factors (such as transforming growth factor-β and vascular endothelial growth factor), activation of protein kinase C, increase in oxidative stress, enhanced formation of advanced glycosylation end products, and increased flux through the aldose reductase pathway.

Clinical Presentation

If untreated, patients initially present with no evidence of renal disease but then progress from microalbuminuria to nephropathy to nephrotic syndrome and, finally, to dialysis-requiring end-stage renal disease.

Differential Diagnosis

In diabetic patients with impaired renal function and/or proteinuria, symptoms of urinary tract obstruction and systemic diseases other than diabetes (such as lupus or hepatitis B or C among others) should be sought. Imaging or biopsy may be considered in selected cases.

Diagnosis

The diagnosis is easily made in long-term (>10 years) T1DM individuals with renal functional impairment and proteinuria, especially if there is concurrent retinopathy, the retinal–renal syndrome. The diagnosis may be less certain in people with T2DM since the actual time of onset of the disease is often not clear, and about one in four patients may not have retinopathy.

A clinical diagnosis of diabetic kidney disease can be made if there is persistent albuminuria and/or persistent decreased glomerular filtration rate (GFR). Screening for proteinuria is conveniently accomplished with a spot urine sample. Because of the well-known variability in day-to-day urinary albumin excretion, the diagnosis should only be made if two specimens are abnormal. An additional diagnostic caveat is that the presence of factors other than renal disease, which can elevate urinary albumin excretion, must be ruled out. These include urinary tract infection, hematuria, acute febrile illness, uncontrolled hypertension, heart failure, vigorous exercise, and short-term pronounced hyperglycemia. Decreased GFR is defined as an eGFR <60 mL/min/1.73 m^2 using a creatinine-based formula. Persistence of these abnormalities for at least 3 months should be confirmed, because transient abnormalities, which can be induced by a variety of unrelated disorders, are common.

It is important to note that albuminuria is not required to make a clinical diagnosis of diabetic kidney disease. A substantial minority of patients with diabetes and decreased eGFR have <30 mg/g of albuminuria, and such patients commonly have histopathologic findings consistent with diabetic kidney disease.

Management/Treatment

Good glycemic control has been shown to protect kidney function and is a major part of therapy. Equally important is blood pressure control. The goal is a blood pressure less than 140/90 (<125/75 if serum creatinine is elevated and proteinuria is >1 gram/24 hours). Therapy should be initiated with angiotensin-converting enzyme inhibitors, angiotensin receptor blockers, renin–angiotensin system (RAS) blockade, or SGLT-2 inhibitors, and many patients will need three to four different agents to achieve goals. Additionally, some GLP-1 receptor agonists have been shown to reduce the incidence of a composite kidney endpoint (consisting of a new onset of albuminuria >300 mg/day, doubling of serum creatinine, ESKD, or kidney death). Since SGL-2 inhibitors and GLP-1 receptor agonists also reduce the rates of cardiovascular disease, they are important agents in diabetes management. There is data suggesting that statin therapy may preserve kidney function, as may dietary protein restriction.

NEUROPATHY

Definition/Overview

Diabetic neuropathy can be subdivided into generalized symmetric polyneuropathies and focal/multifocal mononeuropathies. Symmetric polyneuropathies include three distinct entities: acute sensory, chronic sensorimotor, and autonomic neuropathies. Focal/multifocal neuropathies are further subcategorized into cranial, truncal, focal limb, and diabetic amyotrophy. Chronic distal sensorimotor polyneuropathy (DPN) and autonomic neuropathy (AN) are the two most common forms. A simple definition of DPN is "the presence of symptoms and/or signs of peripheral nerve dysfunction in people with diabetes after the exclusion of other causes". DPN is the most common form of neuropathy. About half the time, DPN is subclinical. AN may manifest itself in one or multiple organ systems. More than 50% of individuals with diabetes may expect to develop a diabetic neuropathy. The duration of diabetes correlates well with the development of neuropathy. Those with T1DM typically begin to develop neuropathies after 5 years, while in individuals with T2DM, the neuropathy may begin prior to the clinical diagnosis of diabetes.

Etiology

The duration of diabetes, as well as the level of hyperglycemia, plays a central role in the development of diabetic neuropathies. Other factors thought to play a role in the development of neuropathy include hypertension, hyperlipidemia, obesity, tobacco use, and alcohol consumption.

Acute sensorimotor neuropathy, although rare, is thought to be a result of marked metabolic derangement including ketoacidosis and rapid fluctuations in glycemic control.

Mononeuropathies have two distinct etiologies. The most common form is entrapment. This can be seen in up to 30% of diabetic people. Microvascular infarcts, whose symptoms are self-limiting, also lead to mononeuropathies and are rare in comparison.

Pathophysiology

Hyperglycemia in DPN and AN leads to the intracellular accumulation of sorbitol, via the actions of the aldose reductase pathway. As a result, cellular osmolality is increased and myoinositol is decreased. Hyperglycemia also leads to the development of advanced glycosylation end products. These factors, coupled with the increased development of reactive oxygen species (multiple pathways) and the decrease in available antioxidants, lead to a functional limitation in axonal transport, impairment of neurotropism, and alteration of gene expression. Ischemia is also thought to play a role in the development of

2.8

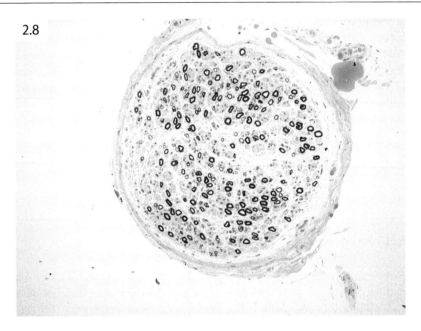

FIGURE 2.8   Diabetic neuropathy in a sural nerve. Note the wedge-shaped areas with axonal loss and a mild overall decrease in axonal number. (Courtesy of Dr. Henry Brown.)

polyneuropathies. Heightened expression of protein kinase C (PKC), PAI-1, transforming growth factor beta (TGF-β), and VEGF in diabetes leads to increases in endothelial injury and micro-/macrovascular occlusion. An example of diabetic neuronal loss in a sural nerve biopsy is shown in Figure 2.8.

Clinical Presentation

DPN most frequently presents as paresthesia, hyperesthesia, deep aching pain, burning, or an electrical sensation. These symptoms are typically worse at night. It is symmetric in distribution. The disease typically affects the distal extremities; most commonly the feet and lower legs. It has a progressive symmetric distal-to-proximal course, leading to the classic stocking-glove distribution. In 50% of instances, DPN is subclinical and may present with calluses or a painless foot ulcer. Acute sensorimotor neuropathy presents with similar findings as DPN. The hallmark is the sudden onset, severity, and typical self-limiting course.

ANs present in a variety of ways, dependent upon the organ systems that are affected. Cardiac AN may present as decreased exercise tolerance, fatigue, weakness with exercise, postural hypotension, dizziness, tachycardia, or overt syncope. In many instances, cardiac AN is silent. Esophageal motility disturbances are not uncommon. These are manifested by either excessive peristaltic contractions (Figure 2.9) or absent contractions (Figure 2.10). The gastric presentation of AN is varied. It ranges from gastroparesis, abdominal pain, vomiting, belching, early satiety, and constipation to diarrhea and incontinence. Genitourinary symptoms include vaginal dryness, erectile dysfunction, nocturia, urinary retention, urinary incontinence, or increased urinary frequency, and striking examples of neurogenic bladders are shown in Figures 2.11 and 2.12. Sudomotor symptoms associated with AN include hyperhidrosis, anhidrosis, heat intolerance, and dry skin.

Focal/multifocal mononeuropathies also have varied presentations. Patients with diabetic amyotrophy will present with unilateral or bilateral severe neuropathic pain. Physical findings include proximal

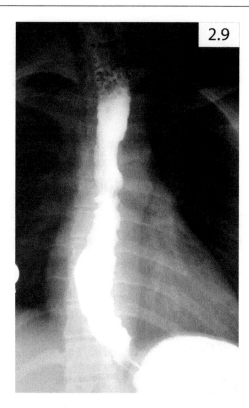

FIGURE 2.9   Tertiary contractions in the esophagus of a diabetic patient. (Courtesy of Dr. Laurie Lomasney.)

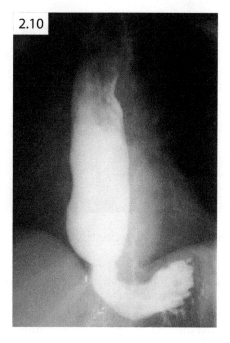

FIGURE 2.10   Absence of contractions in the esophagus of a diabetic patient. (Courtesy of Dr. Laurie Lomasney.)

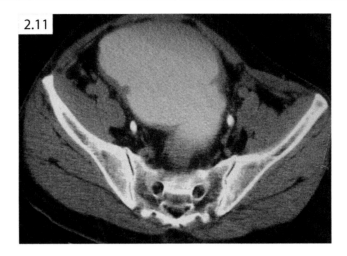

FIGURE 2.11   Neurogenic bladder. (Courtesy of Dr. Laurie Lomasney.)

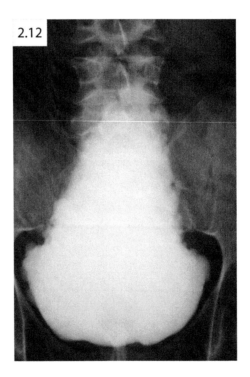

FIGURE 2.12   Neurogenic bladder with diverticula. (Courtesy of Dr. Laurie Lomasney.)

thigh weakness and atrophy. Those with thoracic polyradiculopathy may present with severe pain in a bandlike distribution about the chest or abdomen. Cranial mononeuropathies can affect the oculomotor, trochlear, and abducens nerves, leading to ophthalmoplegia. Patients with diabetic ophthalmoplegia present with unilateral pain, ptosis, and diplopia. Peripheral mononeuropathies may produce effects in the median, ulnar, radial, and peroneal nerves. This has an acute onset and may result in symptoms such as foot drop.

Differential Diagnosis

Chronic inflammatory demyelinating process (CIDP), B_{12} deficiency, spinal stenosis, hypothyroidism, and uremia occur more frequently in the diabetic population. Imaging, laboratory workup, and neurology referral should be used to elucidate the etiology of the neuropathy. In asymmetric polyneuropathies, the diagnosis of systemic vasculitis should be entertained.

Diagnosis

DPN is a clinical diagnosis, and a complete history and physical are essential. Simple inspection of the feet may reveal calluses or ulcerations of an insensate foot. Regularly checking pinprick, temperature perception, vibratory sense (using a 128 Hz tuning fork), pressure sensation (using a 10 g monofilament), and ankle reflexes are recommended. The combination of any two positive tests has an 87% sensitivity for detecting DPN.

Detection of AN involves diverse testing based on the organ system involved, but the details are beyond the scope of this chapter.

Focal/multifocal neuropathies can be diagnosed through a meticulous history and physical. Electrophysiological studies may aid in the determination of the site of nerve entrapment or infarction.

Management/Treatment

There are numerous drugs used to treat DPN. The first goal of therapy (with all neuropathies) should be to improve glycemic control. Regular inspection of the feet may prevent amputation by identifying early foot lesions otherwise missed because of insensate feet. Subsequent therapy should be directed at appropriately controlling blood pressure and following cholesterol guidelines. Medications for symptomatic relief of pain include tricyclic drugs (e.g., amitriptyline), anticonvulsants (gabapentin and topiramate), pregabalin, capsaicin cream, selective serotonin reuptake inhibitors, and duloxetine. Vasodilators have been shown to have limited success. For refractory pain, the use of opioids or pain service consultation may be necessary. Treatment of mononeuropathies may include surgical decompression of entrapped nerves.

Cardiac AN may respond to beta blockers, ACE inhibitors, and supervised exercise therapy. Postural hypotension, after exclusion of other diseases, may respond to the use of midodrine or octreotide. Gastroparesis, chronic abdominal pain, and vomiting may respond to frequent small meals, prokinetic agents (metoclopramide and erythromycin), gastric pacing, pyloric Botox, or enteral feedings. Constipation may be approached with high-fiber diets, bulking agents, and osmotic laxatives. Erectile dysfunction may respond to phosphodiesterase 5 inhibitors (sildenafil, vardenafil, and tadalafil), prostaglandins, or a prosthesis. Bladder dysfunction can be treated with bethanechol or intermittent catheterization.

SKIN MANIFESTATIONS

Overview

Skin manifestations in diabetes mellitus are common. Many skin manifestations seen in association with diabetes mellitus may also be seen in other conditions. These lesions may result from microangiopathy, hyperinsulinemia, hyperlipidemia, reaction to treatments, or immune compromise leading to infections.

NECROBIOSIS LIPOIDICA DIABETICORUM

Definition/Overview

This disease is an uncommon finding affecting 0.3%–1.2% of patients. Necrobiosis is most commonly seen in individuals with T1DM, although it manifests in those with T2DM and patients with insulin resistance. About one in four patients with necrobiosis do not carry a diagnosis of diabetes. Women are three times more likely to develop these lesions

Etiology

This skin lesion may be the result of diabetic microangiopathy, immune complex disease, abnormal production of collagen, and impaired neutrophil migration. The lesions are commonly associated with poor glycemic control, but there is no evidence that necrobiosis is prevented by good glycemic control.

Pathophysiology

Biopsy examination of necrobiosis reveals thinning central dermis, collagen degeneration, and granulomatous inflammation of the subcutaneous tissue, as well as blood vessel wall thickening.

Clinical Presentation

The lesions are most common on the pretibial aspect of the leg and are generally bilateral in presentation (Figure 2.13). Less often they are found on the trunk, arms, and face. Initially, they are seen as small red papules. These eventually coalesce to form a large circular lesion with a waxy yellow center. Telangiectasias are seen in this area of the lesion (Figure 2.14). Mature lesions have been characterized

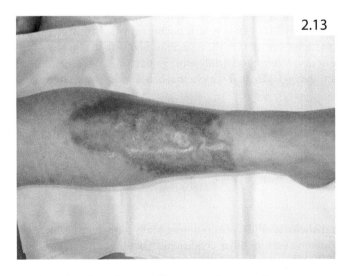

2.13

FIGURE 2.13 Necrobiosis lipoidica diabeticorum. (Courtesy of Drs. Anthony Peterson and David Eilers.)

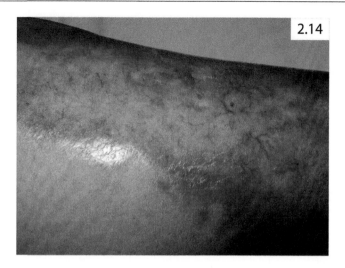

FIGURE 2.14 Necrobiosis lipoidica diabeticorum with telangiectasia. (Courtesy of Drs. Anthony Peterson and David Eilers.)

as having a 'porcelain-like sheen'. The lesions may become ulcerative (35%) and direct trauma to the area should be avoided. These lesions may spontaneously disappear in up to 19% of patients.

Differential Diagnosis

Differential diagnosis of this lesion includes granuloma annulare, necrobiotic xanthogranuloma (associated with paraproteinemia), rheumatoid arthritis nodules, sarcoidosis, stasis dermatitis, lichen sclerosus et atrophicus, Hansen's disease, and erythema nodosum.

Diagnosis

Diagnosis is through history and physical examination as well as familiarity with the lesion.

Management/Treatment

Both medical and surgical treatments of necrobiosis lipoidica have been of limited efficacy. In ulcerative or complicated cases, surgery or split-thickness skin grafts have been used. Medical treatments have included topical or intralesional corticosteroids, fibrinolytic agents, nicotinamide, tacrolimus, pentoxifylline, heparin, antiplatelet agents, ticlopidine hydrochloride, tretinoin, cyclosporine, and thalidomide.

ACANTHOSIS NIGRICANS

Definition/Overview

Acanthosis nigricans is a papillomatosis and hyperkeratosis of the skin. The lesions are commonly associated with T2DM and hyperinsulinemic states. This lesion may be seen in up to 36% of people with

T2DM. Acanthosis has a higher prevalence in Blacks, Hispanics, and Native Americans when compared with Caucasians.

Etiology

Hyperinsulinemic states and obesity are commonly associated with acanthosis nigricans, suggesting that insulin resistance may participate in the genesis of this lesion. The incidence of acanthosis in moderately obese individuals may be as high as 27% and up to 54% in severe obesity.

Pathophysiology

Acanthosis nigricans is characterized as a dermal thickening with hyperpigmentation. Acanthosis is thought to arise from insulin stimulation of insulin-like growth factor-1 receptors in keratinocytes leading to epidermal hyperplasia.

Clinical Presentation

The dermal thickening seen in acanthosis appears as dark, velvety areas (Figure 2.15). They are commonly distributed to the axilla, neck, back, and periumbilical areas. In diabetic dermopathy, groups of small >5 mm red papules occur on the arms and legs of diabetic individuals. These lesions slowly develop shallow centers and characteristically evolve into hyperpigmented scars.

Differential Diagnosis

Rapidly appearing lesions of acanthosis in elderly nonobese patients should prompt the clinician to search for occult malignancy, as there is an association with paraneoplastic syndromes and cancer. Acanthosis

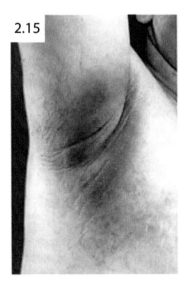

FIGURE 2.15   Acanthosis nigricans. (Courtesy of *Mayo Clinic Proceedings*. With permission.)

nigricans is also associated with polycystic ovarian syndrome, congenital adrenal hyperplasia, Cushing's disease, acromegaly, obesity, and Prader–Willi syndrome.

Diagnosis

Diagnosis is through history and physical examination as well as familiarity with the lesion. Groups of small >5 mm red papules occur on the arms and legs of diabetics. These lesions slowly develop shallow centers and characteristic hyperpigmentation.

Management/Treatment

Reduction of insulin resistance by weight loss and/or use of metformin or thiazolidinediones may lead to amelioration or even disappearance of acanthosis.

CUTANEOUS INFECTIONS

Definition/Overview

Malignant otitis externa is predominantly seen in elderly patients with glucose intolerance or diabetes mellitus. The most common causative bacterium is *Pseudomonas aeruginosa* though it may also, less commonly, be secondary to *Aspergillus*, *Staphylococcus*, *Proteus*, *Klebsiella*, or *Candida*.

Mucormycosis, or zygomycosis, is a rare but rapidly growing infection by the class of fungi Zygomycetes. They are common in nature and are aerosolized as spores. In diabetic patients or patients with metabolic acidosis, the most common and devastating manifestation is rhinocerebral mucormycosis. Almost three-quarters of all cases of rhinocerebral mucormycosis are associated with diabetes.

Pathophysiology

P. aeruginosa is not a common pathogen of the external ear. It is thought to be introduced by contamination of water. Poor tissue perfusion, secondary to microangiopathy, and being immunocompromised increase susceptibility to this infection. The infection may spread to the meninges, brain, or mastoid process.

Rhinocerebral mucormycosis most likely begins with the inhalation of spores and the seeding of the nares. The infection begins in the presence of hyperglycemia or metabolic acidosis. The presence of ketone reductase allows the fungi to proliferate in acidic environments and hyperglycemic states.

Clinical Presentation

Patients with malignant otitis media may present with fever and localized ear pain and drainage. Development of meningitis or osteomyelitis may occur. The initial site of infection in diabetic patients is the nasal turbinates. Presentation is consistent with acute sinusitis. Patients may rapidly develop fever, sinus tenderness and pain, purulent discharge, and severe headaches. Spread is to contiguous areas. Common sites include the orbits, palate, and brain. If the etiology of the infection is fungal, there may be marked tissue destruction and angioinvasion. Nerve palsies, proptosis, facial swelling, and cyanosis of overlying structures may be seen.

Differential Diagnosis

Squamous cell carcinoma of the external ear may mimic signs and symptoms of malignant otitis media.

Diagnosis

Diagnosis of malignant otitis externa is accomplished through history and physicals. Laboratory values may indicate the presence of an infection. The erythrocyte sedimentation rate, although nonspecific, is generally elevated. Biopsy of the ear is the only reliable mechanism to differentiate between squamous cell carcinoma and malignant otitis externa. Culture will help determine the causative organism and direct appropriate antimicrobial therapy.

Diagnosis of mucormycosis is via culture. The aggressive nature of the investigation warrants rapid identification. Direct biopsy and staining of necrotic tissue are appropriate. Clinicians should treat patients immediately if suspicion is high. CT scan or magnetic resonance imaging should be employed to determine the extent of the disease.

Management/Treatment

Malignant otitis externa may be treated with parenteral combination antibiotics or single-agent fluoroquinolone. Current treatment of rhinocerebral mucormycosis includes aggressive and potentially disfiguring debridement. Amphotericin B is the antifungal of choice.

DIABETIC DERMOPATHY

Definition/Overview

Diabetic dermopathy is a common finding in patients with long-standing diabetes mellitus and encompasses many types of skin lesions that are not explained by other classifications of skin lesions. It is a diagnosis of exclusion.

Etiology

Diabetic dermopathy is associated with long-standing disease. The areas affected suggest a relationship with local trauma.

Differential Diagnosis

For dermopathy, cutaneous infections and cancer must be ruled out.

Management/Treatment

There is no specific treatment for diabetic dermopathy.

OTHER INFECTIONS

A more common, though less dramatic, infection is intertrigo (Figure 2.16). This is an infectious or noninfectious inflammatory condition of two closely opposed skin surfaces. Although, when infectious in etiology, it may result from any of a variety of microorganisms; the most common cause is *Candida*. Treatment consists of treating the predisposing factor (e.g., weight loss if possible), topical antifungals, and drying agents.

Tinea infections are fairly common as well (Figure 2.17). They are caused by the organism *Pityrosporum orbiculare* and are treated by topical antifungal agents.

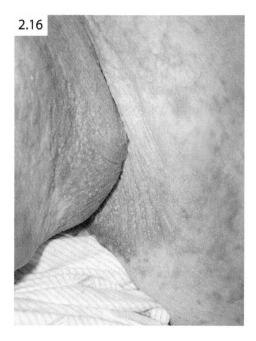

FIGURE 2.16   Axillary intertrigo. (Courtesy of Dr. Eva Parker.)

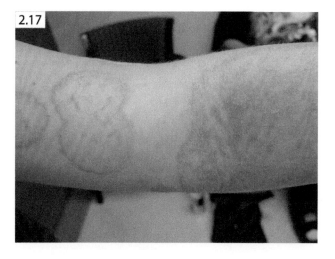

FIGURE 2.17   Tinea. (Courtesy of Drs. Anthony Peterson and David Eilers.)

COMMON DRUG REACTIONS

Definition/Overview

A common finding of drug therapy in diabetes mellitus is localized skin reaction (Figure 2.18). Insulin administration may lead to a variety of localized reactions. Hypersensitivity reactions, lipohypertrophy, lipoatrophy, nodule formation, and cellulitis may be seen in patients administered insulin. The use of sulfonylureas may lead to the development of a wide variety of skin manifestations. Thiazolidinediones, metformin, alpha-glucosidase inhibitors, DPP-4 inhibitors, and SGLT-2 inhibitors have not been associated with significant cutaneous manifestations. GLP-1 agonists can be associated with local skin irritation at the site of injection.

Etiology

Please refer to the following section 'Pathophysiology'.

Pathophysiology

Lipohypertrophy likely results from the localized effects of insulin. Insulin in high concentration leads to the inhibition of lipolysis locally. Lipoatrophy is a localized immunologic reaction to the impurities found within the various insulin preparations. Impurities in insulin preparations may cause hypersensitivity reactions locally or systemically. With the use of indwelling catheters associated with insulin pumps, direct skin trauma may lead to hard nodular formations. Additionally, these chronic sites may lead to a port of entry for infections leading to localized cellulitis.

Differential Diagnosis

In patients with severe systemic allergic reactions, all medications should be evaluated thoroughly. Vasculitis should be considered in patients with significant skin lesions.

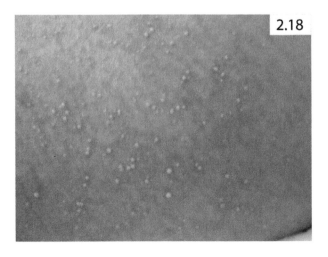

2.18

FIGURE 2.18 Typical drug eruption. (Courtesy of Drs. Anthony Peterson and David Eilers.)

Diagnosis

Diagnosis of lipohypertrophy, lipoatrophy, and pump-related injury is by history, physical examination, and familiarity with the character of the lesion. Deterioration in glycemic control in patients using the insulin pump may indicate skin problems at the site. Localized cellulitis presents with an increasing area of erythema, fever, and pain.

Sulfonylurea allergic reactions are related temporally to the initiation of therapy and are diagnosed through a thorough history and physical. These reactions are typically erythema multiforme, erythema nodosum, morbilliform rash, or simple pruritus. Reactions with the intake of alcohol result in an unpleasant flushing sensation. Jaundice may accompany more severe reactions to sulfonylurea. Photoallergic reactions to ultraviolet B radiation manifest as eruptions on the sun-exposed skin, typically the hands, face, and neck.

Management/Treatment

Treatment of lipohypertrophy, nodules associated with insulin pumps and some GLP-1 agonists, and lipoatrophy is simply to vary the site employed for insulin delivery. Patients utilizing insulin pumps should avoid using single sites for greater than 72 hours at a time. Cellulitis should be treated with an appropriate antibiotic regime. Withdrawal of the sulfonylurea is warranted for significant skin changes. In severe reactions, such as Stevens–Johnson syndrome, hospitalization, and supportive care are necessary.

BULLAE

Bullae are rare and tend to appear spontaneously from normal skin (Figure 2.19). They are usually on the lower extremities but sometimes on the arms, hands, and fingers. They may be intraepidermal or subepidermal. Intraepidermal bullae are sterile and nonhemorrhagic and resolve spontaneously within a few weeks. Subepidermal bullae may be hemorrhagic and may heal with scarring and atrophy. The only therapy is local care to avoid local infection while the lesions resolve spontaneously.

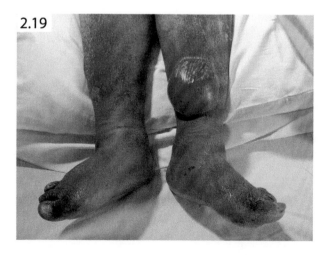

FIGURE 2.19   Diabetic bullae. (Courtesy of Drs. Anthony Peterson and David Eilers.)

THE DIABETIC FOOT

Definition/Overview

A patient with diabetes can have serious foot complications, including ulcers and amputation, largely due to the combined impact of neuropathy and peripheral vascular disease. Diabetic foot ulcers and lower-extremity amputations are serious and expensive complications that may affect as many as 15% of people with diabetes during their lifetime. Simple and inexpensive interventions may decrease the amputation rate by up to 85%.

Etiology

Many etiologic and risk factors can participate in the development of the diabetic foot, especially ulceration. Primarily, diabetic foot disease is a culmination of the combined effects of peripheral neuropathy and peripheral vascular disease. Other factors are associated with increased risk, however. These include increasing duration of diabetes, age, male gender, poor glycemic control, and microvascular and macrovascular diabetic complications. There is a weak association with cigarette smoking (though it should be avoided in any case), and alcohol consumption does not have a clear association with foot ulcerations.

Pathophysiology

Neuropathy leads to ulceration by several mechanisms. First, there is loss of sensation so an individual may not recognize the development of ulceration early. Second, the motor component of neuropathy leads to atrophy of the intrinsic muscles of the foot, resulting in a flexion deformity. This results in increased pressure on the metatarsal heads and tips of toes, common places for ulceration (Figure 2.20). Third, peripheral sympathetic autonomic neuropathy causes dyshidrosis and dry skin, which can readily crack, allowing for the invasion of pathogenic bacteria. Autonomic neuropathy may also be involved with arteriovenous shunting leading to altered skin and bone perfusion. Neuropathy, because of sensory loss, can also lead to the development of Charcot foot and attendant ulceration (Figures 2.21–2.23).

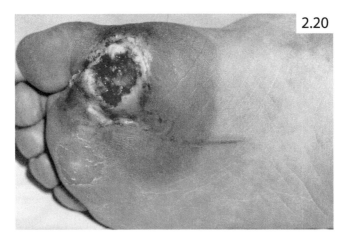

2.20

FIGURE 2.20   Ulcer secondary to chronic focal pressure callus. (Courtesy of Dr. Ronald Sage.)

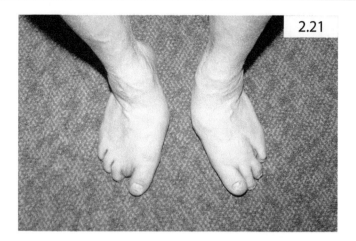

FIGURE 2.21 Chronic Charcot feet with hammer toes. (Courtesy of Dr. Ronald Sage.)

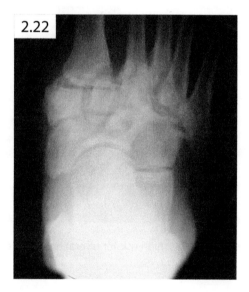

FIGURE 2.22 Radiograph of a Charcot foot. (Courtesy of Dr. Laurie Lomasney.)

Another pathophysiologic factor is limited joint mobility because of glycosylation of the skin, soft tissue, and joints. This limited joint mobility at the subtalar and first metatarsophalangeal joint causes higher plantar pressures than in those with normal mobility and further aggravates the situation caused by the flexion deformity. People with diabetes and neuropathy are more likely to have gait abnormalities making them prone to suffer some kind of injury during ambulation. Calluses may further increase pressure, and hemorrhages and early ulcers can form underneath calluses (Figure 2.24).

Peripheral vascular disease, highly prevalent in people with diabetes, is an infrequent precipitating event but plays a major role in delayed wound healing and gangrene (Figures 2.25–2.27). Infection may ultimately lead to osteomyelitis (Figures 2.28 and 2.29).

In the context of neuropathy, biomechanical problems, and peripheral vascular disease, a definable precipitating event may start the process of ulceration. This is often poorly fitting footwear.

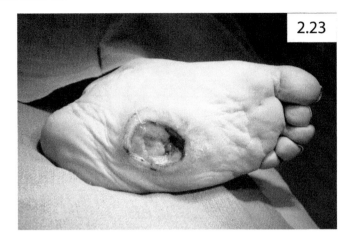

FIGURE 2.23   Neuropathic ulcer in Charcot foot. (Courtesy of Dr. Ronald Sage.)

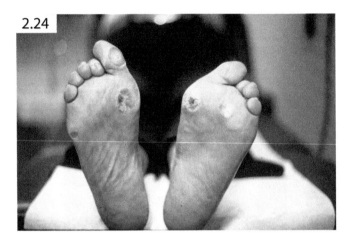

FIGURE 2.24   Plantar focal pressure calluses, high risk for ulceration. (Courtesy of Dr. Ronald Sage.)

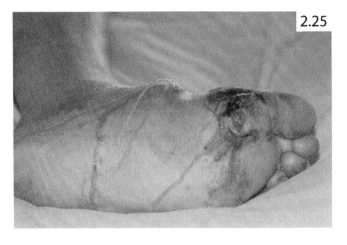

FIGURE 2.25   Extensive limb threatening ascending infection arising from first metatarsal ulcer secondary to chronic focal pressure callus. (Courtesy of Dr. Ronald Sage.)

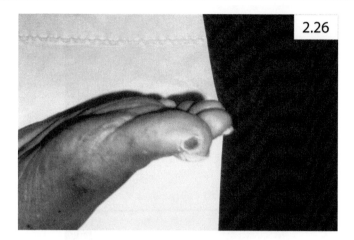

FIGURE 2.26   Distal ischemic ulcer. (Courtesy of Dr. Ronald Sage.)

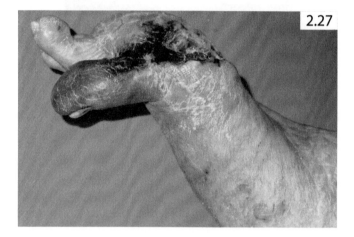

FIGURE 2.27   Severe ischemic ulceration. (Courtesy of Dr. Ronald Sage.)

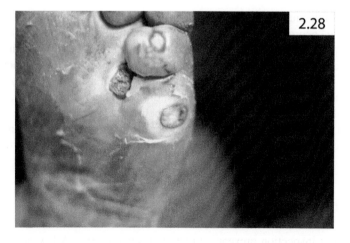

FIGURE 2.28   Ulcer with exposed bone and osteomyelitis. (Courtesy of Dr. Ronald Sage.)

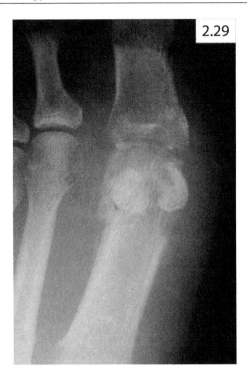

FIGURE 2.29 Radiograph showing osteomyelitis. (Courtesy of Dr. Laurie Lomasney.)

Clinical Presentation

In its most extreme form, patients with diabetic feet present with foot ulcerations, often infected. Short of this, the presentation is that of peripheral neuropathy, peripheral vascular disease, flexion deformities of the toes, interosseous muscle wasting, dry and cracked skin, and toenail deformities.

Diagnosis

A detailed discussion of the many modes of diagnosis of each of the component factors in the development of the diabetic foot (e.g., neuropathy, biomechanical abnormalities, and peripheral neuropathy) is beyond the scope of this chapter. However, in taking the history, attention should be given to classic symptoms of peripheral neuropathy, especially numbness, and classical symptoms of peripheral vascular disease, notably claudication. A previous history of ulceration is important as well. The physical exam includes a foot inspection to assess for obvious foot deformities, dry skin, cracks in the skin, calluses, and toenail deformities. A neurologic examination to ascertain whether there is sensory loss, and palpation of the pulses should be part of the routine. More specialized procedures such as nerve conduction velocity testing, Doppler, or angiograms may be necessary for some individuals and should be decided on a case-by-case basis.

Management/Treatment

The old axiom that foot inspection prevents amputation remains true. A key part of management is to make sure that the patient and/or a family member looks at the feet daily – top, bottom, and between the toes. Patients should be advised to call their physicians immediately at any sign of infection or anything unusual. The importance of daily self-examination should be reinforced by the physician doing this at every clinic visit. Proper-fitting shoes are essential. Patients should be instructed to dry their feet thoroughly after bathing and use skin moisturizers liberally to keep the skin from getting dry and cracked.

The development of peripheral neuropathy can be delayed by good glycemic control, so that is part of the management. Surgical debridement of calluses and good nail care is fundamental. Surgery to correct bony deformities may be indicated. Claudication, a manifestation of peripheral vascular disease, can be managed by a graded exercise program and, in some cases, vascular surgery. Fungal nail infections can be treated with topical and systemic agents.

CARDIOVASCULAR DISEASE IN DIABETES

Definition/Overview

Diabetes mellitus is a well-established independent risk factor for the development and progression of coronary heart disease (CHD), peripheral vascular disease (PVD), and atherosclerotic cardiovascular disease (CVD). CHD is two- to threefold more common in individuals with diabetes than in the general population. Women with diabetes are at a greater risk for the development of CHD than men. The prevalence of symptomatic and silent CHD in this population after age 49 is estimated to be 30%. The cumulative mortality from CHD is approximately 35% at age 55 in people with T1DM. Individuals with T2DM without known coronary disease had a similar rate of developing a myocardial infarction (approximately 20%) compared with nondiabetic patients with a previous history of myocardial infarction. This was independent of other traditional risk factors. Poor glycemic control is well correlated with the increase in the prevalence of CHD and myocardial infarction. Carotid arterial disease development and progression are directly correlated with glycemic control. Despite these relationships, no studies have clearly shown that improved glycemic control prevents coronary or carotid disease in T2DM. Studies have suggested that there might be a delayed macrovascular benefit from periods of antecedent good glycemic control in T1DM. Duration of diabetes mellitus has a significant impact on the development and progression of peripheral arterial disease. Although intensive glycemic control is always advocated, the relationship between glycemic control and peripheral arterial disease treatment has not been well established and no glycemic intervention has been shown to improve PVD.

Etiology

The primary defect in cardiovascular disease is the formation and progression of atherosclerotic plaques, with resultant occlusive or thromboembolic disease. Common risk factors for its development include diabetes mellitus, hypertension, hypercholesterolemia, chronic kidney disease, smoking, obesity, age, and family history.

Pathophysiology

Atherosclerosis development is multifactorial. Central to development and progression is endothelial dysfunction. In some patients, there is likely a genetic predisposition to endothelial dysfunction. In other patients, endothelial dysfunction is triggered by hyperglycemia, hypertension, hyperlipidemia, and the products of smoking. At baseline, there appears to be a reduction in the production and release of nitric oxide, a potent vasodilator that has antiatherosclerotic and antiplatelet properties. Dysfunctional endothelial cells express adhesion molecules that trap circulating monocytes. These are then translocated into the

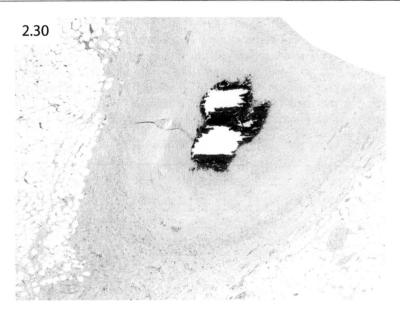

FIGURE 2.30   Coronary artery with atherosclerosis and calcification. (Courtesy of Dr. Henry Brown.)

vessel wall itself where they meet a highly oxidative environment. The environment converts the monocytes to macrophages. LDL cholesterol particles also become oxidized within the vessel wall and this process makes them more easily taken up by macrophages. These lipid-laden macrophages are called foam cells and will eventually rupture leading to development of the earliest identifiable histological feature of atherosclerosis: the fatty streak. The oxidized LDL-C particles additionally stimulate tissue macrophages to release proinflammatory cytokines and adhesion molecules, self-perpetuating the inflammatory process. Hyperglycemia further exacerbates inflammatory cytokine production and oxidative stress. With 60%–70% occlusion of a vessel, the patient is likely to experience symptoms. Plaque rupture results in acute syndromes. This phenomenon is typically associated with plaques occluding less than 50% of the vessel lumen. Plaques may additionally undergo remodeling and calcification. The pathology of plaque, plaque rupture, and subsequent ischemic fibrosis is shown in Figures 2.30–2.32.

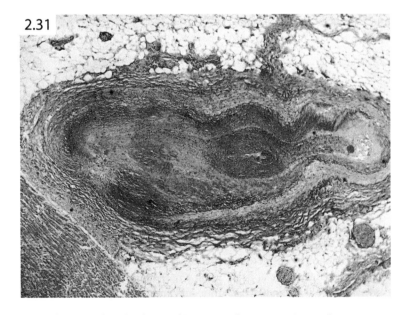

FIGURE 2.31   Ruptured atherosclerotic plaque. (Courtesy of Dr. Henry Brown.)

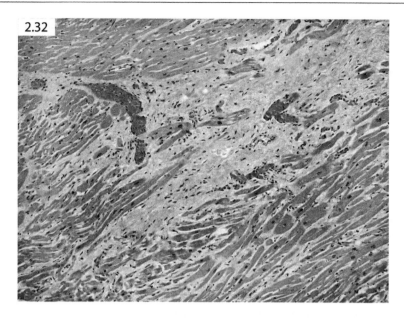

FIGURE 2.32 Postischemic subendocardial fibrosis. (Courtesy of Dr. Henry Brown.)

Clinical Presentation

Cardiovascular disease diagnosis in the diabetic may present as both a straightforward diagnosis or with an insidious onset resulting in disastrous consequences. For example, coronary disease can present as sudden death.

PVD may initially present with the progression of hair loss in the lower extremities, worsening neuropathy, an overall cold sensation in the feet, or claudication. Diabetics with pronounced PVD may be predisposed to the development of ulceration and infection.

Patients with carotid and cerebrovascular disease present with headache, nausea, syncope, symptoms of stroke, or an early harbinger of severe disease, the transient ischemic attack. A physical exam may reveal carotid bruits and subtle neurological deficits.

Diagnosis

A physical examination can guide a clinician in the diagnosis and early treatment of vascular complications of diabetes mellitus. Although powerful imaging and laboratory testing are available, the art of the physical examination remains the cornerstone in the diagnosis and stratification of cardiovascular disease. Details of various diagnostic modalities are beyond the scope of this discussion.

Management/Treatment

Acute coronary, peripheral, and cerebral injuries related to arterial insults in diabetic patients should be treated in an emergent fashion under the care of appropriate surgical and acute care physicians. Access to interventional procedures should not be delayed in favor of medical management in patients with non-ST segment elevation myocardial infarction. Patients should be initially treated with oxygen, nitrates, antiplatelet agents, beta-blockers, and high-dose statins. Patients who have undergone revascularization for CHD should avoid the use of the sulfonylurea glyburide, as in the periprocedural setting this sulfonylurea may reduce the powerful myocardial protection afforded by ischemic preconditioning. Individuals with hyperglycemia, both known diabetics and new onset, admitted to the hospital or intensive care setting should be managed utilizing glycemic protocols. The use of insulin in hyperglycemic patients should be advocated in this setting regardless of their previous medical regimen and regardless of whether the patient has an antecedent history of diabetes. Decreased mortality and morbidity have been demonstrated for cardiovascular patients in the surgical and medical intensive care units in many but not all studies with good glycemic control achieved by insulin.

Therapy should also be directed at controlling cardiovascular risk factors over the long term. Positive lifestyle changes and control of hypertension, microalbuminuria, and lipids should aggressively be instituted. Liberal use of SGLT-2 inhibitors should be instituted given the remarkable cardiovascular benefits of these agents. If not contraindicated by gastrointestinal issues, GLP-1 agents should be frontline therapy once discharged, as these agents also have demonstrated cardiovascular protection.

Secondary Causes of Diabetes

Although uncommon, it is important to not overlook secondary causes of diabetes associated with physical findings, where treatment could ameliorate the underlying insulin resistance and hyperglycemia. These include acromegaly, excess cortisol states, and glucagonoma.

ACROMEGALY

Definition

Acromegaly is almost always caused by a growth hormone (GH)-secreting adenoma of the pituitary gland and is associated with increased morbidity and mortality. Growth hormone excess that occurs before fusion of the epiphyseal growth plates in a child or adolescent is called pituitary gigantism; when the excess GH appears in an adult, soft tissue changes are the clinical clues leading to the diagnosis.

Etiology

Excess GH stimulates hepatic secretion of insulin-like growth factor-I (IGF-I), which causes most of the clinical manifestations of the disease. The clinical diagnosis is often delayed because of the slow progression of the signs of acromegaly over a period of many years.

Pathophysiology

Serum GH concentrations and IGF-I concentrations are increased in virtually all patients with acromegaly. The increases in serum IGF-I are often disproportionately greater than those in GH for two reasons: GH secretion fluctuates more and GH stimulates the secretion of IGF binding protein-3 (IGFBP-3), the major IGF-I binding protein in serum. Other rare causes of acromegaly include pituitary somatotroph carcinoma, hypothalamic tumor secreting growth hormone-releasing hormone (GHRH), nonendocrine tumor secreting GHRH, ectopic secretion of GH by a nonendocrine tumor, and excess growth factor activity.

Clinical Presentation

Clinical clues to acromegaly include visual field defects, cranial nerve palsy, acral enlargement including thickness of soft tissue of hands and feet, prognathism, arthritis, proximal myopathy, hypertrophy of frontal bones, skin tags, macroglossia, thyromegaly, hepatomegaly, and galactorrhea.

Diagnosis

A normal serum IGF-I concentration is strong evidence that the patient does not have acromegaly. If the serum IGF-I concentration is high (or equivocal), serum GH should be measured after oral glucose administration. It is equally acceptable to proceed immediately to MRI after obtaining an elevated level of IGF-I. If the MRI is normal, then studies to identify a GHRH- or GH-secreting tumor should be undertaken. All patients with acromegaly have increased GH secretion. However, the random serum GH concentration is often in the range of 2 to 10 ng/mL during much of the day, values that can be found in normal subjects. Unlike normal subjects, the patient's serum GH concentrations change little during the day or night, and in most patients do not change in response to stimuli such as food or exercise. Nevertheless, because of the variations in serum GH that occur in normal subjects and in patients with other disorders, a high value cannot be interpreted without knowing when the blood sample was obtained and something about the patient. To obviate these problems it is best not to obtain random measurements of serum GH.

The most specific dynamic test for establishing the diagnosis of acromegaly is an oral glucose tolerance test. In normal subjects, serum GH concentrations fall to 1 ng/mL or less within 2 hours after ingestion of 75 g glucose. In contrast, the post-glucose values are greater than 2 ng/mL in acromegaly.

Management/Treatment

Since acromegaly is associated with increased cardiovascular risk, almost all patients should be treated, even those who are asymptomatic and those in whom the disorder does not seem to be progressing. Selective transsphenoidal surgical resection is the treatment of choice for patients. Surgical resection may be followed up with radiotherapy or medical treatment with analogs of somatostatin (growth hormone-inhibitory hormone) that inhibit GH secretion more effectively than native somatostatin because of their greater potency and longer plasma half-life. These are octreotide and lanreotide. Octreotide is available in short- and long-acting forms; lanreotide is available in long-acting forms.

EXCESS CORTISOL STATES: CUSHING'S SYNDROME

Definition

Excess cortisol can be due to exogenous use (iatrogenic Cushing's syndrome) or due to endogenous causes, which include benign and malignant adrenal tumors, pituitary ACTH-dependent Cushing's syndrome (Cushing's disease), and ectopic ACTH from other malignancies. It is crucial to determine the cause of the excess glucocorticoids so that appropriate treatment can be rendered.

Etiology

Excess cortisol due to exogenous use (iatrogenic Cushing's syndrome) is more common than any other cause but is seldom reported. Cushing's syndrome may also be caused by a benign adrenal adenoma, often discovered incidentally in radiographic studies. While adrenal nodules are noted in up to 8.7% of adults, they are usually not associated with any clinical adrenal disease. Excess glucocorticoid production, however, is the most common hormone overproduced. A very rare cause of Cushing's syndrome is adrenal carcinoma, which is estimated to be 0.2 to 2 per million per year. Pituitary ACTH-dependent Cushing's syndrome (Cushing's disease) is due to the hypersecretion of pituitary ACTH by the pituitary corticotrophs and is associated with bilateral adrenocortical hyperplasia. It is five to six times more common than Cushing's syndrome caused by benign and malignant adrenal tumors combined, with women three to eight times more likely than men to develop Cushing's disease. Ectopic ACTH syndrome, although often not diagnosed, can cause Cushing's syndrome; about 1% of patients with small-cell lung cancer have ectopic ACTH syndrome and small-cell lung carcinoma causes half of all cases of the syndrome.

Pathophysiology

ACTH-dependent Cushing's syndrome is due to hypersecretion of pituitary ACTH by the corticotrophs and is associated with bilateral adrenocortical hyperplasia. There is loss of synchrony between ACTH and cortisol secretion, with hypersecretion of cortisol and the loss of normal circadian rhythm. Morning plasma ACTH and serum cortisol concentrations may be normal, but late-evening concentrations are high. Salivary cortisol concentrations reflect those of serum free cortisol. The increased cortisol secretion is reflected by increased urinary excretion of cortisol. The pituitary adenoma cells function at a higher than normal set point for cortisol feedback inhibition, and this characteristic is clinically important because it permits the use of dexamethasone suppression to distinguish between pituitary and ectopic ACTH secretion; the latter is usually very resistant to glucocorticoid negative feedback. Almost all patients with Cushing's disease have a pituitary adenoma, although the tumor is often not demonstrable by imaging; the remainder have corticotroph hyperplasia. The tumors are usually microadenomas; only about 5% are macroadenomas. Patients with macroadenomas are more likely to have high plasma ACTH concentrations than those with microadenomas, and the concentrations are less likely to fall with high doses of dexamethasone. Patients with ectopic ACTH secretion will have persistent cortisol elevation, even with high-dose dexamethasone testing. Adrenal adenomas, which are almost always benign, can also oversecrete cortisol, but the concomitant ACTH level will be suppressed.

Clinical Presentation

Clinical clues to the diagnosis of Cushing's disease are underlying centripetal obesity, facial plethora, impaired glucose tolerance or type 2 diabetes, proximal muscle weakness, hypertension, easy bruising, hirsutism, depression, oligomenorrhea, acne, abdominal striae, and edema.

Diagnosis

The diagnosis of Cushing's disease involves suspecting it based on the patient's symptoms and signs, documenting the presence of hypercortisolemia, and determining its cause.

Management/Treatment

If a patient is taking exogenous steroids, discontinuation is recommended if this is possible. If a cortisol-producing adrenal adenoma is found, surgical removal should be curative. If a pituitary adenoma is responsible (Cushing's disease), then neurosurgical intervention is the procedure of choice often followed by radiation therapy. If ectopic ACTH secretion is determined to be the source, treatment of the underlying malignancy is needed.

GLUCAGONOMA

Definition

Glucagonomas are rare islet cell tumors of the pancreas that oversecrete glucagon. The systemic manifestations make it unique among islet cell tumors and provide visible clues that make early diagnosis possible.

Etiology

Nearly all reported cases of glucagonoma syndrome have been associated with tumors originating in the alpha cells of the pancreas. These tumors demonstrate the typical characteristics of islet cell tumors; they are usually encapsulated, firm nodules, varying in size from 2 cm up to 25 cm, and occur most often in the tail of the pancreas.

Pathophysiology

Glucagonomas consist of cords and nests of well-differentiated islet cells. Characteristic alpha cell granules may be seen on electron microscopy. Despite their benign histologic appearance, most pancreatic glucagonomas are malignant, as defined by their propensity for metastasis, which is usually present at the time of diagnosis.

Clinical Manifestations

Patients typically present in their fifth decade, with an even distribution between males and females. The clinical syndrome classically associated with glucagonoma includes necrolytic migratory erythema, cheilitis, diabetes mellitus, anemia, weight loss, venous thrombosis, and neuropsychiatric symptoms. Weight loss and necrolytic migratory erythema are the most prevalent symptoms, occurring in approximately 65% to 70% of patients by the time of diagnosis. Necrolytic migratory characteristically begins as erythematous papules or plaques involving the face, perineum, and extremities. Over the next 7 to 14 days, the lesions enlarge and coalesce. Central clearing then occurs, leaving bronze-colored, indurated lesions. A rash may occasionally appear, before the onset of systemic symptoms, but most patients with rash usually have weight loss, diarrhea, sore mouth, weakness, mental status changes, or diabetes mellitus. Venous thrombosis occurs in up to 30% of patients with glucagonoma; this association with thromboembolism appears to be unique among endocrine tumors. Neurologic symptoms associated with glucagonoma may include ataxia, dementia, optic atrophy, and proximal muscle weakness. The prevalence of metastatic disease at the time of diagnosis varies from 50% to 100%, with the most common site of metastasis being the liver, followed by regional lymph nodes, bone, adrenal gland, kidney, and lung. Rarely, glucagonoma may be associated with multiple endocrine neoplasia syndrome, type 1 (MEN 1); such patients typically have a family history of pituitary, pancreatic islet cell, or parathyroid tumors.

Diagnosis

The characteristic skin lesions of glucagonoma syndrome are often the clue that leads to the correct diagnosis, and the presence of necrolytic migratory erythema should prompt further workup. A serum glucagon level should be obtained. It is important to recognize, however, that conditions other than glucagonoma can induce 'physiologic' elevations in the serum glucagon concentration. These include hypoglycemia, fasting, trauma, sepsis, acute pancreatitis, abdominal surgery, Cushing's syndrome, and renal and hepatic failure. However, these conditions are associated with only moderate elevations of glucagon, usually less than 500 pg/mL (upper limit of normal <100 pg/mL), while a glucagonoma is associated with markedly elevated glucagon concentrations. This should be followed up with an abdominal CT. Since the tumor is usually large by the time of diagnosis, it is localizable by CT in the majority of cases. Endoscopic ultrasonography can detect pancreatic tumors as small as 2 to 3 mm, provides accurate information on the local extent of disease, and is the modality of choice for detecting and biopsying islet cell tumors too small for CT visualization. Finally, somatostatin receptor scintigraphy using radiolabeled octreotide is very sensitive to glucagonomas, however, since these tumors are usually large by the time of diagnosis, this is rarely required for diagnosis.

Management/Treatment

For the minority of cases in which the tumor remains localized at the time of diagnosis, resection of the primary pancreatic tumor is indicated since it offers the chance of a complete cure. Whether a simple enucleation, focal pancreatic resection, or Whipple procedure is performed is dictated by the site and extent of the tumor. Because patients with glucagonoma syndrome suffer from a prolonged catabolic state, nutritional support of some kind is an integral component of therapy. Treatment for metastatic disease includes somatostatin analogs such as octreotide and lanreotide. Finally, interferon improves symptoms of hormonal hypersecretion in 40% to 50% of patients with pancreatic islet cells.

Therapeutic Options for T2DM

Many options are available to clinicians caring for individuals with diabetes, and it is beyond the scope of this book to review them. A very helpful algorithm is included with the recommendations of the American Diabetes Association for managing outpatient diabetes.

BIBLIOGRAPHY

American Diabetes Association Position Statement Cardiovascular Disease and Risk Management, *Diabetes Care* (2022), PMID 34964815/DOI 10.2337/dc22-S010
Bakris et al., *Diabetes Care* (2014), PMID 24558077/DOI 10.2337/dc13-1870
Boulton et al., *Diabetes Care* (2005), PMID 15793206/DOI 10.2337/diacare.28.4.956
Burke et al., *Diabetes Care* (1999), PMID 10526730/DOI 10.2337/diacare.22.10.1655

Cheung et al., *Kidney International* (2021), PMID 33637203/DOI 10.1016/j.kint.2020.10.026

Chronic Kidney Disease and Risk Management, *Diabetes Care* (2022), PMID 34964813/DOI 10.2337/dc22-er03

de Boer et al., *Diabetes Care* (2017), PMID 28830958/DOI 10.2337/dci17-0026

Finnerup et al., *Lancet Neurology* (2015), PMID 25575710/DOI 10.1016/s1474-4422(14)70251-0

Fong et al., *Diabetes Care* (2004), PMID 15451934/DOI 10.2337/diacare.27.10.2540

Freeman R, *Lancet* (2005), PMID 15811460/DOI 10.1016/S0140-6736(05)74815-7

Gross et al., *Diabetes Care* (2005), PMID 15616252/DOI 10.2337/diacare.28.1.164

KDIGO 2012 Clinical practice guideline for the evaluation and management of chronic kidney disease, *Kidney International Supplement* (2013), 3(1) January 1, 2013.

KDIGO 2021 Clinical practice guideline for the management of blood pressure in chronic kidney disease. *Kidney International* (2021), PMID 33637197/DOI 10.1016/j.kint.2020.11.003

McGuire et al., *JAMA Cardiology* (2021), PMID 33031522/DOI 10.1001/jamacardio.2020.4511

Palmer et al., *British Medical Journal* (2021), PMID 35044930/DOI 10.1136/bmj.o109

Passarella et al., *Diabetes Spectrum* (2018), PMID 30140137/DOI 10.2337/ds17-0085

Retinopathy, Neuropathy, and Foot Care. *Diabetes Care* (2022), PMID 34964887/DOI 10.2337/dc22-S012

Standards of Diabetes Care. Diabetes Care (2022), PMID 34964887/DOI 10.2337/dc22-S012, PMID 34964873/DOI 10.2337/dc22-S011, PMID 34964831/DOI 10.2337/dc22-S009, PMID 34964868/DOI 10.2337/dc22-S006

Vinik et al., *Diabetes Care* (2003), PMID 12716821/DOI 10.2337/diacare.26.5.1553

Waldfogel et al., *Neurology* (2017), PMID 28341643/DOI 10.1212.wnl.0000000000003882

Whelton et al., *Hypertension* (2018), PMID 29743247/DOI 10.1161/HYP.0000000000000076

Zelniker et al., *Lancet* (2019), PMID 30424892/DOI 10.1016/s0140-6736(18)32590-x

Obesity

3

Marriam Ali and Sobia Sadiq

ABSTRACT

Obesity is a disorder involving increased body fat and is associated with metabolic disease. The prevalence of obesity is steadily increasing across the globe with deleterious health implications. There are several factors associated with obesity including genetics, metabolic syndromes, neuroendocrine dysregulation, as well as diet and lifestyle habits. Treatment includes prevention strategies, diet and lifestyle modifications, medical pharmacotherapy and surgical interventions.

INTRODUCTION

Body weight is a physiologically regulated parameter; obesity is a derangement of this regulation.[1] Obesity is a major risk factor for the development of diabetes mellitus, cardiovascular diseases, and certain types of cancer. The disease arises from a chronic positive energy balance that is often due to large caloric intake and an increasingly sedentary lifestyle on the background of a genetic and epigenetic predisposition.[2]

Obesity is defined as a body mass index (BMI) of 30.0 or higher and is subdivided into the following categories:[3]

Class 1: BMI of 30 to <35
Class 2: BMI of 35 to <40
Class 3: BMI of 40 or higher, also categorized as 'severe' obesity

EPIDEMIOLOGY

The prevalence of obesity is steadily increasing across the globe with deleterious health implications worldwide. Obesity has been affecting Americans at an accelerated rate over the past two decades (Figure 3.1). From 1999–2000 to 2017–2018, the prevalence of obesity in the US increased from 30.5% to 42.4%. During the same time, the prevalence of severe obesity nearly doubled from 4.7% to 9.2%.[4]

Data were collected through the Behavioral Risk Factor Surveillance System (BRFSS), an ongoing, state-based, telephone interview survey conducted by state health departments with assistance from the

DOI: 10.1201/9781003100669-3

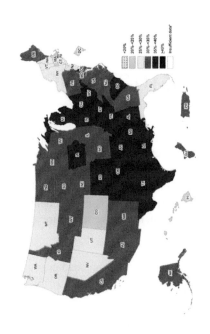

FIGURE 3.1 CDC's Division of Nutrition, Physical Activity, and Obesity (DNPAO) State Adult Obesity Prevalence Map 2011–2018, Behavioral Risk Factor Surveillance System. (Adapted from cdc.gov: https://www.cdc.gov/obesity/data/prevalence-maps.html#overall.)

Centers for Disease Control and Prevention (CDC). Height and weight data used in the BMI calculations were self-reported.

Overweight and obesity are global health issues that affect 68.5% of the adult US population.[5] In most recent years, the category of extreme obesity has seen the greatest proportional change.[5]

PATHOPHYSIOLOGY

Obesity is a disease that involves a long-term positive energy balance in which energy intake is greater than expenditure. Hormonal dysregulation plays an integral part in the pathogenesis and maintenance of excess weight. The set point of the body changes to a higher setting resulting in difficulty maintaining weight loss.[1] The most impactful factor in the development of obesity is calorie intake. Consumption of high-caloric, energy-dense diets promotes excess weight gain. Environmental factors ranging from socio-economic status to exposure to endocrine disruptors to sedentary lifestyles confer further risks of obesity.[1,6] Epigenetic, genetic, and developmental risk factors are still being elucidated with ongoing research (Figure 3.2).

Genetics

Obesity studies among twins, adoptees, and biological versus adoptive parents reveal the presence of genetic factors[7,8] Obesity has been historically divided into two categories: monogenic obesity and polygenic obesity (also known as common obesity) (Figure 3.3).

Common obesity is polygenic and reflects the collective interactions of various genetic predispositions with environmental factors. The FTO (fat mass- and obesity-associated) gene variant has the strongest association hypothesized to be due to increased energy intake.

Monogenic obesity can be subdivided into autosomal dominant or recessive inherited forms. Generally, monogenic forms possess abnormalities in leptin signaling.[9] Chromosomal rearrangements result in syndromic obesity like Prader–Willi syndrome, WAGR syndrome, SIM1 syndrome, and pleiotropic syndromes (including Bardet–Biedl syndrome, fragile X syndrome, and Cohen syndrome).[9]

Neuroendocrine Dysregulation

The ventromedial hypothalamic nucleus (VMH) is regarded as the satiety center, whereas the lateral hypothalamus (LH) is the hunger center.[10] The hormonal signal of satiety and hunger come largely from the adipose tissue, pancreas, and liver. Distention and satiety are signaled to the hindgut by peptide YY, GLP1 from the ileum, and cholecystokinin from the duodenum. The adipocyte, anorexigenic hormone leptin plays a significant role in the relationship between obesity and energy homeostasis. Leptin exerts its effects by inhibiting orexigenic neuropeptide Y/Agouti-related peptide neurons and activating anorexigenic proopiomelanocortin (POMC)/cocaine amphetamine-related transcript neurons in the arcuate nucleus, resulting in decreased food intake and increased energy expenditure.[9] Orexigenic ghrelin from the stomach increases with time after a meal. The development of resistance to leptin and ghrelin, hormones that are crucial for the neuroendocrine control of energy homeostasis, is a hallmark of obesity.[2] A deficiency of leptin causes severe hyperphagia and obesity in both humans and animals.[1] Obese individuals have been found to have high levels of leptin and exogenous administration of leptin has demonstrated a resistance to its anorexigenic effects (Figures 3.4 and 3.5).[11]

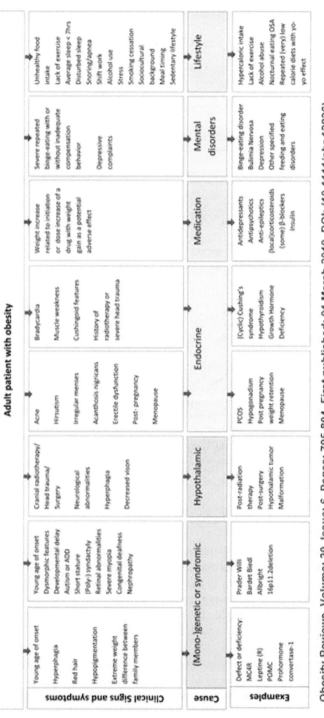

FIGURE 3.2 Distinguishing underlying causes of obesity in adults based on clinical signs and symptoms (From van der Valk, E. S., et al., A Comprehensive Diagnostic Approach to Detect Underlying causes of Obesity in Adults, *Obes. Rev. 20*, 795–804 (2019).)

Obesity Reviews, Volume: 20, Issue: 6, Pages: 795-804, First published: 01 March 2019, DOI: (10.1111/obr.12836)

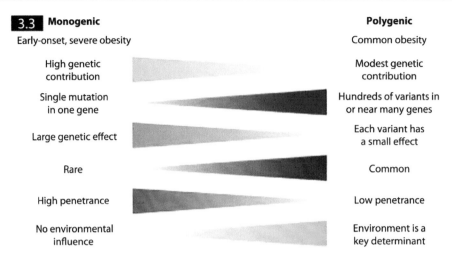

FIGURE 3.3   Key features of monogenic and polygenic obesity (From Loos, R. J. F. & Yeo, G. S. H., The Genetics of Obesity: From Discovery to Biology, *Nat. Rev. Genet.* 1–14 (2021) doi:10.1038/s41576-021-00414-z.)

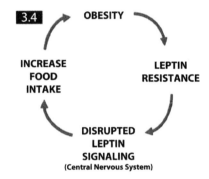

FIGURE 3.4   Schematic representation of different anti-obesity therapies based on the use of leptin. (From Izquierdo, A. G., Crujeiras, A. B., Casanueva, F. F. & Carreira, M. C. Leptin, Obesity, and Leptin Resistance: Where Are We 25 Years Later? *Nutrients* 11, 2704 (2019).)

Development, Age, and Weight Gain

A large body of evidence has shown that intrauterine and early life events are influential in the development of obesity.[12] Multiple reports suggest that endocrine-disrupting chemicals (EDCs) can dysregulate hormonal metabolic processes, particularly in early development, resulting in a propensity to gain weight despite limiting caloric intake and increasing physical activity.[6] An obesogenic perinatal environment contributes to adulthood obesity, and particular maternal factors such as excessive weight gain during pregnancy or preexisting maternal obesity and diabetes can also predispose a person to the development of obesity in adulthood.[13]

Most women experience gestational weight gain and progressive weight gain with multiple pregnancies. Pregnancy was associated with a threefold greater increase in visceral fat deposition compared to non-childbearing women.[14] For some women, this can lead to the development of obesity; women who are overweight or obese at baseline are more likely to gain excessive weight during pregnancy.[15]

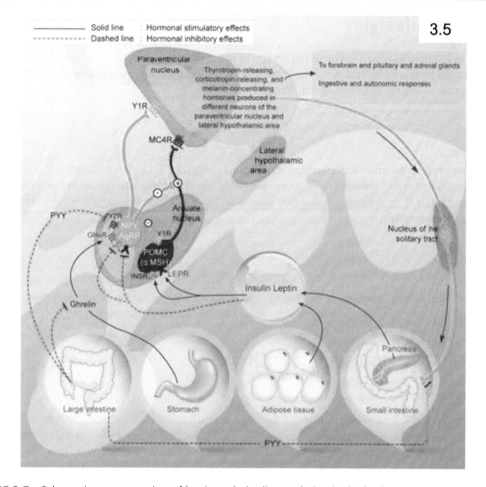

FIGURE 3.5 Schematic representation of leptin and ghrelin regulation in the body.

Aging is associated with weight gain in both genders, although females experience a higher rate of weight gain than men.[16,17] The current literature suggests weight gain in midlife women is due to aging and lifestyle changes rather than menopause, however, estrogen deficiency does lead to an increase in total body fat and a decrease in lean body mass.[18]

Dietary Factors

The availability of energy-dense foods and increased energy intake is sufficient to account for the increase in the prevalence of obesity observed from the 1970s to the 2000s.[19]

Evaluation of dietary macronutrient composition has not shown conclusive evidence that diets high in fats or carbohydrates are consistently associated with weight gain. However, specific food intake has been shown to result in increased weight gain (e.g., french fries, processed red meat) or protection against weight gain (e.g., whole grains and fresh fruit).[20,21]

Sedentary Lifestyles

A reduction in physical activity with aging results in reduced energy expenditure contributing to weight gain. Increased levels of physical activity are associated with the primary prevention of obesity and long-term weight maintenance after intentional weight loss.[21]

Sleep

A reduction in sleep duration has mirrored the obesity epidemic. Trials have shown that reduced sleep leads to altered leptin and ghrelin levels, increased hunger, and a preference for calorie-dense, processed carbohydrate foods.[20,22] Furthermore, reduced sleep also leads to a lower rate of physical activity leading to less energy expenditure.[23]

Drugs

A variety of drugs have been shown to cause weight gain (Table 3.1). Medications can affect energy homeostasis mainly by promoting hunger or by decreasing resting metabolism.[24]

Endocrinopathies Leading to Obesity

Hypothyroidism

Studies have not shown a causal relationship between hypothyroidism and obesity.[25] Overt hypothyroidism does cause modest weight gain. However, subclinical hypothyroidism has not been shown to correlate with weight gain. Current theories hypothesize that changes in TSH may be secondary to obesity. Treating overt hypothyroidism with levothyroxine can cause a modest effect on inducing weight loss, but there is no data supporting levothyroxine use in euthyroid obese patients.[25]

Cushing's Syndrome

A common feature of Cushing's syndrome is progressive central adiposity, fat accumulation in the face and neck, and enlarged dorso- and supraclavicular fat pads with muscle wasting in the extremities.

Hypothalamic Obesity

Hypothalamic obesity is a syndrome resulting from damage to the ventromedial or paraventricular regions of the hypothalamus or amygdala resulting in hyperphagia. It can be seen in patients with resected craniopharyngioma, inflammatory processes such as tuberculosis and sarcoidosis, head trauma, or after cranial irradiation.[24]

Growth Hormone Deficiency

Adults with growth hormone deficiency have an increased body weight compared to age-, sex-, and height-matched adults due to increased fat and reduction in total body water.[26,27]

TABLE 3.1   Medications Associated with Weight Gain by Drug Class.

CATEGORY	DRUG CLASS	WEIGHT GAIN
Psychiatric agents	Antipsychotic	Clozapine Risperidone Olanzapine Quetiapine Haloperidol Perphenazine Quetiapine
	Antidepressants/mood stabilizers: tricyclic antidepressants	Amitriptyline Doxepin Imipramine Nortriptyline Trimipramine Mirtazapine
	Antidepressants/mood stabilizers: SSRIs	Fluoxetine* Sertraline* Paroxetine Fluvoxamine
	Antidepressants/mood stabilizers: MAO Inhibitors	Phenelzine Tranylcypromine
	Lithium	
Neurologic agents	Anticonvulsants	Carbamazepine Gabapentin Valproate
Endocrinologic agents	Diabetes drugs	Insulin (weight gain differs with type and regimen used) Sulfonylureas Thiazolidinediones Sitagliptin* Meglitinides
Gynecologic agents	Oral contraceptives	Progestational steroids Hormonal contraceptives containing progestational steroids
	Endometriosis treatment	Depot leuprolide acetate
Infectious disease agents	Antiretroviral therapy	Protease inhibitors
General	Steroid hormones	Corticosteroids Progestational steroids NSAIDs
	Antihistamines/anticholinergics	Diphenhydramine* Doxepin* Cyproheptadine*

Source: Apovian CM, Aronne LJ, Bessesen DH, et al., Pharmacological Management of Obesity: An Endocrine Society Clinical Practice Guideline, *J. Clin. Endocrinol. Metab*. 100:342 (2015).
* The data supporting the effects of these medications on weight gain are of low quality or conflicting.

TREATMENT

Guidelines for the management of obesity incorporate the presence and severity of weight-related complications as the primary factors that influence the treatment modality. Therapies are aimed at both the prevention and treatment of obesity and its complications through weight loss achieved by lifestyle, pharmacological, and/or surgical interventions. Moderate weight loss, defined as a 5%–10% reduction in baseline weight, is associated with meaningful impacts on obesity-related metabolic risk factors and comorbidities.[28]

Prevention

Strategies aimed at the prevention of obesity include school-based and workplace interventions that focus on learning positive behaviors concerning nutrition and physical activity. Successful interventions include reducing the consumption of weight-promoting foods and refiguring the antiquated food pyramid for plates with healthier proportions, such as adopting a Healthy Plate model in which fruits and vegetables comprise 50% of one's plate and the other half is divided among proteins and fiber-dense carbohydrates (Figure 3.6). Strategies aimed to influence the obesity epidemic via nutrition, however, have been met with several challenges including the expense of and limited access to healthful food options. Additional strategies include improving access to healthful food options as well as encouraging an active lifestyle.

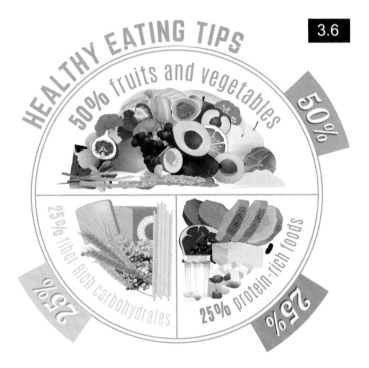

FIGURE 3.6 Healthy Plate Model: components and quantity of a balanced meal focused on 50% intake of fruits and vegetables.

Managing Obesity with Diet, Exercise, and Lifestyle

The cornerstone of all dietary and lifestyle interventions is that energy balance must be negative in order to lose weight. While multiple factors contribute to the degree of weight loss, a calorie deficit of 500 kcal/day and adherence to a dietary program are recommended for successful weight loss. Approaches to exercise include the incorporation of aerobic physical activity building to 150 minutes/week over 3 to 5 days and resistance training two to three times per week. Successful behavioral strategies accompanying diet and exercise include self-monitoring of food intake and physical activity, stimulus control, and goal setting.[29]

Medical Pharmacotherapy

The addition of pharmacotherapy yields greater weight loss and maintenance of weight loss compared with lifestyle therapy alone. Pharmacologic therapies can be implemented in persons with an initial BMI >30 kg/m^2 or >27 kg/m^2 and at least one comorbidity, such as type 2 diabetes mellitus (T2DM), hypertension, or dyslipidemia.[4] The approach to pharmacotherapy should be individualized based on medication efficacy, side effects, and the patient's existing comorbidities. Multiple pharmacologic agents have been approved by the US Food and Drug Administration (FDA) for the treatment of obesity and are reviewed next (also see Figure 3.7).

Orlistat

Branded as Xenical, orlistat selectively inhibits pancreatic lipase, reducing intestinal digestion of fat. It is associated with a maximal weight loss of about −6.65 kg and is the only medication approved by the FDA for use in adolescents with obesity.[30] Orlistat can reduce the absorption of fat-soluble vitamins, and patients should be advised to take vitamin supplements. Rare reports of severe liver injury have been reported, and patients should be monitored for jaundice, anorexia, or change in stool color. More commonly, diarrhea, flatulence, and bloating may occur.

Lorcaserin

Branded as Belviq, lorcaserin reduces food intake by targeting serotonin-2C receptors. It is associated with a maximal weight loss of −5.39 kg (pooled metanalyses of five studies).[5] These studies also demonstrated an improvement in cardiovascular risk factors. Side effects include headache, sinusitis, depression, and anxiety.

Liraglutide or Semaglutide

Branded as Saxenda and Wegovy, liraglutide and semaglutide are GLP-1 agonists administered as a daily or weekly subcutaneous injection respectively. GLP-1 agonists are analogous to GLP-1 with a molecular change that extends its half-life. They improve glycemic control and satiety and reduce body weight. In cardiovascular outcome trials of patients with T2DM, GLP-1 agonists lowered the rate of the first occurrence of death from cardiovascular causes, nonfatal myocardial infarction, or nonfatal stroke. Side effects include nausea, vomiting, and abdominal pain. GLP-1 agonists are contraindicated in patients with a family history of medullary thyroid carcinoma or multiple endocrine neoplasia syndrome type 2 and should not be prescribed in patients with a history of pancreatitis.

Phentermine/Topiramate

Branded as Qsymia, phentermine and topiramate decrease appetite by augmenting norepinephrine and gamma-aminobutyric acid release. This combination produced larger weight loss than observed in

3.7 KEY: ■ PREFERRED DRUG ■ USE WITH CAUTION ■ AVOID

CLINICAL CHARACTERISTICS OR CO-EXISTING DISEASES		MEDICATIONS FOR CHRONIC WEIGHT MANAGEMENT				
		Orlistat	Lorcaserin	Phentermine/ topiramate ER	Naltrexone ER/ bupropion ER	Liraglutide 3 mg
Diabetes Prevention (metabolic syndrome, prediabetes)			Insufficient data for T2DM prevention		Insufficient data for T2DM prevention	
Type 2 Diabetes Mellitus						
Hypertension				Monitor heart rate	Monitor BP and heart rate. Contraindicated in uncontrolled HTN	Monitor heart rate
Cardiovascular Disease	CAD			Monitor heart rate	Monitor heart rate, BP	Monitor heart rate
	Arrhythmia		Monitor for bradycardia	Monitor heart rate, rhythm	Monitor heart rate, rhythm, BP	Monitor heart rate, rhythm
	CHF	Insufficient data	Insufficient data	Insufficient data	Insufficient data	Insufficient data
Chronic Kidney Disease	Mild (50–79 mL/min)					
	Moderate (30–49 mL/min)			Do not exceed 7.5 mg/46 mg per day	Do not exceed 8 mg/90 mg bid	
	Severe (<30 mL/min)	Watch for oxalate nephropathy	Urinary clearance of drug metabolites	Urinary clearance of drug	Urinary clearance of drug	Avoid vomiting and volume depletion
Nephrolithiasis		Calcium oxalate stones		Calcium phosphate stones		
Hepatic Impairment	Mild-Moderate (Child-Pugh 5–9)	Watch for cholelithiasis	Hepatic metabolism of drug	Do not exceed 7.5 mg/46 mg per day	Do not exceed 8 mg/90 mg in AM	Watch for cholelithiasis
	Severe (Child-Pugh >9)	Not recommended	Not recommended	Not recommended	Not recommended	Not recommended
Depression			Insufficient safety data. Avoid combinations of serotonergic drugs	Avoid maximum dose: 15 mg/92 mg per day	Insufficient safety data. Avoid in adolescents and young adults	
Anxiety				Avoid max dose: 15 mg/92 mg per day		
Psychoses		Insufficient data	Insufficient data	Insufficient data	Insufficient data	Insufficient data
Binge Eating Disorder			Insufficient data, however, possible benefit based on reduction in food cravings	Insufficient data, however, possible benefit based on studies with topiramate	Insufficient data, though possible benefit based on studies with bupropion. Avoid in patients with purging or bulimia nervosa	Insufficient data
Glaucoma				Contraindicated, may trigger angle closure	May trigger angle closure	
Seizure Disorder				If discontinuing from max dose, taper slowly	Bupropion lowers seizure threshold	
Pancreatitis		Monitor for symptoms				Monitor for symptoms. Avoid if prior or current disease
Opioid Use					Will antagonize opioids and opiates	
Women of Reproductive Potential	Pregnancy	Use contraception and discontinue orlistat should pregnancy occur	Use contraception and discontinue lorcaserin should pregnancy occur	Use contraception and discontinue phentermine/topiramate should pregnancy occur (perform monthly pregnancy checks to identify early pregnancy)	Use contraception and discontinue naltrexone ER/bupropion ER should pregnancy occur	Use contraception and discontinue liraglutide 3 mg should pregnancy occur
	Breast-feeding	Not recommended	Not recommended	Not recommended	Not recommended	Not recommended
Age ≥65 years [a]		Limited data available	Insufficient data	Limited data available	Insufficient data	Limited data available
Alcoholism/ Addiction			Might have abuse potential due to euphoria at high doses	Insufficient data, though topiramate might exert therapeutic benefits	Avoid due to seizure risk and lower seizure threshold on bupropion	
Post-Bariatric Surgery		Insufficient data	Insufficient data	Limited data available	Insufficient data	Data available at 1.8 – 3.0 mg/day

[a] Use medications only with clear health-related goals in mind; assess patient for osteoporosis and sarcopenia.

Abbreviations: BP = blood pressure; CAD = coronary artery disease; CHF = congestive heart failure; HTN = hypertension; T2DM = Type 2 Diabetes Mellitus.

FIGURE 3.7 Chronic weight medical management selection.[33] (Adapted from American Association of Clinical Endocrinology.)

clinical trials with single drugs with a maximal weight loss of 15.6 kg.[5,31] Improvements were also seen in glycemic and blood pressure parameters. Contraindications include pregnancy (due to an increased risk of cleft lip/palate in infants), glaucoma, hyperthyroidism, and monoamine oxidase inhibitors. Additional concerns include an increased risk of kidney stones and tachycardia.

Naltrexone/Bupropion

Branded as Contrave, naltrexone and bupropion work together to reduce food intake by stimulating adrenergic and dopaminergic receptors, and inhibiting a feeding stimulus *B*-endorphin, respectively. Maximal weight loss was −13.2 kg in a meta-analysis of six studies.[5] Bupropion is approved as a single agent for depression and smoking cessation, and thus may be a favorable choice should they coexist. Contraindications include uncontrolled hypertension, seizure disorders, drug or alcohol withdrawal, and long-term opioid use.

Selection and Duration of Pharmacotherapy

Although there are few head-to-head trials comparing pharmacologic interventions, meta-analyses of randomized trials have identified that all drug interventions were effective at weight loss when compared to placebo and lifestyle therapy alone.[32] Therefore, simultaneous initiation of lifestyle therapies and pharmacotherapy should be considered. Pharmacotherapy should be considered as chronic disease management, as short-term treatment (under 6 months) did not demonstrate long-lasting health benefits.

Initiation of specific weight-loss pharmacotherapy for patients must include consideration of side effects, mechanism of action, comorbidities, and contraindications. Therefore, selection must be individualized, but a generalizable algorithm does not currently exist. A few disease-specific considerations are reviewed next.

Hypertension
In patients with coexisting hypertension, orlistat, lorcaserin, phentermine/topiramate ER, liraglutide, or semaglutide are preferred. Naltrexone/bupropion combinations are contraindicated in uncontrolled hypertension.[29]

Diabetes
All weight-loss drugs should be considered in patients with coexisting diabetes. Liraglutide and semaglutide may be preferred due to improved glucose-dependent insulin release and associated glycemic outcomes.

Renal Impairment
Weight-loss medications should be avoided in advanced renal failure (GFR <30). However, orlistat, liraglutide, or semaglutide can be considered with caution and discontinued in volume depletion. Additionally, orlistat or phentermine/topiramate ER should not be utilized in patients at risk of nephrolithiasis.[29]

Hepatic Impairment
All weight-loss medications should be avoided in severe hepatic impairment (Child–Pugh score >9) with dose adjustments in hepatic impairment. Similarly, clinicians should have awareness of the increased risk of cholelithiasis in patients undergoing weight-loss therapy, particularly GLP-1 agonists.[29]

SURGICAL THERAPY

Bariatric surgery remains the most effective management option for severe obesity and the management or resolution of comorbidities (Figures 3.8–3.10).[34] The mechanisms by which various bariatric procedures

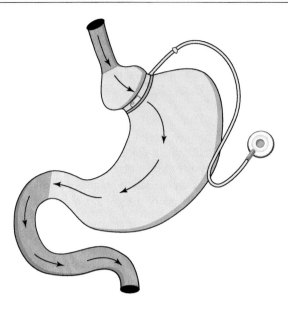

FIGURE 3.8   Adjustable gastric banding. An external ring with an inflatable balloon is placed around the proximal stomach. The balloon can be adjusted to modulate gastric restriction. It is less effective than other bariatric procedures, particularly in sustaining weight loss, and is thus falling out of favor.[36]

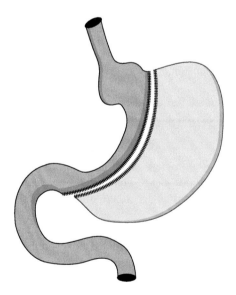

FIGURE 3.9   Sleeve gastrectomy. A tube-like stomach is created by excising a majority of the greater curvature resulting in a marked reduction in gastric capacity. Emerging evidence supports neurohormonal modulation and is associated with better weight loss and metabolic outcomes than purely restrictive approaches.[9]

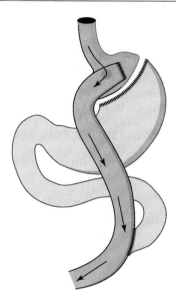

FIGURE 3.10 Roux-en-Y gastric bypass (RYGB). The stomach is divided to create a small gastric pouch that is connected through a gastrojejunostomy to a distal segment of the jejunum. The remainder of the stomach drains into the bypassed portion of the bowel and continuity is resorted by a jejunojejunostomy. Along with neurohormonal effects and impacts on nutrient signaling, RYGB involves an intrinsic malabsorptive and restrictive component.[9] Patients should be followed by a nutritionist to replenish macronutrient and micronutrient stores.

exert their benefits include primarily restrictive, malabsorptive, and/or neurohormonal effects. Indications for surgical management of severe obesity include adults with an initial BMI >40 kg/m^2 or >35 kg/m^2 with at least one serious comorbidity.[35] Patients should also participate in a comprehensive program focused on nutrition, behavior, and medical support, both preoperatively and on follow-up.

REFERENCES

1. Schwartz, M. W. et al. Obesity Pathogenesis: An Endocrine Society Scientific Statement. *Endocr. Rev.* 38(4), 267–296 (2017).
2. Cui, H., López, M. & Rahmouni, K. The Cellular and Molecular Bases of Leptin and Ghrelin Resistance in Obesity. *Nat. Rev. Endocrinol.* 13(6), 338–351 (2017).
3. CDC. Defining Adult Overweight and Obesity. *Centers for Disease Control and Prevention* (2021). https://www.cdc.gov/obesity/adult/defining.html.
4. Hales, C. M., Carroll, M.D., Fryar, C.D. & Ogden, C.L. Prevalence of Obesity and Severe Obesity Among Adults: United States, 2017–2018. *NCHS Data Brief* 360, 1–8 (2020). PMID: 32487284.
5. Bray, G. A. et al. The Science of Obesity Management: An Endocrine Society Scientific Statement. *Endocr. Rev.* 39(2), 79–132 (2018).
6. Heindel, J. J., Newbold, R. & Schug, T. T. Endocrine Disruptors and Obesity. *Nat. Rev. Endocrinol.* 11(11), 653–661 (2015).
7. Wardle, J., Carnell, S., Haworth, C. M. & Plomin, R. Evidence for a Strong Genetic Influence on Childhood Adiposity despite the Force of the Obesogenic Environment. *Am. J. Clin. Nutr.* 87(2), 398–404 (2008).

8. Loos, R. J. F. & Yeo, G. S. H. The Genetics of Obesity: from Discovery to Biology. *Nat. Rev. Genet.* 1–14 (2021) doi:10.1038/s41576-021-00414-z.

9. Tirthani, E., Said, M. S. & Rehman, A. Genetics and Obesity. In: *StatPearls* (StatPearls Publishing, 2021).

10. Obradovic, M. et al. Leptin and Obesity: Role and Clinical Implication. *Front. Endocrinol.* 12, 585887 (2021).

11. Izquierdo, A. G., Crujeiras, A. B., Casanueva, F. F. & Carreira, M. C. Leptin, Obesity, and Leptin Resistance: Where Are We 25 Years Later? *Nutrients* 11(11), 2704 (2019).

12. Fernandez-Twinn, D. S., Hjort, L., Novakovic, B., Ozanne, S. E. & Saffery, R. Intrauterine Programming of Obesity and Type 2 Diabetes. *Diabetologia* 62(10), 1789–1801 (2019).

13. Josefson, J. L. et al. The Joint Associations of Maternal BMI and Glycemia with Childhood Adiposity. *J. Clin. Endocrinol. Metab.* 105(7), 2177–2188 (2020).

14. Gunderson, E. P. et al. Childbearing May Increase Visceral Adipose Tissue Independent of Overall Increase in Body Fat. *Obes. Silver Spring Md* 16(5), 1078–1084 (2008).

15. Mannan, M., Doi, S. A. R. & Mamun, A. A. Association between Weight Gain during Pregnancy and Postpartum Weight Retention and Obesity: A Bias-Adjusted Meta-Analysis. *Nutr. Rev.* 71(6), 343–352 (2013).

16. Karvonen-Gutierrez, C. & Kim, C. Association of Mid-life Changes in Body Size, Body Composition and Obesity Status with the Menopausal Transition. *Healthcare (Basel)* 4(3), 42 (2016).

17. Poehlman, E. T. et al. Physiological Predictors of Increasing Total and Central Adiposity in Aging Men and Women. *Arch. Intern. Med.* 155(22), 2443–2448 (1995).

18. Kapoor, E., Collazo-Clavell, M. L. & Faubion, S. S. Weight Gain in Women at Midlife: A Concise Review of the Pathophysiology and Strategies for Management. *Mayo Clin. Proc.* 92(10), 1552–1558 (2017).

19. Swinburn, B., Sacks, G. & Ravussin, E. Increased Food Energy Supply Is More than Sufficient to Explain the US Epidemic of Obesity. *Am. J. Clin. Nutr.* 90(6), 1453–1456 (2009).

20. Mozaffarian, D., Hao, T., Rimm, E. B., Willett, W. C. & Hu, F. B. Changes in Diet and Lifestyle and Long-Term Weight Gain in Women and Men (2011) doi:10.1056/NEJMoa1014296.

21. Hruby, A. et al. Determinants and Consequences of Obesity. *Am. J. Public Health* 106(9), 1656–1662 (2016).

22. Reutrakul, S. & Cauter, E. V. Sleep Influences on Obesity, Insulin Resistance, and Risk of Type 2 Diabetes. *Metab. Clin. Exp.* 84, 56–66 (2018).

23. Ogilvie, R. P. & Patel, S. R. The Epidemiology of Sleep and Obesity. *Sleep Health* 3(5), 383–388 (2017).

24. van der Valk, E. S. et al. A Comprehensive Diagnostic Approach to Detect Underlying Causes of Obesity in Adults. *Obes. Rev.* 20(6), 795–804 (2019).

25. Sanyal, D. & Raychaudhuri, M. Hypothyroidism and Obesity: An Intriguing Link. *Indian J. Endocrinol. Metab.* 20(4), 554–557 (2016).

26. Binnerts, A., Deurenberg, P., Swart, G. R., Wilson, J. H. & Lamberts, S. W. Body Composition in Growth Hormone-Deficient Adults. *Am. J. Clin. Nutr.* 55(5), 918–923 (1992).

27. Rosén, T., Bosaeus, I., Tölli, J., Lindstedt, G. & Bengtsson, B. A. Increased Body Fat Mass and Decreased Extracellular Fluid Volume in Adults with Growth Hormone Deficiency. *Clin. Endocrinol. (Oxf.)* 38(1), 63–71 (1993).

28. Heymsfield, S. B. & Wadden, T. A. Mechanisms, Pathophysiology, and Management of Obesity (2017) doi:10.1056/NEJMra1514009.

29. Garvey, W. T. et al. American Association of Clinical Endocrinologists and American College of Endocrinology Comprehensive Clinical Practice Guidelines for Medical Care of Patients with Obesity. *Endocr. Pract.* 22, 1–203 (2016).

30. Dong, Z. et al. Comparative Efficacy of Five Long-Term Weight Loss Drugs: Quantitative Information for Medication Guidelines. *Obes. Rev.* 18(12), 1377–1385 (2017).

31. Garvey, W. T. et al. Two-Year Sustained Weight Loss and Metabolic Benefits with Controlled-Release Phentermine/Topiramate in Obese and Overweight Adults (SEQUEL): A Randomized, Placebo-Controlled, Phase 3 Extension Study. *Am. J. Clin. Nutr.* 95(2), 297–308 (2012).

32. Khera, R. et al. Association of Pharmacological Treatments for Obesity With Weight Loss and Adverse Events: A Systematic Review and Meta-Analysis. *JAMA* 315(22), 2424–2434 (2016).

33. Garvey, W. T. et al. American Association of Clinical Endocrinologists and American College of Endocrinology Comprehensive Clinical Practice Guidelines for Medical Care of Patients with Obesity. *Endocr. Pract.* 22, 1–203 (2016).

34. Schauer, P. R. et al. Bariatric Surgery versus Intensive Medical Therapy for Diabetes – 3-Year Outcomes (2014) doi:10.1056/NEJMoa1401329.

35. Mechanick, J. I. et al. Clinical Practice Guidelines for the Perioperative Nutritional, Metabolic, and Nonsurgical Support of the Bariatric Surgery Patient – 2013 Update: Cosponsored by American Association of Clinical Endocrinologists, The Obesity Society, and American Society for Metabolic & Bariatric Surgery. *Obes. Silver Spring Md* 21 S1 (2013).
36. Albaugh, V. L., Flynn, C. R., Tamboli, R. A. & Abumrad, N. N. Recent Advances in Metabolic and Bariatric Surgery. *F1000Research* 5, 978 (2016).

Metabolic Bone Disorders

4

Natasha S. Kadakia, Caroline Poku,
Rod Marianne Arceo-Mendoza, and Pauline Camacho

OSTEOPOROSIS

Definition/Overview

Osteoporosis is a chronic progressive disease characterized by low bone density, microarchitectural bone deterioration, and decreased bone strength, leading to increased bone fragility and increased fracture risk. In 1994, the World Health Organization (WHO) published criteria for the diagnosis of osteoporosis based on bone mineral density (BMD). Normal BMD is defined as a BMD value within 1 standard deviation of the young adult female reference mean and is designated as a T-score ≥−1. The young adult female reference mean is calculated from the mean BMD of healthy females aged 20–29 of a single ethnicity. Low bone mass (osteopenia) is defined as a BMD that is between 1 and 2.5 standard deviations below the young adult mean and is designated as a T-score <−1 and >−2.5. Osteoporosis is defined as a BMD 2.5 standard deviations or more below the young adult mean designated as a T-score <−2.5. Last, severe osteoporosis is defined as a BMD 2.5 standard deviations or more below the young adult mean in the presence of one or more fragility fractures. The diagnosis of osteoporosis is based either upon the aforementioned WHO criteria or the presence of fragility fractures. These types of fractures occur with low-impact trauma, such as falling from a standing position, excluding fractures of the fingers, toes, skull, and face.

In addition, per the 2020 guidelines of the American Association of Clinical Endocrinologists and American College of Endocrinology (AACE/ACE), osteoporosis may also be diagnosed in patients who have osteopenia with a high FRAX® (Fracture Risk Assessment Tool) score. FRAX uses clinical history and, optionally, dual-energy X-ray absorptiometry (DXA) scores to calculate fracture risk. The AACE/ACE diagnosis of osteoporosis in postmenopausal women includes a T-score of −2.5 or lower in the lumbar spine, femoral neck, total proximal femur, or 1/3 radius; low-trauma spine or hip fracture (regardless of bone mineral density); or a T-score between −1.0 and −2.5 with a fragility fracture of the proximal humerus, pelvis, or distal forearm.

DOI: 10.1201/9781003100669-4

Etiology

Osteoporosis is the most common bone disease in humans. Approximately 33.6 million Americans have osteopenia or low bone mass, and 10 million have osteoporosis, of whom 80% are females and 20% are males. The disease affects people of all ethnicities to varying degrees. Non-Hispanic White and Asian people have the greatest incidence of osteoporosis followed by Hispanics and then non-Hispanic Blacks. Osteoporosis is responsible for more than 1.5 million fractures annually. One in two women and one in four men over the age of 50 will have an osteoporosis-related fracture during their lifetime. The national health care costs for osteoporosis exceed $20 billion annually, with projected total costs of care in 2040 to exceed $95 billion. Osteoporosis can be classified as either primary or secondary. Primary osteoporosis is bone loss associated with menopause and the aging process. Secondary osteoporosis can occur as a result of multiple conditions (Table 4.1).

Pathophysiology

Bone is dynamic. It is constantly undergoing formation and breakdown under the coordinated actions of osteoblasts and osteoclasts. Approximately 5%–10% of the adult skeleton is replaced annually through a process called remodeling. Remodeling occurs at focal sites termed 'bone remodeling units'. At these sites, osteoclasts and osteoblasts function in concert to replace old bone with new bone (Figure 4.1).

The process begins with bone resorption by osteoclasts. Mononuclear cells proceed to line the resorption lacunae and deposit a cement line. Osteoprogenitor cells replace the mononuclear cells in the bone remodeling unit. These cells differentiate into osteoblasts and begin to lay down the organic matrix. This is then followed by the deposition of minerals. Osteoporosis occurs due to aberrancy in bone remodeling in that there is an increase in osteoclast activity with a concomitant decrease in osteoblast activity. There is also an increase in the total number of bone remodeling units. Therefore, bone resorption is occurring at more sites than usual and in the presence of impaired bone formation. The actions occurring at the bone remodeling unit are under the influence of multiple factors such as estrogen, testosterone, and cytokines. Wnt/β-catenin signaling stimulates osteoblastic activity by promoting the progression of Osterix1 (Osx1)-expressing cells to osteoblasts. In addition, the Wnt pathway prevents the cellular death of mature osteoblasts, thereby prolonging their lifespan. Wnt/β-catenin signaling also decreases osteoclast differentiation by stimulating the production and secretion of osteoprotegerin (OPG), an antagonist of the receptor activator of nuclear factor-B ligand (RANKL). RANKL is secreted by osteocytes and is necessary for bone resorption. During the process of osteoclast generation, RANKL and macrophage colony–stimulating factors provide a very important step leading to osteoclast differentiation. Overall, if there is a deletion of this Wnt/β-catenin signaling pathway, there is a subsequent increase in osteoclast number with an increase in bone resorption, leading to a decrease in bone mass.

Clinical Presentation

Osteoporosis is often called a 'silent disease' because bone loss occurs without symptoms. It usually presents as either a fragility fracture or is discovered on radiographic imaging. There are several risk factors associated with osteoporosis including advanced age, being female, an estrogen-deficient state or early menopause, family history of osteoporosis, prior history of low-trauma fractures, cigarette smoking, being thin, anorexia nervosa, low calcium intake, vitamin D deficiency, low testosterone, inactive

TABLE 4.1 Causes of Secondary Osteoporosis

ENDOCRINE	RHEUMATOLOGIC	DRUGS	GASTROINTESTINAL	HEMATOLOGIC DISEASES	OTHER
Hyperthyroidism	Rheumatoid arthritis	Glucocorticoids	Celiac sprue	Multiple myeloma	Renal insufficiency
Primary hyperparathyroidism	SLE	Anticonvulsants	IBD	Mastocytosis	End-organ failure
Cushing's syndrome			Other malabsorptive syndromes		Organ transplantation
Hypogonadism		Lithium	Whipple procedure		Malnutrition
Vitamin D deficiency		Cytotoxic drugs	Gastric bypass surgery		Alcoholism
Calcium deficiency		Heparin			HIV
		Aromatase inhibitors			COPD
		Gonadotropin-releasing hormone agonist			Prolonged non-weight-bearing states
		Immunosuppressants			

COPD, chronic obstructive pulmonary disease; HIV, human immunodeficiency virus; IBD, inflammatory bowel disease; SLE, systemic lupus erythematosus.

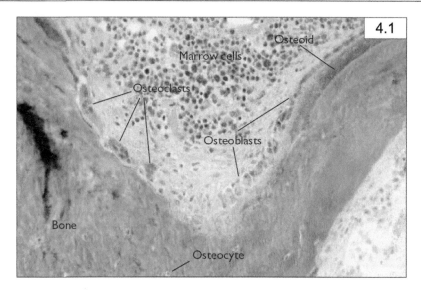

FIGURE 4.1   Photomicrograph of bone consisting of a bone remodeling unit composed of osteoclasts and osteoblasts. (Courtesy of Dr. Susan Ott, http://courses.washington.edu/bonephys/ophome.html.)

lifestyle, excessive use of alcohol, being Caucasian or Asian, chronic illness, and various medications. On examination, the patient may have severe back pain, loss of height, or spinal deformities, such as kyphosis or stooped posture. Other findings may point toward osteoporosis risk factors leading to further diagnostic workup for osteoporosis.

Osteoporosis is associated with increased bone fragility and increased fracture risk. Hip fractures are the most devastating complication of osteoporosis, and 90% of hip fractures occur in patients over the age of 50. One out of every six Caucasian women will have a hip fracture during their lifetime. There is a 30% excess mortality in the first year after a hip fracture. The diagnosis, treatment, and prevention of osteoporosis result in a considerable decrease in the incidence of fractures and, therefore, a decrease in mortality and morbidity.

Differential Diagnosis

The differential diagnosis for low bone mass and fractures includes osteomalacia, malignancy, and the myriad of secondary causes of osteoporosis.

Diagnosis

A DXA scan of the lumbar spine and femoral neck is the most common way to diagnose osteoporosis. Other imaging modalities include quantitative ultrasound, quantitative computed tomography (CT), and radiography. Compared to DXA scanning, a quantitative ultrasound looks at the calcaneus as the primary site of measurement. In terms of fracture risk discrimination, this modality is equivalent to that of DXA. However, ultrasonography cannot be used for monitoring skeletal changes or evaluating response to therapy. Quantitative CT allows for selective assessment of both cortical and trabecular bone. This is important since due to its high turnover rate, trabecular bone enables prediction of spinal fractures. However, quantitative CT is more expensive and involves greater radiation exposure. Radiography is less sensitive. DXA provides information regarding bone mineral density and using reference means can

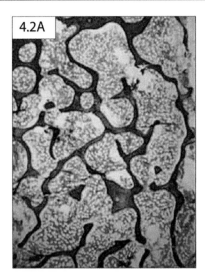
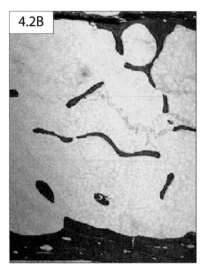

FIGURE 4.2   Bone biopsies. (A) Normal trabecular bone, (B) osteoporosis. (Courtesy of Dr. Susan Ott, http://courses.washington.edu/bonephys/ophome.html.)

provide both T-scores and Z-scores. Z-scores compare the individual's bone density with age-matched controls. In postmenopausal women and in men over age 50, T-scores have the greatest validity. In premenopausal women and men under age 50, Z-scores have the most validity. The reference mean for Z-scores should be age and ethnicity appropriate, particularly in children. The trabecular bone score, or TBS, is an analytical tool that looks at measurements and trabecular bone architecture from lumbar spine images.

Histopathologic findings in osteoporosis include cortical thinning, increased cortical porosity, and thin trabeculae (Figure 4.2), and bone densitometry reveals decreased bone mineral density (Figures 4.3 and 4.4). Radiography may reveal compression fractures of the spine (Figure 4.5).

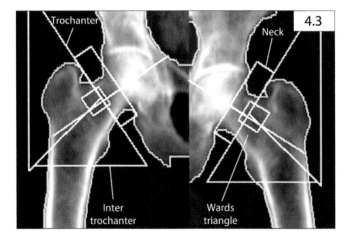

FIGURE 4.3   Dual-energy X-ray absorptiometry of the left and right hip from a patient with severe osteoporosis. The regions are labeled. The total hip is the sum of the regions.

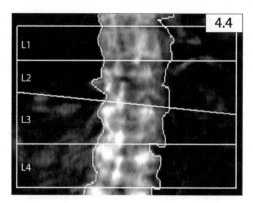

FIGURE 4.4 Dual-energy X-ray absorptiometry of the lumbar spine. The yellow and white lines are added to the image to guide the scanner software in calculating the bone density.

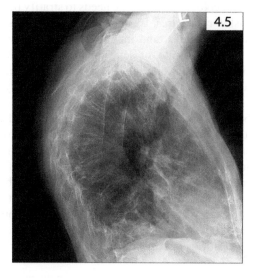

FIGURE 4.5 Lateral radiograph of a patient with severe osteoporosis revealing kyphosis secondary to multiple vertebral fractures.

Management/Treatment

The treatment and prevention of osteoporosis begins with nonpharmacologic therapies. Daily calcium and vitamin D intake should be optimized. In premenopausal women, the daily elemental calcium intake should be 1,000 mg/d. At menopause that should be increased to 1,200 mg/d. Similarly, men should optimize their elemental calcium intake to 1,000 mg/d until age 71 and then increase it to 1,200 mg/d. Current AACE recommendations show an intake of at least 1,000–2,000 IU of vitamin D per day to maintain optimal vitamin D levels. If patients have risk factors such as obesity or malabsorption, or are on medications affecting vitamin D metabolism, then they may need a higher dose. The optimal 25 OHD is 30–50 ng/ml.

Exercise is recommended in the treatment and prevention of osteoporosis. Weight-bearing exercise helps to maintain or increase bone mass. Regular exercise improves strength and coordination, which reduces the risk of falls. Fall prevention is important in reducing fall-related fractures. Interventions that reduce the risk of falls are essential. Risk factors for falls include visual impairment, poor balance or gait, neuromuscular and musculoskeletal disabilities, muscle weakness, postural hypotension, medications, cognitive impairment, and environmental hazards. Cessation of habits such as cigarette smoking and excessive alcohol consumption is suggested in the treatment and prevention of osteoporosis.

Indications for pharmacologic therapy are low T-score, high FRAX score, or a previous fragility fracture. It is also important to risk-stratify these patients, as their fracture risk determines the initial choice of therapy as well as the duration of treatment. Examples of very high fracture risk include recent fractures (e.g., ≤12 months), fractures while on approved therapy, multiple fractures, fractures while on medications causing skeletal harm, T-score <–3.0, high risk of falls, and high FRAX score.

Medications used in the treatment of osteoporosis include antiresorptive agents such as oral and IV bisphosphonates, selective estrogen agonists/antagonists, estrogen/progesterone replacement therapy, nasal calcitonin, denosumab, and anabolic agents, including teriparatide and abaloparatide. Lastly, romosozumab, which is a humanized monoclonal antibody against osteocyte-derived sclerostin, has both anabolic and anti-resorptive activity. The primary goal in the treatment of osteoporosis is to reduce the incidence of fractures. A secondary goal is to maintain and, if possible, normalize the BMD.

When recommending pharmacologic therapy, one needs to stratify patients into those who are high risk or those with very high risk for fractures. Examples of very high risk fractures include advanced age, frailty, steroid use, very low T-scores, and increased fall risk. For patients who are high risk, one can start with oral or IV bisphosphonate, or denosumab. For the initial treatment option for very high risk patients, the recommendation is for abaloparatide, teriparatide, denosumab, zoledronate, or romosozumab. Once started on therapy, the clinician is to reassess yearly for response to therapy and fracture risk.

Bisphosphonates inhibit bone resorption by decreasing the number and activity of osteoclasts. Strong clinical trial evidence supports the use of alendronate, risedronate, ibandronate, and zoledronic acid for preventing fractures in women with postmenopausal osteoporosis and in men with osteoporosis. These agents have been shown to reduce vertebral fractures by 50%–70% and hip fractures by 40% in postmenopausal women. Per AACE guidelines, for oral bisphosphonates, consider a bisphosphonate holiday after 5 years of treatment if fracture risk is no longer high, but continue treatment up to an additional 5 years if fracture risk remains high. If there is a very high fracture risk and if using oral bisphosphonate, consider a bisphosphonate holiday after 6 to 10 years of stability. For IV zoledronic acid, consider a bisphosphonate holiday after 3 years in high-risk patients or until fracture risk is no longer high, and continue for up to 6 years in very high risk patients.

Oral bisphosphonates are contraindicated in patients with esophageal irritation or stricture, hypocalcemia, hypersensitivity to bisphosphonates, the presence of gastrointestinal (GI) malabsorption (gastric bypass procedures, celiac disease, Crohn's disease, etc.), or renal insufficiency (creatinine clearance <30 mL/min). Rare adverse events of prolonged bisphosphonate therapy include osteonecrosis of the jaw and atypical fractures of the femur. These occur at a rate of 1/10,000–100,000 patient-years. These adverse events are mitigated by bisphosphonate holidays for risedronate.

Raloxifene is a selective estrogen receptor modulator that is approved for both the treatment and the prevention of postmenopausal osteoporosis. In clinical studies, raloxifene has been shown to decrease vertebral fractures by about 50%. However, no evidence is currently available for raloxifene that assesses nonvertebral or hip fracture reduction. When raloxifene is discontinued, there is a loss of skeletal protection in the following 1–2 years.

The use of estrogen/progesterone replacement therapy remains controversial in the treatment of osteoporosis. Estrogen alone or in combination with progesterone decreases bone turnover, bone loss, and fractures. Due to the risks associated with estrogen/progesterone therapy, it is recommended that other proven therapies are used in the treatment and prevention of osteoporosis. If estrogen/progesterone therapy is desired, the lowest possible dose over the shortest possible time is suggested.

Calcitonin inhibits bone resorption by osteoclasts. It is usually administered as a nasal spray. In clinical studies, nasal calcitonin has been shown to prevent bone loss and vertebral fractures, but not nonvertebral or hip fractures. Because of its modest effect on osteoporosis treatment and the absence of a BMD increase (except for in the spine), this drug is mostly used as an alternative agent.

Teriparatide is a recombinant human parathyroid hormone (PTH) analog. It is a potent bone anabolic agent that increases bone turnover. Studies show that teriparatide increases bone density, and reduces vertebral fractures by 65% and nonvertebral fractures by 53%. Its use is recommended in postmenopausal women with severe bone loss who are at high risk for fracture, as well as for the treatment of hypogonadal or primary osteoporosis in men at high risk for fracture. It is also approved for the treatment of glucocorticoid-induced osteoporosis. When treatment with teriparatide is stopped, there is a decline in bone density in the following year. Fracture reduction may persist for 1 or 2 years after termination of therapy. Use of bisphosphonates or denosumab after teriparatide therapy prevents bone mineral density loss and may result in a further increase in BMD. Teriparatide should not be used in patients with a history of bone malignancy, Paget's disease of bone, unexplained hypercalcemia, skeletal radiation exposure, or those younger than 18 years.

Abaloparatide, a modified PTH-related peptide 1–34, is an anabolic agent approved for the initial treatment of women with postmenopausal osteoporosis who are at high risk of fracture or have failed/developed an intolerance to other therapies. Just like teriparatide, it is contraindicated in patients with Paget's disease. When looking at data comparing abaloparatide to teriparatide, gains in BMD were greater with abaloparatide, especially in the femoral neck, total hip, and 1/3 radius. Fracture reduction was also greater with abaloparatide than with teriparatide. Side effects of both abaloparatide and teriparatide include nausea, orthostatic hypotension, and leg cramps. Both abaloparatide and teriparatide have warnings regarding the occurrence of osteosarcomas in rats treated with very high doses. Also, abaloparatide and teriparatide are limited to no longer than 2 years in total duration. The initiation of alendronate after discontinuation with abaloparatide has been studied with results showing an increase in BMD. Current data shows that treatment with either teriparatide or abaloparatide should be followed by antiresorptive therapy, typically with either a bisphosphonate or denosumab.

Denosumab is a humanized monoclonal antibody that works on reducing the rate of differentiation of precursor cells into mature osteoclasts. It also decreases the survival of activated osteoclasts. In the FREEDOM trial, which looked at postmenopausal women with osteoporosis, denosumab showed an antifracture efficacy as early as 1 year after starting therapy. Studies showed persistent fracture protection and a good safety profile with a duration of up to 10 years. It is important to note that when treatment is stopped, after 2–8 years, BMD rapidly declines. There have also been case reports of multiple vertebral fractures after stopping denosumab. Thus patients who are being discontinued from denosumab need to be transitioned to an antiresorptive agent and closely watched. There have been cross-over studies with exploratory analysis showing stable BMD 2 years posttransition from denosumab to oral bisphosphonates. There are also studies showing stabilization of BMD with IV zoledronic acid.

Romosozumab is a humanized monoclonal antibody that inhibits sclerostin. This is a protein that is secreted by osteocytes to reduce bone formation. This pharmacological agent was approved in April 2019. Its indication for use is in the postmenopausal population who are at high risk of fracture or who have failed/developed an intolerance to other therapeutic agents. This therapy is limited to 12 months. The FRAME trial looked at postmenopausal women and compared romosozumab to placebo and saw a 73% lower risk of new vertebral fractures after 1 year of using romosozumab when compared to placebo. With this medication, there is a risk of myocardial infarction, stroke, and cardiovascular death. It is contraindicated in patients who had a myocardial infarction or stroke in the previous year prior to initiation of therapy.

Combination therapy with an anabolic and an antiresorptive therapy, shows some BMD benefit but no fracture reduction data has been demonstrated yet. There is evidence to support sequential use of anabolic followed by antiresorptive therapy, and conflicting evidence on combination therapy.

PRIMARY HYPERPARATHYROIDISM

Definition/Overview

Hyperparathyroidism is a disease defined by the overproduction of PTH. It can be classified as primary, secondary, or tertiary. Primary hyperparathyroidism (PHP) is characterized by hypercalcemia due to the autonomous overproduction of PTH, either as a result of parathyroid cell proliferation or impaired calcium-sensing ability. Secondary hyperparathyroidism is the overproduction of PTH due to hypocalcemia and vitamin D deficiency. Tertiary hyperparathyroidism is the development of autonomous parathyroid function manifested as hypercalcemia and elevated PTH in patients with long-standing secondary hyperparathyroidism. Recently there has been recognition, which has a high PTH level, and normal total serum calcium and ionized calcium. There is a risk of progression to hypercalcemic primary hyperparathyroidism.

Etiology

PHP is present in about 1% of the adult population. The incidence of the disease increases to 2% or higher after age 55. PHP is two to three times more common in women than in men, with postmenopausal women having the highest incidence. Approximately 80%–85% of cases of PHP are caused by a single parathyroid adenoma. The remainder is due to multiple gland hyperplasia affecting all parathyroid glands (10% of cases), double adenomas (4% of cases), and rarely parathyroid carcinoma (1% of cases). PHP is most commonly due to a sporadic parathyroid adenoma but may be inherited in endocrine syndromes such as MEN type 1, MEN type 2A, familial hyperparathyroidism, and hyperparathyroidism jaw tumor syndrome. Associated risk factors include neck irradiation and treatment with lithium.

Pathophysiology

Solitary parathyroid adenomas are monoclonal or oligoclonal tumors most frequently arising from somatic or germline mutations in parathyroid precursor cells. Several genes that develop mutations in PHP have been identified. The MEN type 1 gene is a tumor suppressor gene and the gene known to most frequently have somatic mutations in both copies in parathyroid adenomas. Activating mutations of the cyclin D1 gene resulting in the overexpression of the protein cyclin D1 have been identified in parathyroid adenomas. Activating mutations in the RET protooncogene have also been identified in parathyroid adenomas. Of note, although the calcium-sensing receptor and the vitamin D receptor mediate inhibition of the parathyroid gland, no mutations of these genes have been isolated in parathyroid adenomas.

In secondary hyperparathyroidism, the elevated PTH is a physiologic response to hypocalcemia. Hypocalcemia can be due to chronic renal disease. In chronic renal disease, hyperphosphatemia impairs the ability of the kidneys to reabsorb calcium, resulting in hypercalciuria and hypocalcemia. Additionally, there is impaired conversion of 25-hydroxyvitamin to 1,25-dihydroxyvitamin D in the diseased kidney, the active form of vitamin D. It is a calcemic agent regulating calcium and phosphate transport as well as a cell differentiating agent important for a number of cell types including the osteoclast, enterocyte, and keratinocyte. Ultimately, a deficiency of 1,25-dihydroxyvitamin D results in hypocalcemia, which is a stimulus to the parathyroid cells to produce PTH.

Hypocalcemia can also be due to vitamin D deficiency. Vitamin D, although termed a vitamin, is in fact better described as a prohormone. The term 'vitamin D' includes a large group of closely related secosteroids. Cholecalciferol is the form of vitamin D obtained when radiant energy from the sun strikes the skin and converts 7-dehydrocholesterol into vitamin D_3. Vitamin D deficiency can occur when there is decreased exposure to the sun, decreased dietary intake of foods containing vitamin D, or decreased absorption of vitamin D from the diet due to malabsorption syndromes such as celiac sprue. Whatever the cause for the low vitamin D, as described earlier, it is essential for calcium homeostasis.

Clinical Presentation

In the past, the classic clinical presentation of PHP consisted of 'stones, moans, and groans', i.e., nephrolithiasis, osteoporosis, fractures, gout, peptic ulcer disease, pancreatitis, fatigue, anxiety, depression, and cognitive dysfunction. Other manifestations of PHP include muscle weakness, fatigue, renal insufficiency, hypomagnesemia, hypophosphatemia, hypertension, left ventricular hypertrophy, valvular calcifications, vascular stiffness, chondrocalcinosis, pseudogout, normochromic and normocytic anemia, and band keratopathy (Figure 4.6). Essentially, clinical manifestations of PHP are all secondary to induced hypercalcemia, hypercalciuria, and increased bone turnover. With the inclusion of total calcium on the basic metabolic panel, most patients are diagnosed early in the course of PHP secondary to hypercalcemia. Consequently, if calcium levels increase over time, patients are often asymptomatic or have subtle neurobehavioral symptoms such as fatigue and weakness.

As most patients with PHP are asymptomatic, the physical examination often fails to lead to a definitive diagnosis. Careful examination may reveal proximal muscle weakness or illicit nonspecific symptoms, such as depression, lethargy, and vague aches and pains. Diagnosis is usually dependent upon biochemical tests.

Differential Diagnosis

The differential diagnosis of hypercalcemia mainly includes cancer, milk-alkali syndrome, granulomatous disease, hyperthyroidism, thiazide diuretics, lithium, and familial hypocalciuric hypercalcemia.

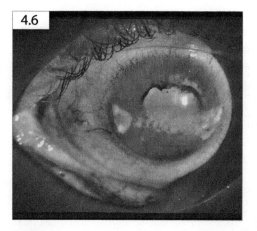

FIGURE 4.6 Band keratopathy in a patient with hyperparathyroidism. The name is derived from the distinctive appearance of calcium deposition in a band across the central cornea. (Courtesy of Dr. Glen Sizemore.)

A normal or elevated PTH excludes malignancy, calcium and vitamin D toxicity, and granulomatous diseases.

Diagnosis

The diagnosis of PHP requires the determination of serum total or ionized calcium and intact PTH. A 24-hour urinary calcium should be obtained to rule out familial hypocalciuric hypercalcemia, a disorder of the renal calcium-sensing receptor. A calcium-to-creatinine clearance ratio below 0.01 differentiates patients with familial hypocalciuric hypercalcemia from those with PHP. Associated laboratory abnormalities include decreased serum phosphate levels, high normal or increased serum chloride levels, elevated levels of blood urea nitrogen, elevated levels of creatinine, and elevated levels of bone-specific alkaline phosphatase. Patients with PHP should have a bone densitometry scan performed to ascertain the presence or absence of osteopenia or osteoporosis. Parathyroid imaging has no role in the diagnosis of PHP, but ultrasonography or sestamibi scanning of the parathyroid glands should be used for operative planning. Imaging can aid in localizing the parathyroid adenoma(s) to particular parathyroid glands (Figure 4.7).

Patients may satisfy the diagnosis of normocalcemic PHP if they have elevated parathyroid hormone but normal levels of serum and ionized calcium. To diagnose this, the clinician must rule out secondary causes of elevated parathyroid hormone. These include primary hypercalciuria, malabsorption syndromes, kidney disease, or medication induced (loop diuretics, bisphosphonates, or denosumab therapy). Elevated serum parathyroid hormone with multiple values of normal albumin-adjusted calcium and ionized calcium in the setting of a normal serum 25-hydroxyvitamin D, and appropriate renal function (eGFR >60 mL/min/1.73 m^2) supports the diagnosis of normocalcemic PHP. Over time, normocalcemic PHP can progress to primary hyperparathyroidism.

Histology of the parathyroid gland in hyperparathyroidism can distinguish between malignancy and hypercellular causes such as adenoma and hyperplasia. Histologically, normal parathyroid tissue shows a cell-to-fat ratio of 1:1. Hypercellular parathyroid tissue is typified by the loss of the normal amount of fat. The classic radiographic findings in PHP include nephrolithiasis (Figure 4.8), subperiosteal resorption (Figure 4.9), thinning of the distal third of the clavicle (Figure 4.10), and osteitis fibrosa cystica (Figure 4.11).

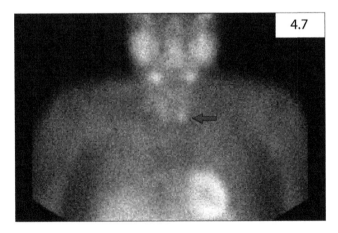

FIGURE 4.7 Sestamibi scan of a patient with a left lower parathyroid adenoma (arrow). The patient's salivary glands (parotid, submandibular, and sublingual) represent the bright areas around the jaw.

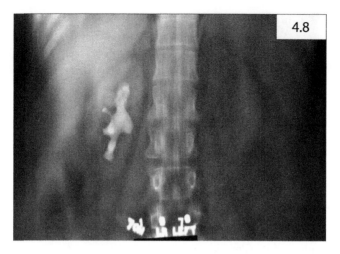

FIGURE 4.8 Abdominal radiograph showing nephrolithiasis in the right renal medulla in a patient with hyperparathyroidism. (Courtesy of Dr. Glen Sizemore.)

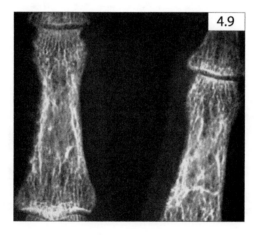

FIGURE 4.9 Radiograph of the hands revealing subperiosteal bone resorption of the digits in a patient with hyperparathyroidism. (Courtesy of Dr. Glen Sizemore.)

Management/Treatment

Surgery is the first-line treatment for PHP in symptomatic patients. The best management for asymptomatic patients with PHP is more controversial. The 2016 Guidelines for the Management of Primary Hyperparathyroidism as suggested by the American Association of Endocrine Surgery recommends surgery for patients who fulfill the following criteria:

1. Serum calcium >1.0 mg/dl (0.25 mmol/l) above the upper limit of normal.
2. Creatinine clearance <60 mg/min, or 24-hour urine for calcium >400 mg/day and increased stone risk by biochemical stone risk analysis, or nephrolithiasis or nephrocalcinosis on imaging study.
3. T-score <–2.5 at any site and/or previous fracture fragility.
4. Age <50 years.

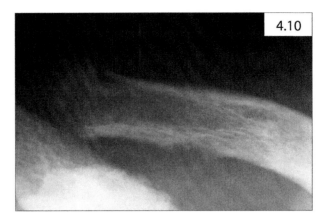

FIGURE 4.10   Radiograph of the shoulder revealing thinning of the distal third of the clavicle in a patient with hyperparathyroidism. (Courtesy of Dr. Glen Sizemore.)

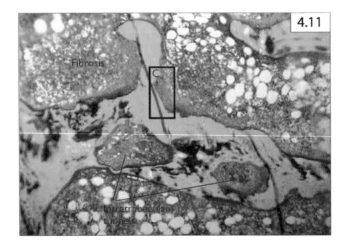

FIGURE 4.11   A photomicrograph of a bone biopsy revealing osteitis fibrosis. This occurs in patients with hyperparathyroidism from increased osteoclastic resorption of calcified bone with replacement by fibrous tissue resulting in softened and deformed bone that may develop cysts.

Preoperative localization is optional in patients without previous neck surgery. There is an improvement in localization accuracy when combining thyroid ultrasonography with technetium 99m sestamibi imaging, with sensitivities of 60%–70%. Intraoperative PTH monitoring (IPM) guides surgeons while doing minimally invasive parathyroid surgeries. IPM provides a more focused approach with cure rates as high as 97%–99%. Repeat surgery may be necessary for up to 5% of patients who develop persistent PHP due to incomplete resection of tissue. In these patients, a diagnosis of familial hypocalciuric hypercalcemia (FHH) should be ruled out before repeat surgery.

Medical management is used for those patients who do not meet surgical criteria or who refuse surgery. BMD tests should be performed every 1–2 years and biochemical profiles should be assessed yearly. Patients are instructed to maintain adequate hydration, avoid thiazide diuretics, and limit their dietary intake of calcium to less than 1,000 mg/day. Several medications are of benefit in treating PHP. Based on current guidelines, cinacalcet has been shown to lower serum calcium in patients with PHP. Calcium-sensing receptor agonists act directly on parathyroid cells by way of the calcium-sensing receptor to inhibit the secretion of PTH. It has not been shown to affect BMD, kidney stones, or quality of life. These calcimimetic agents may prove beneficial in the treatment of PHP. Currently, they are approved for the treatment of secondary hyperparathyroidism and parathyroid cancer.

Alternatively, bisphosphonates inhibit bone resorption, but a persistent lowering of serum calcium has not been shown. Thus far, pharmacological treatment has not been shown to improve both BMD and serum calcium levels. Estrogen/progesterone has been shown to increase bone density in postmenopausal women with PHP, and some studies indicate that it can decrease serum calcium levels. However, the risks of hormone therapy must be weighed against the benefits of the treatment of PHP. Estrogen/progesterone are not first-line agents. In secondary hyperparathyroidism, the goal is to reduce PTH levels to appropriate goals depending on kidney function. In vitamin D deficiency, treatment with ergocalciferol or cholecalciferol usually results in the normalization of the vitamin D level and the concomitant normalization of the calcium and PTH. In renal disease, the administration of calcium salts and 1,25-dihydroxyvitamin D_3 or calcitriol usually results in the normalization of the serum calcium level. The calcium salts increase the calcium available for absorption and also chelate the phosphate in the intestines. Calcitriol acts at the kidneys, intestines, and bone to decrease calcium renal loss, increase calcium absorption, and increase bone mobilization. As the calcium normalizes, the PTH level also normalizes. Calcimimetic agents, as described earlier, are currently approved for treatment of secondary hyperparathyroidism. In some cases of severe secondary hyperparathyroidism and tertiary hyperparathyroidism in renal failure, parathyroidectomy may be required.

HYPOPARATHYROIDISM AND PSEUDOHYPOPARATHYROIDISM

Definition/Overview

Hypoparathyroidism is a rare entity defined by reduced levels of parathyroid hormone, leading to hypocalcemia, hyperphosphatemia, and inappropriately low or normal PTH. Pseudohypoparathyroidism results from resistance to parathyroid hormone resulting in similar biochemical features as hypoparathyroidism, except the PTH is elevated.

Etiology

The most common cause of hypoparathyroidism is an injury to or removal of the parathyroid glands during neck surgery, which accounts for about 75% of cases. The incidence of hypoparathyroidism after neck surgery is about 8%. Postsurgical hypoparathyroidism may be transient, permanent, or even intermittent. Other causes of hypoparathyroidism can be categorized by developmental defects in the parathyroid gland, defects in the PTH molecule, defective regulation of PTH secretion, autoimmune hypoparathyroidism, defects in the type 1 PTH receptor, or defects of the stimulatory guanine nucleotide-binding protein.

Pathophysiology

Defects in the PTH molecule have been shown to result in hypoparathyroidism. A few cases of familial hypoparathyroidism have been described in which the cause is a mutation in the gene for PTH. The mutation results in the synthesis of a defective PTH molecule and undetectable amounts of PTH in serum.

DiGeorge syndrome, the most common genetic etiology, is a congenital defect resulting in the agenesis of the parathyroid glands. DiGeorge syndrome is associated with rearrangements and microdeletions affecting genes on the long arm of chromosome 22. This in turn affects the protein that is necessary for the development of the thymus and parathyroids. The manifestations of this syndrome include conotruncal cardiac defects, facial malformations, learning disability, and incomplete development of the brachial arches, resulting in varying degrees of parathyroid and thymic hypoplasia.

Hypoparathyroidism can also arise from defective regulation of PTH secretion. Autosomal dominant hypercalciuric hypocalcemia is caused by activating mutations of the parathyroid and renal calcium-sensing receptors that result in hypocalcemia and hypercalciuria. The mutations cause excessive calcium-induced inhibition of PTH secretion. The hypocalcemia is usually mild and asymptomatic.

Hypoparathyroidism can occur as a consequence of autoimmunity. Autoimmune polyglandular syndrome type 1 consists of hypoparathyroidism, mucocutaneous candidiasis, adrenal insufficiency, and primary hypogonadism, as well as the less common features of malabsorption, gastrointestinal disorders, hypothyroidism, and diabetes. The syndrome is inherited as an autosomal recessive trait and is caused by mutations in an autoimmune regulator (AIRE) gene. The mutation in AIRE is postulated to lead to a loss of self-immune tolerance, thus leading to destruction of the parathyroids, adrenals, and other endocrine glands.

Defects in the type 1 PTH receptor can result in low PTH levels. Jansen's chondrodystrophy is caused by activating mutations of the type 1 PTH receptor. It is characterized by short limbs, mild hypercalcemia, and low serum PTH concentrations. Since the serum calcium level is mildly elevated, it does not fulfill the definition of hypoparathyroidism.

Pseudohypoparathyroidism occurs due to PTH resistance as a consequence of defects in the PTH receptor-associated stimulatory guanine nucleotide-binding protein. It is characterized by hypocalcemia and hyperphosphatemia due to resistance to PTH. There are several forms of pseudohypoparathyroidism. Patients with type 1a have hypocalcemia, hyperphosphatemia, elevated PTH levels, hormone resistance to thyrotropin and gonadotropins, and display characteristic physical features that are collectively termed 'Albright's hereditary osteodystrophy (AHO)'. Maternal transmission of the mutation is required for the manifestations of this mutation. Typically, patients have short stature, round facies, brachydactyly (Figures 4.12 and 4.13), obesity, and ectopic soft tissue or dermal ossification(s). In the calvaria, this may manifest as hyperostosis frontalis interna. Intracranial calcification(s) (Figure 4.14), cataracts, band keratopathy, subcutaneous calcifications, and dental hypoplasia (Figure 4.15) are also common but are likely the consequences of long-standing hypocalcemia. Type 1b patients present predominantly with renal PTH resistance and lack any features of AHO. Patients with type 1c present with both AHO and PTH resistance

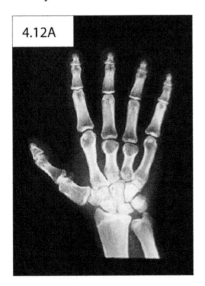
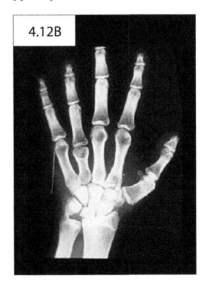

4.12A

4.12B

FIGURE 4.12   Radiographs of a patient's hands. A: Brachydactyly of the third and fourth digits; B: brachydactyly of the fourth digit. (Courtesy of Dr. Glen Sizemore.)

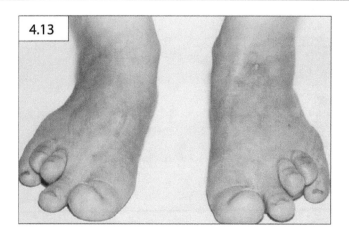

FIGURE 4.13 Photograph of the feet of a patient revealing brachydactyly of the third and fourth digits. (Courtesy of Dr. Glen Sizemore.)

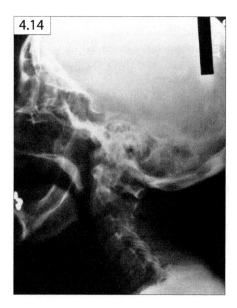

FIGURE 4.14 Basal ganglia calcification of a patient with hypoparathyroidism. (Courtesy of Dr. Glen Sizemore.)

but have normal stimulatory guanine nucleotide-binding protein function. Type 2 patients present with a normal urinary cyclic adenosine monophosphate (cAMP) response to PTH but lack a phosphaturic response. Furthermore, they lack any signs of AHO or resistance to other hormones. Last, patients with type 2 disease do not display a familial origin.

Clinical Presentation

The clinical findings associated with hypoparathyroidism are primarily due to the level and rate of change of serum calcium. When hypocalcemia occurs acutely, clinical manifestations include tetany, muscle cramps, muscle spasms, myopathy, paresthesia, seizures, fatigue, anxiety, and lethargy. When hypocalcemia occurs more chronically, patients may have very few symptoms apart from a history of cataracts.

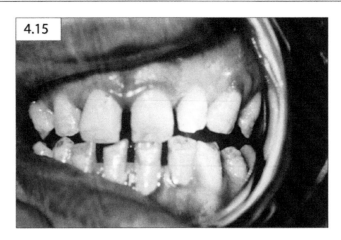

FIGURE 4.15   Dental hypoplasia in a patient with pseudohypoparathyroidism. (Courtesy of Dr. Glen Sizemore.)

The examination findings are also somewhat dependent upon the degree and duration of hypocalcemia. Findings include hypotension, a positive Trousseau's sign (carpal spasm with inflation of the blood pressure cuff above systolic), a positive Chvostek's sign (facial muscle contraction when the facial nerve is tapped on the ipsilateral side anterior to the ear), papilledema, congestive heart failure, dry and coarse skin and hair, and brittle hair and nails. The clinician should also look for any depigmentation in the skin and any signs of fungal infection. One should always inspect the neck for any signs of anterior neck surgery. Patients with pseudohypoparathyroidism present with the findings of hypoparathyroidism. Some patients will also display the clinical findings of short stature, rounded face, foreshortened fourth metacarpals, obesity, and subcutaneous calcifications characteristic of AHO.

Differential Diagnosis

The differential diagnosis of hypoparathyroidism includes iatrogenic from neck surgery, infiltration of the parathyroid as seen in hemochromatosis, Wilson's disease, granulomas, metastatic cancer, idiopathy, human immunodeficiency virus (HIV) infection, hypermagnesemia, and acute severe hypomagnesemia.

Diagnosis

Hypoparathyroidism is diagnosed based on biochemical tests with initial screening to include serum calcium, blood urea nitrogen/creatinine, serum phosphate, and magnesium levels. In hypoparathyroidism, serum calcium concentrations are decreased and serum phosphate levels are increased. Serum PTH is inappropriately normal, low, or undetectable. Usually, serum 1,25-dihydroxyvitamin D is low. Alkaline phosphatase activity is normal. Intestinal calcium absorption and bone resorption are both suppressed. The renal filtered load of calcium is decreased, and the 24-hour urinary calcium excretion is reduced. Renal tubular reabsorption of phosphate is elevated. A bone densitometry scan in patients with chronic hypoparathyroidism shows defects in the mineralization of new bone and can help with determining the onset of the disease. Abdominal imaging can also be used to look for nephrolithiasis or nephrocalcinosis. In pseudohypoparathyroidism, diagnosis is generally made based on the measurement of low cAMP and phosphate levels in the urine following an infusion of synthetic PTH (1–34). The exception is in pseudohypoparathyroidism type 2 in which there is a normal increase in cAMP levels in response to synthetic PTH but no phosphaturic response.

Management/Treatment

Treatment for hypoparathyroidism includes therapies targeted to the underlying cause when possible, as well as the normalization of the serum calcium level. Calcium salts, 1,25-dihydroxyvitamin D, vitamin D analogues, and magnesium are the mainstay of therapy. For patients with symptoms such as seizures, tetany, and electrocardiographic changes, as well as those in which hypocalcemia suddenly develops, intravenous calcium should be administered. Calcium gluconate is preferred and should be continued until the patient is stabilized with monitoring of calcium every 4–6 hours. Oral treatment with calcium salts is directed to maintain serum calcium in the low normal range to prevent hypercalciuria. In patients with hypoparathyroidism, the PTH-dependent renal production of 1,25-dihydroxyvitamin D is impaired. Therefore, patients require supplementation with calcitriol. Last, hypomagnesemia can contribute to hypoparathyroidism. Therefore, in patients with hypoparathyroidism, hypomagnesemia, and normal renal function, magnesium replacement should be initiated. Patients with hypoparathyroidism have been successfully treated with recombinant human PTH (1–84); however, in September 2019 the drug was recalled by the US Food and Drug Administration (FDA) due to a defect in the mechanism of delivery of the medication. Treatment of pseudohypoparathyroidism is similar to that of hypoparathyroidism and consists largely of calcium replacement and calcitriol. Requirements for vitamin D supplementation are usually lower than in patients with hypoparathyroidism. Supplementation with 1,25-dihydroxyvitamin D is ideal, but patients can be treated with vitamin D analogs as well. Patients with AHO may require specific treatment for problems related to their developmental and skeletal abnormalities. Patients with pseudohypoparathyroidism type 1a may require therapy for associated hypogonadism or hypothyroidism.

PAGET'S DISEASE

Definition/Overview

Paget's disease is a metabolic disorder of the bone featuring aggressive osteoclast-mediated bone resorption and impaired osteoblast-mediated bone formation, resulting in disorganized skeletal remodeling causing pain, deformities, and fractures.

Etiology

The estimated prevalence of Paget's disease in the US is about 1% per the National Health and Nutrition Examination Survey. It occurs most commonly in the countries of Great Britain, Australia, New Zealand, North America, and Western Europe, where there is a prevalence of about 3%. It rarely affects Africans, Asians, or people from the Indian subcontinent. Some studies suggest that there is a slight male preponderance. It rarely occurs in individuals under the age of 20. The exact etiology of Paget's disease is currently unknown. Family history of Paget's disease is identified in 15%–30% of patients, suggesting a possible genetic component. Heterozygous mutations affecting either of two genes have been shown in affected families to be linked to Paget's disease. Most of these genes are involved in osteoclast differentiation and function. The first group consists of 11 different mutations, all of which are clustered around the ubiquitin-binding domain of the sequestosome 1 protein. This protein modulates activity of the NF-κ β pathway, an important mediator of osteoclast function. The second group of mutations consists of domain-specific defects within valosin-containing proteins that predispose to Paget's disease in a rare syndrome also associated with late-onset inclusion body myopathy and dementia. Further evidence of the heterogeneity of the genetics of Paget's disease has come from studies reporting linkage of the disease with candidate loci at chromosome 5q31, chromosome 2, and chromosome 10. Once the genes associated with these loci are identified, a fuller understanding of the pathogenesis of familial Paget's disease should follow.

Another possible etiology for Paget's disease comes from observational studies that suggest the involvement of virus particles. Particles resembling paramyxovirus nucleocapsids, as well as antigens and nucleic acid sequences of measles virus, canine distemper virus, and respiratory syncytial virus have been identified in the nuclei and cytoplasm of pagetic osteoclasts.

Pathophysiology

Paget's disease occurs as a result of overactive osteoclasts coupled with an increase in osteoblastic function in a focal manner (Figure 4.16). The woven bone that is formed at a fast rate is structurally weaker and abnormal, increasing the risk of fracture. It typically involves just one bone or a few bones. The bones most often involved include the axial skeleton: skull, pelvis, vertebra, femur, or tibia. Osteolytic fronts progress approximately 1 cm yearly. The subsequent 'mixed stage' disease features cortical thickening, disorganized coarse trabeculae, and bone expansion. In cases of advanced disease, bones are widened and heterogeneously ossified. This pagetic process does not spread spontaneously to adjacent bones. However, there currently is no cure.

Clinical Presentation

Paget's disease is usually asymptomatic and discovered incidentally. The prevalence of the signs and symptoms of Paget's disease is uncertain, but the disease usually manifests in the skeleton. The most common presenting symptom is bone pain, seen in approximately 40% of patients. Other symptoms include bone deformity, warmth of the skin overlying an affected bone, secondary arthritis, and headaches or hearing loss if Paget's disease of bone affects the skull. If the disease involves the skull, jaw, clavicle, or a long bone of the leg, then skeletal expansion or distortion may be obvious. Mild to moderate, deep, aching bone pain characteristically begins late in the clinical course, persists throughout the day and at rest, and seems worse at night. Weight bearing often intensifies the pain, especially if there are osteolytic lesions. A sudden fracture, a new mass, or constant or worsening bone pain may herald malignant transformation. Osteosarcomas, or other skeletal sarcomas, develop in less than 1% of patients with Paget's disease but are more common and aggressive than in age-matched controls. Several neurologic findings may be present.

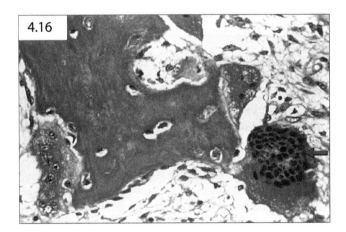

FIGURE 4.16 Hematoxylin and eosin decalcified stained section from a bone biopsy revealing an active lesion of Paget's disease with large multinucleated osteoclasts as well as osteoblasts that are repairing bone previously resorbed by the osteoclasts. The arrow points to a giant osteoclast. (Courtesy of Dr. Glen Sizemore.)

Hearing loss may result from skull involvement. Less commonly basilar impressions, hydrocephalus with headache and dizziness, and cranial nerve deficits may occur. In the spine, compression or ischemia may cause pain, dysesthesias, or paralysis.

Differential Diagnosis

The differential diagnosis includes Paget's disease, bone metastases, fibrous dysplasia, renal osteodystrophy, fluorosis, mastocytosis, tuberous sclerosis, and osteomalacia.

Diagnosis

Paget's disease is generally diagnosed using biochemical tests. Elevated serum total or bone-specific alkaline phosphatase (ALP) levels are present in patients with Paget's disease and reflect increased bone formation. Gamma-glutamyl transferase (GGT) can be used to help further differentiate the source of ALP and bone-specific ALP can confirm the diagnosis. Other less specific markers of bone formation include osteocalcin. Markers of bone resorption such as serum and urinary c-telopeptide and n-telopeptide are elevated in Paget's disease. The disease can be confirmed using radiographs and bone scans, which can also detect asymptomatic areas of disease. The radiographic features of Paget's disease include osteolytic, osteosclerotic, and mixed lesions.

Histologically, Paget's disease can be divided into two phases. The active phase features disorganized bone architecture. There are clusters of numerous, large, multinucleated osteoclasts adjacent to many osteoblasts. The osteoblasts synthesize matrix so rapidly that collagen forms an immature woven or lamellar pattern with faint cement lines. The stroma is vascular and fibrous. The late phase features thick trabeculae with a mosaic pattern of prominent cement lines at the interfaces of the numerous past episodes of bone resorption followed by bone formation (Figure 4.17). Osteoblast activity remains apparent with pale osteoid deposition.

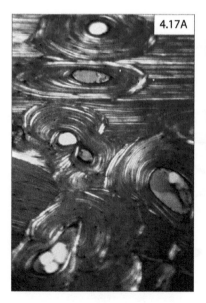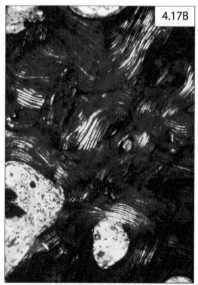

FIGURE 4.17   Polarized views of (A) normal bone and (B) pagetic bone. The normal bone has a highly organized lamellar structure, whereas the pagetic bone displays a chaotic picture of lamellar and woven bone with disorganized structure, often termed the 'mosaic pattern'. (Courtesy of Dr. Glen Sizemore.)

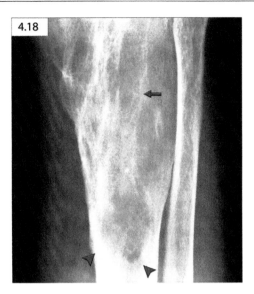

FIGURE 4.18   Radiograph of the tibia and fibula of a patient with Paget's disease revealing an area of severe osteolytic activity (arrow) associated with a small degree of bony expansion in the distal region of the tibia (arrowheads). (Courtesy of Dr. Glen Sizemore.)

Radiographs of affected areas show cortical thickening and irregular areas of lucency and sclerosis (Figures 4.18 and 4.19). Skull involvement in Paget's disease is characterized by bony enlargement as well as cotton wool areas (Figures 4.20 and 4.21). Involvement of the long bones often results in bowing deformities (Figures 4.22 and 4.23). On a plain radiograph, the leading edge of an osteolytic front in the appendicular bones often appears shaped like a flame, a letter V, or a blade of grass (Figure 4.24). Bone scans in patients with Paget's disease reveal intense uptake at pagetic areas. Usually, the bone scan reveals lesions throughout the body, particularly in areas such as the pelvis, vertebra, and scapula (Figure 4.25).

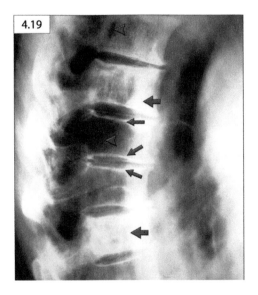

FIGURE 4.19   Radiograph of the lateral spine of a patient with Paget's disease revealing cortical thickening (small arrows) and irregular areas of lucency (arrowheads) and sclerosis (large arrows). (Courtesy of Dr. Glen Sizemore.)

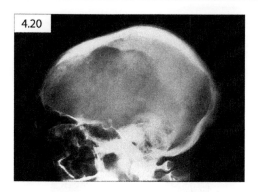

FIGURE 4.20   Radiograph of the skull showing Paget's disease as characterized by a large circumscribed area of bone loss, termed 'osteoporosis circumscripta', a common finding in Paget's disease. (Courtesy of Dr. Glen Sizemore.)

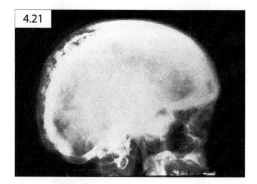

FIGURE 4.21   Radiograph of the skull showing the late sclerotic phase of Paget's disease as characterized by tremendous thickening of the cranial vault with chaotic bone structure. (Courtesy of Dr. Glen Sizemore.)

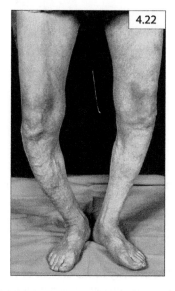

FIGURE 4.22   Photograph of a Paget's disease patient with bowing of the long bones of the leg. (Courtesy of Dr. Glen Sizemore.)

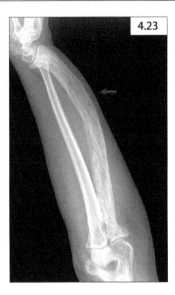

FIGURE 4.23 Radiograph of the arm of a patient with Paget's disease revealing bowing of the radius as well as cortical thickening and irregular areas of lucency and sclerosis (arrow).

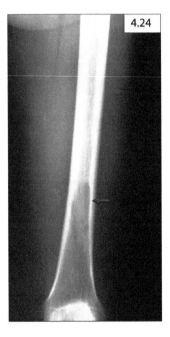

FIGURE 4.24 Radiograph of a long bone in a patient with Paget's disease showing the leading edge of an osteolytic front appearing shaped like a flame, a letter V, or a blade of grass. (Courtesy of Dr. Glen Sizemore.)

Management/Treatment

There is no cure for Paget's disease. The severity of the disease is variable. Morbidity and mortality come from the pain, deformity, fracture, and sarcomatous degeneration of pagetic bone. The goal of therapy is to slow osteoclastic bone resorption. There are several indications for the treatment of patients with Paget's disease. Treat if (1) the serum alkaline phosphatase is at least three or four times the upper limit of

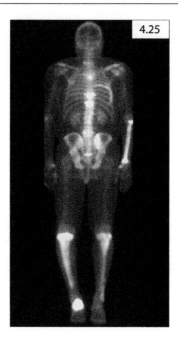

FIGURE 4.25 Bone scan of a patient with Paget's disease revealing lesions throughout the body, particularly in the pelvis, vertebra, long bones, and scapula.

normal; (2) there are fractures or pain in the pagetic bone; (3) there is skull involvement with hearing loss or headaches; (4) there is monostotic disease of weight-bearing bones; (5) there is involvement of critical sites that may lead to complications such as arthritis or fractures; and (6) there is a need to pretreat patients prior to surgery to reduce hypervascularity and blood loss.

The most commonly used agents for the treatment of Paget's disease are bisphosphonates. These agents are synthetic analogs of inorganic pyrophosphate that are not biodegradable. They have skeletal half-lives measured in years and adhere to mineralized surfaces. Osteoclasts selectively take up bisphosphonates resulting in the disruption of energy metabolism and specific enzymatic pathways. Both the oral and intravenous agents have been proven effective, with intravenous zoledronic acid showing a superior response rate and longer duration of remission. After a first course of treatment, these agents can normalize markers of bone turnover in most patients with moderate to severe Paget's disease. Furthermore, most patients report relief from pain. After a single course, biochemical remission can persist for 6–18 months with oral bisphosphonates and several years with zoledronic acid. A major side effect of oral bisphosphonates is upper gastrointestinal irritation. The Endocrine Society recommends a single 5 mg intravenous dose of zoledronic acid as the treatment of choice. This is based on two clinical trials that compared zoledronic acid with oral risedronate. At 6 months, therapeutic response, ALP levels, onset of action, pain relief, and quality of life were significantly better in the zoledronic acid group.

Intravenous pamidronate or zoledronic acid avoids this side effect, but after an infusion, patients may develop an acute phase reaction characterized by transient mild fever, myalgias, headache, and malaise that lasts 1–3 days and is responsive to analgesics and antipyretics. This, however, is uncommon and is not seen in more than 15% of patients. Transient iritis develops in some patients treated with intravenous pamidronate. With all bisphosphonates, there is a risk for osteonecrosis of the jaw and atypical femur fractures. Hypocalcemia may develop in patients treated with intravenous bisphosphonates. This risk can be minimized by correcting vitamin D deficiency and calcium deficiency before the infusion. After treatment, the patient should continue appropriate vitamin D and calcium supplementation.

Paget's disease can be treated with subcutaneous calcitonin as a second-line agent. Treatment with calcitonin remains an option if bisphosphonates are not tolerated or contraindicated. Calcitonin has been shown to decrease markers of bone turnover by 50%. It also often decreases bone pain and warmth, improves neurologic complications, and can heal osteolytic lesions. One drawback is that soon after cessation of therapy, disease reactivation is likely. About 25% of patients acquire resistance to calcitonin. Side effects include nausea and flushing.

OSTEOMALACIA

Definition/Overview

'Osteomalacia' is a term that encompasses several disorders all of which are characterized by defective bone matrix mineralization. The term 'rickets' is often used interchangeably with osteomalacia. Rickets generally refers to defective bone matrix mineralization of the newly formed bone and growth plate cartilage present in children. Osteomalacia generally refers to defective bone matrix mineralization at the sites of bone remodeling present in both children and adults.

Etiology

The prevalence of osteomalacia is dependent upon the criteria used for diagnosis, i.e., clinical, biochemical, bone histology, or quantitative bone histomorphometry. On a global scale, vitamin D deficiency is by far the most common cause of osteomalacia. It can be assumed that osteomalacia is prevalent in regions where nutritional rickets is common. It is difficult to approximate the prevalence since histological confirmation of osteomalacia in children and adolescents with rickets is lacking. In studies describing bone histomorphometry of the femoral head or iliac crest biopsy in patients with hip fracture, the frequency of osteomalacia was shown to range from none to more than 30%. Defective bone matrix mineralization can be caused by (1) calcium deficiency (hypocalcemic osteomalacia), (2) phosphorous deficiency (hypophosphatemic osteomalacia), or (3) primary defects in local bone processes (osteomalacia with normal mineral homeostasis). Hypocalcemic osteomalacia is essentially due to vitamin D deficiency. Vitamin D deficiency can occur as a result of inadequate nutritional intake, lack of exposure to sunlight, and intestinal malabsorption syndromes such as celiac sprue or inflammatory bowel disease. Osteomalacia caused by vitamin D deficiency is seen in three stages. Initially, patients will present with normal serum calcium and phosphate levels with elevated alkaline phosphatase, serum PTH, and 1,25-dihydroxyvitamin D levels. At this stage, bone histomorphometry reveals only the effects of excess PTH without a mineralization defect. In the second stage, serum calcium levels tend to decline, and both serum PTH and alkaline phosphatase values increase further. At this point, there is some evidence of impaired mineralization seen on bone histomorphometry. In the third stage, hypocalcemia and hypophosphatemia are seen with further exacerbation of secondary hyperparathyroidism and cessation of bone matrix mineralization.

Pseudovitamin D deficiency has also been described. It consists of two syndromes caused by congenital errors in vitamin D metabolism. Pseudovitamin D deficiency type I is an autosomal recessive disorder resulting in a defect in renal tubular 25(OH)D-1-alpha hydroxylase and thereby 1,25-dihydroxyvitamin D deficiency. Pseudovitamin D deficiency type II is a hereditary condition resulting in defects in the calcitriol receptor effector system leading to resistance to 1,25-dihydroxyvitamin D.

Hypophosphatemic rickets is an X-linked disorder that results in decreased renal tubular absorption of phosphorus. The disease affects males and is characterized by hypophosphatemia, growth retardation, and lower limb deformities. A milder case can occur in females who are heterozygous for the gene. Osteomalacia with normal mineral homeostasis is seen in hypophosphatasia. This rare disorder results from decreased tissue-specific alkaline phosphatase activity. Clinical presentation can vary and is generally more severe during childhood than adulthood. Hypophosphatasia is characterized by low alkaline phosphatase levels, normal or high calcium and phosphate levels, and high serum pyridoxal 5'-phosphate.

Pathophysiology

The causes of osteomalacia from vitamin D deficiency can be classified as extrinsic or intrinsic. Vitamin D derived from endogenous production in the skin or absorbed from the gut is a prohormone. It is transformed into its active form by two successive steps: hydroxylation in the liver to 25-hydroxyvitamin D followed by I α-hydroxylation in the renal proximal tubule to 1,25-dihydroxyvitamin D. The 25-hydroxylation of vitamin D in the liver is not tightly regulated. The principal determinant of the rate of 25-hydroxylation is the circulating level of vitamin D. In contrast, the renal I α-hydroxylase enzyme is under tight regulation by PTH, calcitonin, 1,25-dihydroxyvitamin D, calcium, and phosphorus. Once in its active form, the effects of 1,25-dihydroxyvitamin D are mediated via a high-affinity intracellular vitamin D receptor. The vitamin D receptor acts as a ligand-modulated transcription factor that belongs to the steroid, thyroid, and retinoic acid receptors gene family.

1,25-Dihydroxyvitamin D is the most powerful physiologic agent that stimulates the active transport of calcium and to a lesser degree phosphorus and magnesium, across the small intestine. Disorders in vitamin D action result in a decrease in the net flux of minerals to the extracellular compartment causing hypocalcemia and secondary hyperparathyroidism. Prolonged vitamin D deficiency decreases serum calcium, causing an increase in serum PTH levels. The increased PTH levels, which act on bone and kidney, cause an increase in serum calcium levels toward normal. As such, elevated serum PTH levels can be considered a pathognomonic hallmark in many patients with vitamin D deficiency. Increased renal phosphate clearance due to secondary hyperparathyroidism and reduced absorption of phosphorus due to deficient 1,25-dihydroxyvitamin D action on the gut result in hypophosphatemia. Low concentrations of calcium and phosphorus in the extracellular fluid lead to defective mineralization of the organic bone matrix.

Clinical Presentation

The clinical features of rickets are weakness, bone pain, bone deformity, and fragility fractures. The most rapidly growing bones show the most striking abnormalities. Thus, the clinical features will depend on the age of onset. Rickets is not present at birth, as calcium and phosphorus levels in fetal plasma are sustained by placental transport from maternal plasma that is not regulated by the fetal vitamin D system. Children with hereditary disorders of vitamin D action usually develop the characteristic features of rickets within the first 2 years of life. The rib cage may be deformed, contributing to respiratory failure. Dental eruption is delayed. Muscle weakness and hypotonia are severe and result in a protuberant abdomen and further contributing to respiratory failure. This may also cause the inability to walk without support. After the first year of life with the acquisition of erect posture and rapid linear growth, the deformities are most severe in the legs, causing the bowing of long bones of the lower extremities. The clinical features of osteomalacia are subtle and may include bone pain or low back pain of varying severity. Severe muscle weakness and hypotonia may be prominent features in adults with osteomalacia. Improvement of myopathy occurs after very low doses of 1,25-dihydroxyvitamin D. The first clinical presentation of osteomalacia may be an acute fracture of the long bones, pubic rami, ribs, or spine. Because of the reduction in the mineral content of the bones, fractures can occur in the axial and appendicular skeleton. The clinical presentation of a pseudofracture can be diagnostic of osteomalacia.

In patients with rickets occurring before the age of 2 years, physical examination often reveals widened cranial sutures, frontal bossing, posterior flattening of the skull, widening of the wrists, bulging of the costochondral junction, and indentation of the ribs at the diaphragmatic insertion. The teeth usually show enamel hypoplasia. Bow legs and knock knee deformities as well as widening of the end of long bones develop as the patient becomes weight bearing. Examination findings of patients with osteomalacia are often more subtle. Patients often have bone pain, muscle weakness, hypotonia, and fractures.

Differential Diagnosis

The differential diagnosis includes osteoporosis, vitamin D deficiency, liver disease, renal disease or renal osteodystrophy, 1-alpha hydroxylase deficiency, vitamin D resistance, X-linked hypophosphatemic rickets, autosomal dominant hypophosphatemic rickets, renal phosphate loss, excessive antacid intake, hereditary hypophosphatemic rickets with hypercalciuria, drug toxicities including anticonvulsants, cholestyramine, glucocorticoids, fluoride, etidronate, parenteral aluminum, imatinib, hypophosphatasia, acidosis, and oncogenic osteomalacia.

Diagnosis

Diagnosis is primarily made through biochemical evaluation. The underlying cause can usually be determined by measuring the 25-hydroxyvitamin D, 1,25-dihydroxyvitamin D, serum calcium, 24-hour urinary calcium, serum phosphorus, intact PTH, urinary cAMP, urinary phosphate, bone-specific alkaline phosphatase, and osteocalcin. The characteristic biochemical features of vitamin D deficiency are low to low normal concentrations of serum calcium, low urinary calcium excretion, hypophosphatemia, increased serum intact PTH levels, increased urinary cAMP excretion, and decreased tubular reabsorption of phosphate. Biochemical markers associated with increased osteoid production such as bone-specific alkaline phosphatase and osteocalcin will be elevated in states of rickets and osteomalacia. If unable to make a definitive diagnosis based on the clinical and biochemical evaluation, then the most reliable way to establish the diagnosis is with an undecalcified bone biopsy.

The characteristic histologic feature of rickets and osteomalacia is deficiency or lack of mineralization of bone matrix (Figure 4.26). In clinical practice, the bone specimen obtained is from the iliac crest. Therefore, the histologic picture is osteomalacia. Osteomalacia is defined as excess osteoid and a quantitative dynamic proof of defective bone matrix mineralization obtained by analysis of time-spaced tetracycline labeling.

The specific radiographic features of rickets reflect the failure of cartilage calcification and endochondral ossification and, therefore, are best seen in the metaphysis of rapidly growing bones. The metaphyses are widened, uneven, concave, or cupped, and because of the delay in or absence of calcification, the metaphyses become partially or totally invisible (Figures 4.27–4.29). In more severe forms, rarefaction and thinning of the cortex of the entire shaft, sparse bone trabeculation, and bone deformities will become evident. Greenstick fractures may appear as well. The radiographic features of osteomalacia are either

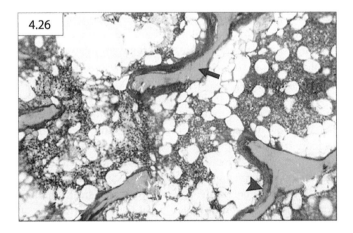

FIGURE 4.26   Bone biopsy revealing osteomalacia as defined as excess osteoid (arrow) and defective bone matrix mineralization (arrowhead). (Courtesy of Dr. Susan Ott, http://courses.washington.edu/bonephys/ophome.html.)

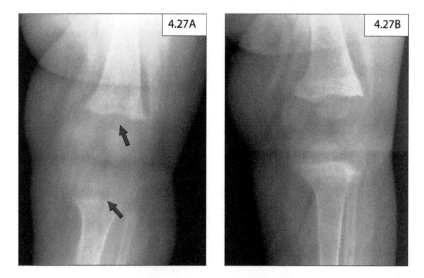

FIGURE 4.27 Radiograph of the lower extremity of a patient with rickets (A) before and (B) after treatment. The metaphyses are widened, uneven, concave, or cupped and partially invisible (arrows). (Courtesy of Dr. Glen Sizemore.)

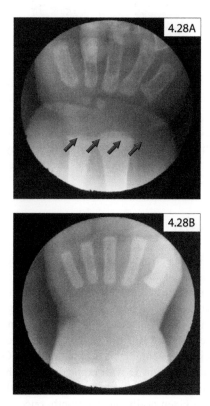

FIGURE 4.28 Radiograph of the hand of a patient with rickets (A) before and (B) after treatment. The metaphyses are widened, uneven, concave, or cupped and partially invisible (arrows). (Courtesy of Dr. Glen Sizemore.)

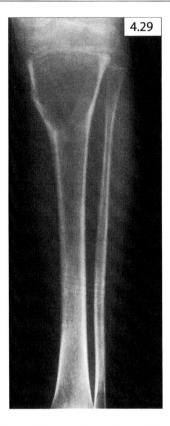

FIGURE 4.29 Radiograph of the tibia and fibula of a patient with rickets. The metaphyses are widened, uneven, concave, or cupped and partially invisible. (Courtesy of Dr. Glen Sizemore.)

mild, such as generalized, nonspecific osteopenia, or more specific, such as pseudofractures, commonly seen at the medial edges of the shaft of long bones (Figure 4.30). In hypocalcemic osteomalacia, radiographic features of secondary hyperparathyroidism, such as subperiosteal resorption and cysts of the long bones, may exist.

Management/Treatment

Rickets and osteomalacia comprise a spectrum of diseases. The prognosis is dependent upon age at presentation and the severity of the disease. Patients with rickets often have lifelong morbidity and mortality. In contrast, patients with asymptomatic osteomalacia in adulthood may have complete resolution of the disease with treatment. Treatment depends in large part on the etiology of the osteomalacia. The goals of therapy for vitamin D–deficiency osteomalacia are to ease the symptoms, foster an environment for fracture healing, and improve bone strength, all while correcting any biochemical abnormalities. The goal with treatment of vitamin D–deficiency osteomalacia is to maintain 25(OH)D levels >30 ng/ml. Typically, treatment consists of replacement of vitamin D with ergocalciferol, cholecalciferol, or, in severe cases, calcitriol. Because vitamin D is stored in fat and released slowly and the half-life of 25-hydroxyvitamin D is 2–3 weeks, the vitamin can be given orally once a month, once every 6–12 months, or once a year by injection. Calcitriol (1,25-dihydroxyvitamin D) is given in cases where there is impaired renal conversion of 25-hydroxyvitamin D to 1,25-dihydroxyvitamin D, such as in 1-alpha hydroxylase deficiency or when there is severe malabsorption and secondary hyperparathyroidism. Patients with hypophosphatemic

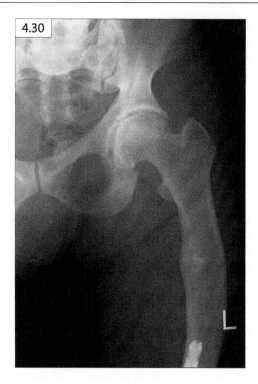

FIGURE 4.30 Radiograph of the left pelvis, hip, and proximal half of the lower extremity with a pseudofracture at the medial edges of the femur. (Courtesy of Dr. Glen Sizemore.)

rickets benefit from treatment with phosphorus and 1,25-dihdroxyvitamin D. In the case of drug-induced osteomalacia, treatment is the discontinuation of the offending agent.

SCLEROTIC BONE DISORDERS

Definition/Overview

Sclerotic bone disorders consist of a group of illnesses characterized by impaired osteoclast resorption and/or increased osteoblast-mediated bone formation, ultimately resulting in thickening of cortical and lamellar bone.

Epidemiology and Etiology

Osteopetrosis is a heterogeneous group of sclerotic bone disorders defined by defects in proteins in differentiated osteoclasts, resulting in impaired osteoclast resorption. They are rare and can be grouped into three main variants: (1) the autosomal dominant benign form that occurs in adulthood, termed 'osteopetrosis tarda'; (2) the autosomal recessive malignant form that occurs in infancy, termed 'osteopetrosis congenita'; and (3) the autosomal recessive intermediate form that occurs in childhood, termed 'marble bone disease'.

Sclerotic bone disease also occurs as a consequence of prostate and breast cancer bone metastases that induce increased osteoblast activity. Bone metastases occur in up to 70% of patients with advanced breast or prostate cancer. The exact incidence of bone metastasis is unknown, but it is estimated that 350,000 people die from bone metastases annually in the United States. Metastases to the bone are a poor prognostic sign, as only 20% of patients with breast cancer are still alive 5 years after the discovery of bone metastasis.

Pathophysiology

Osteopetrosis is characterized by impaired osteoclastic bone resorption. The osteoclast is a multinucleated cell with a typical ruffled border that is capable of breaking down both the inorganic and organic matrix of bone. Osteoclastic bone resorption requires the establishment of a pH gradient across the ruffled membrane and the synthesis and release of lysosomal enzymes, in particular tartrate-resistant acid phosphatase (TRAP) and cysteine proteinases such as the cathepsins, which are capable of degrading collagen. Multiple genes are involved in the etiology and pathophysiology of osteopetrosis. The gene mutations range from autosomal recessive to autosomal dominant. The severity of the mutations ranges from moderate to malignant. It should be noted that a substantial percentage of patients with osteopetrosis have no identifiable gene defect.

The mechanisms of osteoblastic metastasis and the factors involved are unknown. Endothelin-1 has been implicated in osteoblastic metastasis from breast cancer. It stimulates the formation of bone and the proliferation of osteoblasts in bone organ cultures, and serum endothelin-1 levels are increased in patients with osteoblastic metastasis from prostate cancer. In addition to endothelin-1, platelet-derived growth factor, a polypeptide produced by osteoblasts in the bone microenvironment, urokinase, and prostate-specific antigen (PSA) may also be involved. Prostate cancer cells also release PSA, a kallikrein serine protease. PSA can cleave PTH-related peptides at the N-terminus, which could block tumor-induced bone resorption. It may also activate osteoblastic growth factors released in the bone microenvironment during the development of bone metastases.

Clinical Presentation

Clinical history in sclerotic bone disease is dependent upon the etiology. Autosomal recessive osteopetrosis presents in infancy and is associated with failure to thrive and growth retardation. This form of osteopetrosis is very severe and usually results in death by 2 years of age. Proptosis, blindness, deafness, and hydrocephalus occur in these patients as bone encroaches on the cranial foramina. A critical feature of autosomal recessive osteopetrosis is severe bone marrow failure resulting in pancytopenia. Thrombocytopenia, leukoerythroblastic anemia, elevated serum acid, and alkaline phosphatase levels are also usually present. Hypocalcemia may or may not be present. Death from autosomal recessive osteopetrosis occurs as a result of severe anemia, bleeding, and/or infection. In rare instances, patients survive into adulthood. They present with severe anemia, recurrent fractures, growth retardation, deafness, blindness, and massive hepatosplenomegaly.

Intermediate autosomal recessive osteopetrosis is not characterized by bone marrow failure and survival rates are better. Patients are usually of short stature and present with intracranial calcifications, sensorineural hearing loss, and psychomotor retardation.

Autosomal dominant osteopetrosis is asymptomatic in about 50% of cases and detected by a family history of bone disease or as an incidental radiologic finding. About 40% of patients present with fractures related to brittle osteopetrotic bones or with osteomyelitis, especially of the mandible. There is sufficient retention of the marrow cavity for normal hematopoiesis to occur in patients with autosomal dominant osteopetrosis.

The consequences of bone metastases are often devastating. Patients with osteoblastic metastases have bone pain and pathologic fractures because of the poor quality of bone produced by the osteoblasts.

Differential Diagnosis

The differential diagnosis of sclerotic bone disease includes malignant autosomal recessive osteopetrosis, intermediate autosomal recessive osteopetrosis, autosomal dominant osteopetrosis, severe osteoclast poor osteopetrosis, transient infantile osteopetrosis, osteopetrosis with renal tubular acidosis, osteopetrosis with neuronal anomalies, osteopetrosis with anhidrotic ectodermal dysplasia, immunodeficiency, lymphedema, osteopetrosis with Glanzmann thrombasthenia, and metastatic breast or prostate cancer.

SCLEROSING BONE DISORDER	ONSET (AGE)	AFFECTED SKELETAL REGION	TYPICAL FINDINGS
Osteopetrosis	Autosomal dominant, adulthood	Skull, long bones, spine	Symmetric increase in bone mass with a 'bone within a bone' appearance
Pycnodyostosis	Early childhood	Skull, long bones, orbital region	Recurrent fractures, disproportionate short stature with narrow thorax and large cranium
Osteomalacia	Middle-aged, more predominant in males	Spine and pelvis	Coarsening of trabecular bone resembling osteomalacia
Osteopoikilosis	Childhood	Long bones, hands, feet	Spotty and patchy texture
Paget's disease		Axial skeleton	Coarse trabecular thickening with bone enlargement

Diagnosis

The diagnosis of sclerotic bone disease is derived from a combination of clinical findings, as well as radiologic evidence of dense, deformed, and diffusely sclerotic bone. Generalized osteosclerosis is apparent radiographically, often with a 'bone within a bone' appearance (Figure 4.31). Transverse radiolucent bands may be observed, and it may be difficult to discern the marrow cavity. The decrease in osteoclast activity also affects the shape and structure of bone by altering its capacity to remodel during growth (Figure 4.32). In severely affected patients, the medullary cavity is filled with endochondral new bone, with little space remaining for hematopoietic cells. Osteosclerosis in patients with prostate or breast metastases is similar in appearance radiographically to that seen in osteopetrotic patients (Figure 4.33).

Management/Treatment

Few therapies have proven effective in sclerotic bone disease. Bone marrow transplantation has been shown to be curative in autosomal recessive infantile osteopetrosis. It effectively treats both bone marrow failure and metabolic disturbances. Zoledronic acid, a potent inhibitor of osteoclast activity, differentiation, and survival, has been shown to decrease the risk of skeletal complications in males with androgen-independent prostate cancer and bone metastases. The efficacy of zoledronic acid may extend to other metastatic cancers such as metastatic breast cancer. The remaining options include treatment of

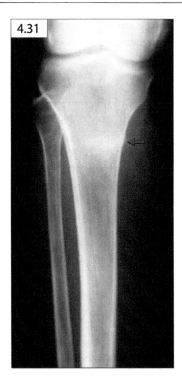

FIGURE 4.31   Radiograph of the tibia with a sclerotic pseudofracture (arrow) as well as the typical 'bone within a bone' appearance. (Courtesy of Dr. Glen Sizemore.)

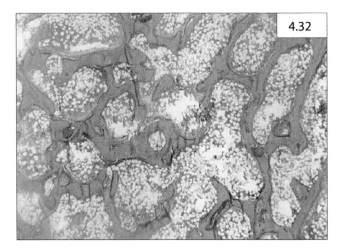

FIGURE 4.32   Biopsy of sclerotic bone revealing increased new bone, increased disorganization, and decreased marrow cellularity. (Courtesy of Dr. Susan Ott, http://courses.washington.edu/bonephys/ophome .html.)

associated symptoms. Current guidelines recommend calcium and vitamin D as first-line therapy for the treatment of hypocalcemia and secondary hyperparathyroidism in patients with osteopetrosis. The lack of published studies on noninfantile osteopetrosis makes the development of evidence-based guidelines for the clinical management of these patients difficult.

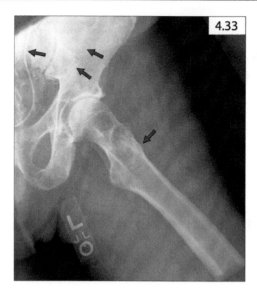

FIGURE 4.33   Radiograph of the pelvis and hip revealing sclerotic osteoblastic metastatic prostate neoplasms (arrows) involving the sacrum, right and left innominate bones, and the left greater trochanter.

REFERENCES

AACE/AAES Task Force on Primary Hyperparathyroidism. The American Association of Clinical Endocrinologists and the American Association of Endocrine Surgeons position statement on the diagnosis and management of primary hyperparathyroidism. *Endocr Prac* 2005;11(1):49–54.

Balemans W, Van Wesenbeeck L, Van Hul W. A clinical and molecular overview of the human osteopetroses. *Calcified TissueInt* 2005;77:263–74.

Bastepe M, Juppner H. GNAS locus and pseudohypoparathyroidism. *Hormone Res* 2005;63:65–74.

Dawson-Hughes B, Gold DT, Rodbard HW, Bonner FJ Jr, Khosla S, Swift SS. Physician's guide to the prevention and treatment of osteoporosis. National Osteoporosis Foundation, 2003. www.nof.org/physguide/index.htm.

Leib ES, Lewiecki EM, Binkley N, Hamdy RC, International society for clinical densitometry: Official positions of the International Society for clinical densitometry. *J Clin Densit* 2004;7:1–6.

Lyles KW, Siris ES, Singer FR, Meunier PJ. A clinical approach to the diagnosis and management of Paget's disease of bone. *J Bone Min Res* 2001;16:1379–87.

Marx SJ. Hyperparathyroid and hypoparathyroid disorders. *N Engl J Med* 2000;343(25):1863–75.

Mauck KF, Clarke BL. Diagnosis, screening, prevention, and treatment of osteoporosis. *Mayo Clin Proc* 2006;81(5):662–72.

Nelson HD, Helfand M, Woolf SH, Allan JD. Screening for postmenopausal osteoporosis: A review of the evidence for the US preventive services task force. *Ann Intern Med* 2002;137:529–41.

NIH Consensus Development Panel. Osteoporosis prevention, diagnosis, and therapy. *JAMA* 2001;285:785–95.

Ott S. Osteoporosis and bone physiology. 2006. http://courses.washington.edu/bonephys/ophome.html

Roodman GD. Mechanisms of bone metastasis. *N Engl J Med* 2004;350(16):1655–64.

Roodman GD, Windle JJ. Paget disease of the bone. *J Clin Investig* 2005;115(2):200–8.

Sambook P, Cooper C. Osteoporosis. *Lancet* 2006;367:2010–18.

Silverberg SJ, Shane E, Jacobs TP, Siris E, Bilezikian JP. A 10-year prospective study of primary hyperparathyroidism with or without parathyroid surgery. *N Engl J Med* 1999;341(17):1249–55.

Tolar J, Teitelbaum SL, Orchard PJ. Osteopetrosis. *N Engl J Med* 2004;351(27):2839–49.

White MP. Paget's disease of the bone. *N Engl J Med* 2006;355(6):593–600.

WHO. *Scientific Group on the prevention and management of osteoporosis. Prevention and Management of Osteoporosis: Report of a WHO Scientific Group.* Publications of the World Health Organization, Geneva, 2003.

Hypothalamic-Pituitary Disorders

5

S. Sethu K. Reddy, Pruthvi Goparaju, and Maria Fleseriu

INTRODUCTION

The pituitary gland is divided into two lobes: anterior (developed from Rathke's pouch) and posterior (developed as a diverticulum growing downward from the base of the hypothalamus). It weighs less than a gram and sits in the sella turcica, which is surrounded by bony walls and floor and a roof made up of dura, and then the optic chiasma, hypothalamus, and third ventricle. The optic chiasma may be anterior (15%), above (80%), or behind the sella (5%). Laterally on each side are the cavernous sinus; internal carotid artery; and cranial nerves III, IV, V1, V2, and VI.

The median eminence is an intensely vascular component at the base of the hypothalamus that forms the floor of the third ventricle. The pituitary stalk arises from the median eminence. The hypothalamus extends anteriorly to the optic chiasm and posteriorly to the mamillary bodies.

Most of the anterior pituitary hormones have associated stimulatory releasing hormones: luteinizing hormone-releasing hormone (LHRH) for both luteinizing hormone (LH) and follicle-stimulating hormone (FSH); corticotrophin-releasing hormone (CRH) for adrenocorticotrophic hormone (ACTH); thyrotropin-releasing hormone (TRH) for thyroid-stimulating hormone (TSH); and growth hormone-releasing hormone (GHRH) for growth hormone (GH). Of note, prolactin (PRL) is under tonic inhibitory influence, with dopamine acting as a PRL release-inhibiting factor (Table 5.1). Magnetic resonance imaging (MRI)

TABLE 5.1 Pituitary Hormones, Hypothalamic Hormones, and Other Regulatory Factors

PITUITARY HORMONE	HYPOTHALAMIC HORMONE	OTHER REGULATORY FACTORS
Thyrotropin (TSH)	TRH	T4, T3, dopamine, Pit 1
ACTH	CRH	ADH, adrenaline, cortisol
LH	LHRH	Estrogen, progesterone, testosterone
FSH	LHRH	Activin, estrogen, inhibin, follistatin, testosterone
GH	GHRH	Somatostatin, estrogens, T4, Pit 1
PRL	PRF	Dopamine, TRH, Pit 1, estrogen, serotonin, vasoactive intestinal peptide, GnRH-associated peptide

ACTH, adrenocorticotrophic hormone; CRH, corticotrophin-releasing hormone; FSH, follicle-stimulating hormone; GH, growth hormone; GHRH, growth hormone-releasing hormone; GnRH, gonadotropin-releasing hormone; LH, luteinizing hormone; LHRH, luteinizing hormone-releasing hormone; PRF, prolactin-releasing factor; PRL, prolactin; TRH, thyrotropin-releasing hormone.

DOI: 10.1201/9781003100669-5

is the best method for visualization of hypothalamic–pituitary anatomy, optic chiasm, vascular structures, and tumor extension to cavernous sinuses.

PITUITARY ADENOMAS

Definition/Overview

Pituitary adenomas are tumors that may present with either hypofunction or hyperfunction, as well as symptoms directly related to mass effect (Table 5.2). Since the advent of computed tomography (CT), microadenomas have been arbitrarily designated as equal or less than 10 mm (Figure 5.1) in diameter and macroadenomas as greater than 10 mm in diameter (Figure 5.2). They are invariably benign, with no sex predilection. Pituitary adenomas are rarely associated with parathyroid and pancreatic hyperplasia or neoplasia as part of the multiple endocrine neoplasia type 1 (MEN1) syndrome. Pituitary carcinomas are rare, but metastases from other solid malignancies (e.g., breast, lung most common) can occur more frequently. The fifth edition of the *WHO Classification of Endocrine and Neuroendocrine Tumors* suggests that pituitary adenomas should be labeled pituitary neuroendocrine tumors (PitNETs).

Etiology

About 50% of pituitary adenomas are prolactinomas, 15% GH-producing, 10% ACTH-producing, and less than 1% secrete TSH. Nonfunctioning pituitary adenomas, or more appropriately named nonsecretory

TABLE 5.2 Clinical Manifestations of Pituitary Tumors

MASS EFFECTS	ENDOCRINE EFFECTS	
	HYPERPITUITARISM	HYPOPITUITARISM
Headaches	GH: acromegaly	GH: short stature in children; increased fat mass, decreased strength, and well-being in adults
Chiasmal syndrome	PRL: hyperprolactinemia	
Hypothalamic syndrome	ACTH: Cushing disease	
• Disturbances of thirst, appetite, satiety, sleep, and temperature regulation	Nelson's syndrome	PRL: failure of postpartum lactation
	LH/FSH: gonadal dysfunction or silent α-subunit secretion	ACTH: hypocortisolism
		LH or FSH: hypogonadism
• Diabetes insipidus	TSH: hypothyroidism	TSH: hyperthyroidism
• SIADH		
Obstructive hydrocephalus		
Cranial nerves III, IV, V1, V2, and VI dysfunction		
Temporal lobe dysfunction Nasopharyngeal mass		
• CSF rhinorrhea		

ACTH, adrenocorticotrophic hormone; CSF, cerebrospinal fluid; FSH, follicle-stimulating hormone; GH, growth hormone; LH, luteinizing hormone; PRL, prolactin; SIADH, syndrome of inappropriate antidiuretic hormone secretion; TSH, thyroid-stimulating hormone.

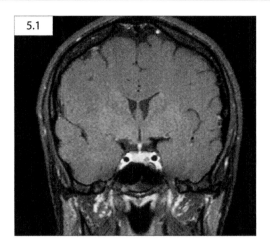

FIGURE 5.1   Pituitary microadenoma. Scan of a 40-year-old male with a 4 mm hypodense lesion in the left lateral pituitary. There was no evidence of any pituitary hypo- or hyperfunction. Pituitary adenomas tend to be hypointense on T1-weighted images and more likely to be hyperintense on T2-weighted images. With gadolinium contrast, the pituitary adenoma is initially hypointense and later hyperintense.

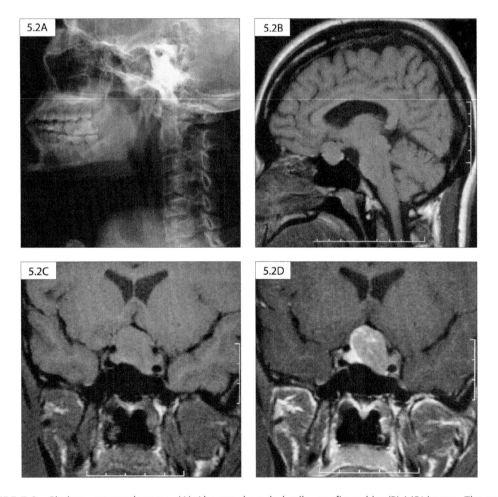

FIGURE 5.2   Pituitary macroadenoma. (A) Abnormal eroded sella, confirmed by (B) MRI image. The coronal images, (C) precontrast and (D) postcontrast, show the true extent of the tumor with evidence of wrapping around the carotid vessel.

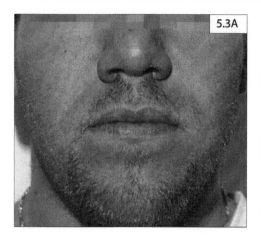
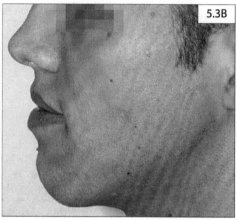

FIGURE 5.3   GH-secreting adenoma. (A) Young male showing some prominence of the frontal sinus and prognathism of lower jaw. Of note, one should always compare with historical images to confirm a change over time. (B) Young male demonstrating herpetegenous forehead wrinkling and prognathism.

adenomas, represent about 25% of pituitary tumors. Most of these adenomas on morphologic examination reveal granules containing hormones, typically components of glycoprotein hormones (Figure 5.3).

Impingement on the chiasma or its branches by pituitary pathology may result in visual field defects, with the most common being bitemporal hemianopsia. Lateral extension of the pituitary mass to the cavernous sinuses may result in diplopia, ptosis, or altered facial sensation. Among the cranial nerves, third nerve palsy is the most common.

Autopsy studies suggest that up to 20% of normal individuals harbor incidental pituitary microadenomas that are pathologically similar in distribution to those that present clinically. The initial workup should be limited and include serum prolactin and insulin-like growth factor-1 (IGF-1) levels. Other screening tests may be performed depending on clinical features. The adenoma can be followed yearly by MRI, with increasing duration between imaging studies, if the size is stable.

PROLACTINOMA

Definition/Overview

Hyperprolactinemia is the most common pituitary disorder. Observational studies in patients with microadenomas indicate that serum PRL concentration or adenoma size increase in only a minority of patients and, indeed, serum PRL decreases in the majority of cases over time. Estrogen therapy in the past has been suggested as a cause of prolactinoma formation, but careful case–cohort studies have found no evidence that oral contraceptives induce development of prolactinomas. Clonal analysis of tumor deoxyribonucleic acid (DNA) indicates that prolactinomas are monoclonal in origin.

Pathophysiology and Clinical Presentation

Hyperprolactinemia impairs pulsatile gonadotropin release (LH and FSH), likely through alteration in hypothalamic LHRH secretion. Women of reproductive age usually present with oligomenorrhea,

TABLE 5.3   Clinical Presentation of Hyperprolactinemia

	MEN	WOMEN
Early		Irregular menses
		Polycystic ovary syndrome
		Reduced fertility
		Galactorrhea
Late	Hypogonadism	Osteoporosis
	Erectile dysfunction	
	Reduced energy	
	Galactorrhea	
	Headaches	
	Impaired visual field	
	Gynecomastia	

amenorrhea, galactorrhea, and infertility. Those with long-standing amenorrhea are less likely to have galactorrhea, likely secondary to long-standing estrogen deficiency. Men and postmenopausal women usually seek medical attention because of mass effect such as headaches and visual field defects. Many men with hyperprolactinemia do not report any sexual dysfunction, but once treated effectively for hyperprolactinemia, the majority realizes the previous presence of problems including decreased libido and erectile dysfunction (Table 5.3). Men with long-standing hypogonadism may have decreased facial and body hair, and soft but usually normal-sized testicles (if hypogonadism starts before completion of puberty, testicles will be small). Patients with microadenomas have a higher frequency of headaches compared to control subjects.

Premenopausal women tend to present earlier with hyperprolactinemia than men or postmenopausal women. Thus, the latter often present with macroadenomas and symptoms of anterior hormone deficiency and local mass effect in the sella. Prolactinomas are four times more common in women.

Differential Diagnosis

It is critical to evaluate drug history carefully since some medications are associated with hyperprolactinemia, and their discontinuation (if possible) will avoid any further, often expensive, workup. Other common conditions associated with elevated PRL levels include pregnancy and hypothyroidism (Table 5.4).

Diagnosis

The PRL level usually correlates well with the size of the tumor. A serum PRL level above 200 μg/L is almost always indicative of a PRL-producing pituitary tumor. Conversely, a serum PRL level below 200 μg/L in the presence of a large pituitary adenoma is usually suggestive of stalk compression. However, one must be wary of the 'hook effect' phenomenon, which leads to modest elevations in PRL (below 200 μg/L) despite the presence of a large tumor. This occurs when extremely elevated levels of PRL interfere with the assay by saturating both the capture and signal antibodies, thus preventing binding. If suspected, the test should be repeated with a 1:100 dilution of the serum. Stimulatory tests, including TRH stimulation tests, are nonspecific and rarely used at present.

TABLE 5.4 Differential Diagnosis of Hyperprolactinemia

PHYSIOLOGIC	PATHOLOGIC	PHARMACOLOGIC
Pregnancy	Prolactinoma	TRH
Postpartum	Acromegaly (25%)	Psychotropic medications
Newborn	Hypothalamic disorders	Phenothiazines
Stress	Chiari–Frommel syndrome	Reserpine
Hypoglycemia	Craniopharyngioma	Methyldopa
Sleep	Metastatic disease	Estrogen therapy
Postprandial hypoglycemia	Pituitary stalk secretion or compression	Metoclopramide, cimetidine (especially intravenous)
Intercourse	Hypothyroidism	Opiates
Nipple stimulation	Renal failure	Verapamil
	Liver disease	Some SSRIs including fluoxetine and fluvoxamine
	Chest wall trauma (burns, shingles)	

SSRI, selective serotonin reuptake inhibitor; TRH, thyrotropin-releasing hormone.

Management/Treatment

Medical therapy with dopamine agonists is now the first-line treatment, since surgical resection is curative only in a minority of patients and is associated with risk of recurrence in all patients. Cabergoline twice weekly, bromocriptine mesylate, and pergolide mesylate are potent inhibitors of PRL secretion and often result in tumor shrinkage. Suppression of prolactin secretion by dopamine agonists depends on the number and affinity of dopamine receptors on lactotrope adenoma. There is usually a substantial decrease in prolactinoma size even when serum PRL levels do not normalize. These medications should be slowly initiated, since side effects often occur at the beginning of treatment. The most common side effects include nausea, headache, dizziness, nasal congestion, and constipation. It is important to remember that it may take up to 6 months before testosterone increases and normal sexual function is restored in men successfully treated for prolactinomas. PRL appears to have an independent effect in men on libido, since exogenous testosterone works poorly in restoring libido in those who continue to have elevated PRL levels.

Although patients with microadenomas or patients without evidence of a pituitary tumor can sometimes be followed without therapy, patients with macroadenomas always need to be treated. Occasionally, a patient with microadenoma or no definite pituitary tumor will have stable PRL levels after dopamine agonist discontinuation. For this reason, it would be reasonable to try a 'drug holiday' after several years of therapy with close follow-up.

Despite early concerns of cardiac valve disease with the use of pergolide and cabergoline, most follow-up studies have not demonstrated an increase in valvular regurgitation. The clinician may order an echocardiogram if clinically suspected. Medical therapy during pregnancy often stirs debate about the continuation of bromocriptine. Tumor-related complications are seen in about 15% of pregnancies and in only 5% of women with microadenomas. A sensible approach would be to stop bromocriptine when pregnancy begins, and then follow the clinical status with MRI and visual field examinations. PRL levels may be misleading in pregnancy. If there is significant worsening in clinical status, bromocriptine could be reinstituted. A large review of over 2,500 pregnancies with bromocriptine use did not reveal any increase in maternal or fetal complications related to therapy. In a follow-up study of over 900 children exposed to bromocriptine in utero, there were no developmental delays observed. Macroprolactinomas are more likely to worsen during pregnancy with symptomatic growth observed in up to 40% of pregnancies. Breastfeeding has not been associated with tumor growth.

Even in the presence of mass effect symptoms such as visual field defects, dopamine agonists are the first line of therapy, since a rapid improvement in symptoms is observed in the majority of patients. Transsphenoidal resection is preferred and reserved for patients with disease refractory to medical therapy. The main advantage of surgery is avoidance of chronic medical therapy. Radiation therapy may be considered for patients who poorly tolerate dopamine agonists and will likely not be cured by surgery (e.g., tumor invasion of cavernous sinuses).

ACROMEGALY

Definition/Overview

Acromegaly is a disease that results from excessive GH secretion usually from a pituitary tumor (Figure 5.4). It occurs at a rate of three to four cases per million per year with mean age at diagnosis of 40 years in males and 45 years in females.

Etiology and Differential Diagnosis

Acromegaly is caused by GH-secreting pituitary tumors (95%) and, rarely, by ectopic GHRH secretion by carcinoids or pancreatic islet cell tumors. Somatotrope adenomas are monoclonal in origin. A Gsp mutation in a $Gsp_{1\alpha}$ subunit in GH cells, leading to continuous GH secretion, has been shown to result in acromegaly. Ectopic GH secretion has been documented in extracts of lung adenocarcinoma, and breast and ovarian cancers. None of these conditions, except one case of pancreatic tumor, has been reported to cause acromegaly.

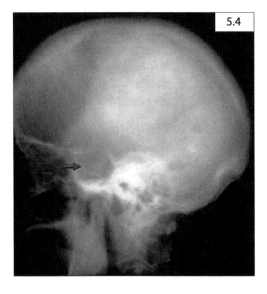

FIGURE 5.4   Acromegaly due to a pituitary tumor. (Courtesy of Dr. Donald Gordon.)

Clinical Presentation

The GH-secreting tumors tend to be more aggressive in younger patients. Classic clinical features include:

- Coarsening of facial features (Figure 5.5)
- Prominent jaw and frontal sinus (Figure 5.6)
- Broadening of hands and feet (Figures 5.7–5.9)
- Hyperhidrosis
- Macroglossia (Figure 5.5C)
- Signs of hypopituitarism
- Diabetes mellitus (10%–25%)
- Skin tags (screening for colonic polyps required)
- Hypertension (25%–30%)
- Cardiomyopathy (50%–80%)
- Carpal tunnel syndrome
- Sleep apnea (5%)

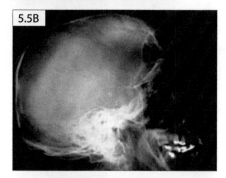
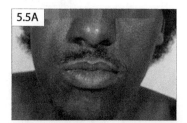
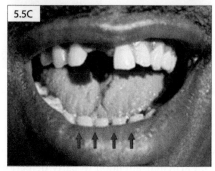

FIGURE 5.5   Coarse facies due to bone overgrowth in acromegaly. (Courtesy of Dr. Donald Gordon.)

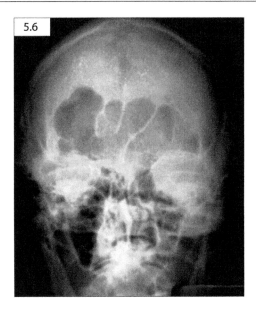

FIGURE 5.6   Enlarged sinuses in acromegaly. (Courtesy of Dr. Donald Gordon.)

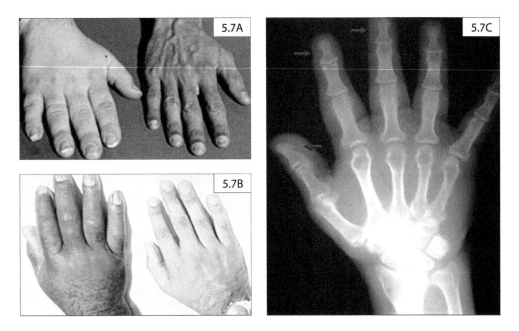

FIGURE 5.7   Hands in acromegaly: (A) thick fingers, (B) spade-like hands, (C) tufting of terminal phalanges. (Courtesy of Dr. Donald Gordon.)

Other features include overgrowth of vertebrae (Figure 5.10), degenerative arthritis (Figure 5.11), and acanthosis nigricans (Figure 5.12). Particular attention to early detection of cardiovascular disease is of paramount importance. Patients with acromegaly have a 3.5-fold increased mortality rate, often due to cardiovascular disease. In addition, acromegalic patients have an increased risk of colon polyps with the potential for an increased risk of malignancy, affecting their life expectancy. For this reason, they should

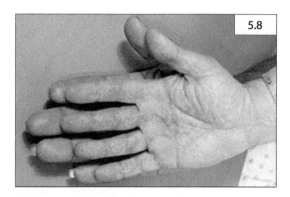

FIGURE 5.8   Hand in acromegaly: thickening of fingers and palm. (Courtesy of Dr. Donald Gordon.)

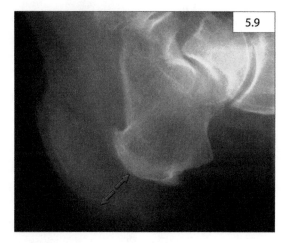

FIGURE 5.9   Thick heel pad in acromegaly.

undergo a colonoscopy every 3–5 years until more data about the frequency of such screening tests are available. It is not clear if more rigorous screening for a variety of cancers, including breast, lung, and prostate cancer, is indicated in these patients.

Diagnosis

Random GH levels can overlap in acromegalic patients and controls, due to GH's pulsatility. Therefore, a single GH level is inadequate to establish the diagnosis. IGF-1 has a longer plasma half-life than GH and is an excellent initial screening test for those suspected to have acromegaly. An elevated IGF-1 level in a clinical setting suggestive of acromegaly almost always confirms the diagnosis. One should be aware that concomitant poorly controlled diabetes or malnutrition could be associated with low IGF-1 levels. The oral glucose tolerance test remains the gold standard test to confirm the diagnosis. Normal individuals suppress their GH level to less than 1 µg/L (using chemiluminescent assays) within 2 hours after ingestion of 100 g oral glucose solution.

In the case of ectopic acromegaly, elevated GHRH can be measured in blood to confirm the diagnosis (usually >300 ng/mL). In the rare patient with a hypothalamic GHRH-secreting tumor, peripheral GHRH levels may be normal. In patients with a GH-secreting pituitary adenoma, the GHRH level is

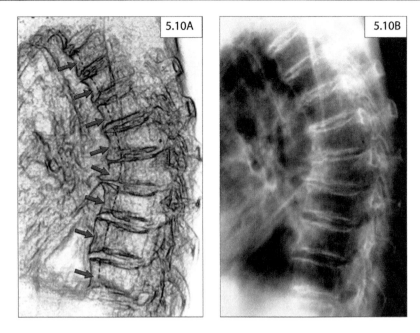

FIGURE 5.10   Overgrowth of vertebrae in acromegaly. (Courtesy of Dr. Donald Gordon.)

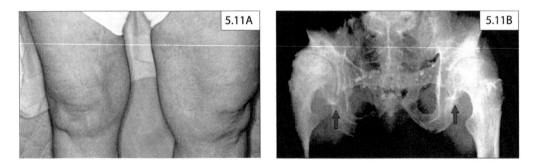

FIGURE 5.11   Degenerative arthritis in acromegaly. (Courtesy of Dr. Donald Gordon.)

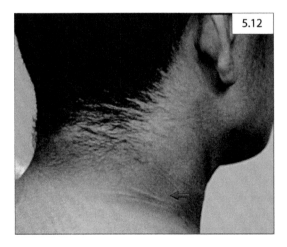

FIGURE 5.12   Acanthosis nigricans in acromegaly. (Courtesy of Dr. Donald Gordon.)

low or undetectable. About 70% of patients with acromegaly have been shown to display a paradoxical GH response to TRH, but unfortunately, with the lack of availability of TRH, this test is no longer easily accessible.

Management/Treatment

The primary aims of treatment include relieving the symptoms, reducing tumor bulk, normalization of IGF-1 and GH dynamics, and preventing tumor regrowth. Medical treatment of acromegaly has improved over the last three decades, since the limitations of radiation and surgical therapy have become evident. Analogs of somatostatin are the most effective medical therapy available for acromegaly. Octreotide therapy has been shown to lower and normalize IGF-1 in 90% and 65% of patients, respectively. It is usually given as a subcutaneous injection three times per day. Long-acting octreotide (Sandostatin LAR) can be given monthly intramuscularly. Long-term observations of patients on somatostatin analogues have shown no evidence of tachyphylaxis. Some degree of tumor shrinkage in up to 50% of patients is expected, although in most cases there is less than 50% shrinkage in tumor size. The most common side effects are gastrointestinal, including diarrhea, abdominal pain, and nausea. The most serious side effect of Sandostatin analogues is cholelithiasis, seen in up to 25% of patients. Its management is similar to those with cholelithiasis in the general population, and routine ultrasonographic screening is not indicated. This type of therapy may be quite useful as an adjunct to radiotherapy since radiotherapy may take several years to significantly reduce GH levels. Recently, an oral formulation of octreotide has been approved for use in those who have responded to GH reduction to injectable octreotide or lanreotide.

Normalization of IGF-1 is seen in only 10%–15% of patients treated with dopamine agonists and is more likely with pituitary tumors secreting both GH and PRL. Pegvisomant, a GH receptor antagonist, is a novel addition to the list of pharmacologic agents for acromegaly. This is administered as a daily subcutaneous injection. IGF-1 is significantly reduced and clinical symptoms improve; however, growth of the tumor is not inhibited and rare cases of tumor enlargement have been reported. In refractory scenarios, a combination of somatostatin receptor ligands with GH receptor antagonists may be considered. Cabergoline has also been used in doses higher than those used for prolactinomas.

The surgical approach is the treatment of choice in those presenting with pituitary microadenomas or when the tumor is confined to sella, with a cure rate of up to 90%. For those with macroadenomas, surgical cure is observed in less than 50% of cases. Even in those not cured by surgery, tumor debulking usually results in the improvement of symptoms and lowering of IGF-1 levels. Radiation therapy almost always induces a decrease in the size of the tumor and GH level, but often fails to normalize IGF-1 levels. Given low efficacy, high risk of hypopituitarism, and lack of knowledge about long-term effects on neuropsychiatric functions, radiation therapy should be reserved for those not responsive to other treatment modalities. Radiosurgery (gamma knife) seems to be superior to conventional radiation therapy, but large studies with strict cure criteria including the normalization of IGF-1 and long-term safety profile are lacking. GH antagonists are currently being investigated.

CUSHING DISEASE AND ECTOPIC ACTH SYNDROME

Definition/Overview

Cushing disease and ectopic ACTH syndrome are associated with excess cortisol secretion caused by ACTH from the pituitary or a nonpituitary tumor, respectively. ACTH-secreting pituitary adenoma is the

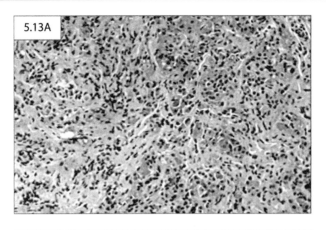

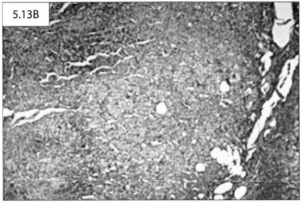

FIGURE 5.13   ACTH-producing adenoma resulting in adrenal hyperplasia in Cushing syndrome.

most common cause of endogenous Cushing syndrome (CS) (60%) with the rest being adrenal (25%) or ectopic (15%) in origin (Figures 5.13 and 5.14).

Clinical Presentation

The following findings are suggestive of a hypercortisolism state:

- Central obesity
- Muscle wasting with proximal muscle weakness
- Thinning of skin and connective tissue
- Osteopenia/osteoporosis
- Spontaneous ecchymosis
- Purplish wide striae (>1 cm) (Figure 5.15)
- Hypokalemia

Other findings, which are less helpful in discriminating patients with and without Cushing, are hypertension, abnormal glucose tolerance, menstrual irregularities, and psychiatric disturbances including depression. Women with Cushing disease typically have fine facial lanugo hair and may have acne and temporal scalp hair loss secondary to increased adrenal androgen secretion. There is usually a 3- to 6-year delay

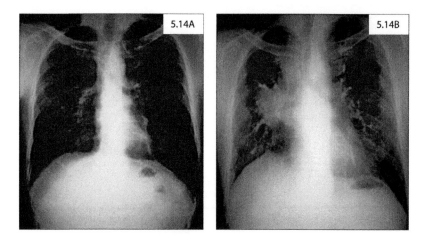

FIGURE 5.14   Small-cell carcinoma of lung with ectopic ACTH overproduction in Cushing syndrome.

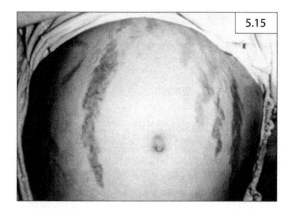

FIGURE 5.15   Clinical features in Cushing syndrome: purple striae.

in diagnosis of patients with Cushing disease, and it may be possible to date the onset of the disease by determining, which scars are pigmented due to excess secretion of ACTH and other melanotropins.

Diagnosis

Twenty-four–hour urinary free cortisol measurement is the single best test for diagnosis of CS. Because of the significant overlap between normal individuals and those with Cushing, random serum cortisol has no role in the diagnosis of Cushing syndrome. A 1 mg overnight dexamethasone suppression test with a morning cortisol level below 1.8 µg/dL virtually rules out the disease but has an up to 40% false-positive rate. The combination of a low-dose dexamethasone suppression test and CRH stimulation test has been shown to have 100% diagnostic accuracy in a study by the National Institutes of Health (NIH). This test may have a significant value in establishing the diagnosis in those with pseudo-Cushing and elevated 24-hour urinary free cortisol. Other tests useful in establishing the diagnosis of Cushing disease include midnight serum and salivary cortisol (Figure 5.16).

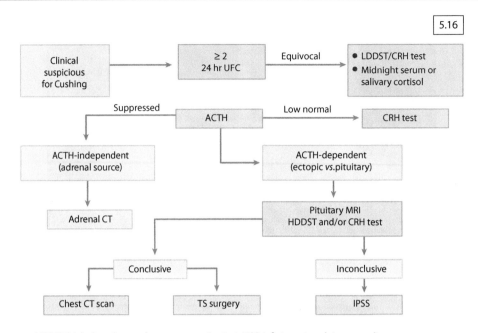

HDDST: high-dose dexamethasone suppresion test; IPSS: inferior petrosal sinus sampling;
LDDST: low-dose dexamethasone suppresion test; TS: trans-sphenoidal; UFC: urinary free cortisol.

FIGURE 5.16   Cushing evaluation: workup algorithm.

Once the diagnosis of CS has been established, the next step is to find out whether it is ACTH dependent (Figure 5.16). Whereas undetectable or low ACTH are consistent with adrenal etiology, low-normal ACTH may be seen in both ectopic Cushing and those with an ACTH-secreting pituitary tumor. A CRH stimulation test is used for differentiation between the two. Although ACTH levels tend to be higher in those with ectopic CS compared to patients with pituitary disease, there is considerable overlap. High-dose dexamethasone test and/or CRH stimulation test are helpful in the differentiation of the two. Cortisol levels are not suppressed with the high-dose (8 mg) dexamethasone test in patients with ectopic ACTH syndrome and CRH stimulation may not lead to a further rise in ACTH. The gold standard test to differentiate pituitary Cushing from an ectopic ACTH-producing tumor is inferior petrosal sinus sampling. This test should be performed by an experienced neuroradiologist and it is essential to note that it cannot be used to make the diagnosis of CS.

Ectopic ACTH syndrome is the most frequent and best studied of the ectopic hormone syndromes. Most tumors associated with ectopic ACTH syndrome are carcinomas and have a poor prognosis. They usually present as a rapid onset syndrome (within 6 months) associated with profound muscle weakness, hyperpigmentation, hypertension, hypokalemia, and edema. Hyperpigmentation is thought to be due to cosecretion of β-melanocyte stimulating hormone (β-MSH), one of the byproducts of ACTH synthesis. Some benign tumors, such as carcinoids or islet cell tumors, have been shown to cause ectopic ACTH syndrome and are difficult to differentiate from pituitary causes of Cushing syndrome. This difficulty is exaggerated by radiologic investigations of the sella that are often negative or show a microadenoma, which is seen in up to 20% of autopsy series in normal individuals.

Management/Treatment

Surgical (transsphenoidal) removal of the ACTH-secreting pituitary tumor is the treatment of choice. Availability of an experienced surgeon is crucial with an 80%–90% remission rate following surgery. An undetectable cortisol level postoperatively off steroid is considered to be an excellent marker for long-term cure. There is a period of temporary adrenal insufficiency following successful surgery, usually of 6–8 months, but may be as long as 2 years in duration. For those not cured by the surgery, other options include a second operation and radiation therapy. Patients whose tumor is unresponsive to these therapies may then be offered medical or surgical adrenalectomy. Ectopic ACTH-producing tumors should be resected if possible. Octreotide may inhibit ectopic ACTH secretion. Mitotane is perhaps the most effective adrenolytic agent. Other medications, such as aminoglutethimide, ketoconazole, or metyrapone, are useful as temporizing agents only. The glucocorticoid antagonist mifepristone has been US - FDA approved therapy that appears to have few side effects. One difficulty is that one cannot rely on cortisol measurements to follow the effect of mifepristone.

OTHER PITUITARY ADENOMAS

Nonfunctioning or Glycoprotein-Secreting Tumors and TSH Adenomas

Definition/Overview

Nonfunctioning or glycoprotein-secreting tumors are usually clinically silent because they are inefficient in secreting hormones and lack a clinically recognizable syndrome. TSH-secreting adenomas are the most uncommon.

Clinical Presentation

Glycoprotein (LH or FSH) secreting adenomas usually come to attention because of manifestations of mass lesions including headache and visual field defect. Patients may present with varying degrees of hypopituitarism due to mass effect. Rarely, an FSH adenoma may cause amenorrhea in a woman, or an LH adenoma may cause precocious puberty in a boy.

The clinical picture in patients with TSH-secreting pituitary adenomas includes pituitary mass lesion, hyperthyroidism, and goiter.

Diagnosis

Diagnosis of an LH or FSH adenoma is confirmed by measurement of either intact glycoprotein hormones or their α and β subunits. Levels of the α subunit tend to be inappropriately elevated, compared with those of the intact hormone itself. The most important biochemical feature of a TSH adenoma is the elevation of thyroid hormone levels in the presence of normal or elevated TSH levels. For this reason, any patient presenting with endogenous hyperthyroidism and an elevated or normal TSH should be further evaluated for the presence of a TSH-secreting pituitary adenoma. Elevated serum PRL and α subunit are in favor of a thyrotrope adenoma and against thyroid hormone resistance syndrome.

Management/Treatment

The transsphenoidal surgical approach is standard, especially if visual function is abnormal. Surgery is rarely curative because of the size of the adenoma on presentation, and radiation therapy is usually needed as an adjunct. Octreotide may help reduce hormone secretion, but further studies are required to assess if it has any effect on tumor size. Dopamine agonists, such as bromocriptine, have been used in high doses, but clinical responses (i.e., changes in tumor size or visual symptoms) occur in less than 10% of patients. Long-acting gonadotropin-releasing hormone (GnRH) agonists and antagonists may reduce secretion of FSH and LH by tumors but do not reduce tumor size. In summary, the efficacy of the medical therapy in patients with nonfunctional or glycoprotein-secreting pituitary adenoma is not established but is used in an attempt to reduce tumor hypersecretion and size following unsuccessful surgery.

Lymphocytic Hypophysitis

Definition/Overview

Lymphocytic hypophysitis is a disease characterized by lymphocytic infiltration of the pituitary gland which may lead to hypopituitarism.

Etiology

Hypophysitis is usually an autoimmune phenomenon, but other etiologies include inflammation secondary to sella tumors or cysts, systemic diseases, and infection or drug-induced causes. More recently, other etiologies, including immunoglobulin G4 (IgG4)-related disease, immunotherapy-induced hypophysitis, and paraneoplastic pituitary-directed autoimmunity, have been described.

Pathophysiology

Lymphocytic infiltration leads to mass effect and eventually hypofunction of the pituitary.

Clinical Presentation

This is often seen in females during or after pregnancy. The clinical manifestations are secondary to hypopituitarism or adrenal insufficiency and/or due to a pituitary mass effect.

Diagnosis

Serum PRL is elevated in half of patients but may be decreased. Antipituitary antibodies are present in some patients and other autoimmune endocrine disorders, including Hashimoto's thyroiditis and Addison's disease have been seen in others. MRI and CT scans of the sella reveal a pituitary mass and, in some cases, thickening of the stalk. MRI shows diffuse and homogeneous contrast enhancement of the anterior pituitary area. Although the diagnosis may be suspected on clinical grounds in a pregnant or postpartum woman, a surgical biopsy is occasionally needed for confirmation of the diagnosis.

Management

Some patients recover fully, while others may need selective hormone replacement. For this reason, patients need to be assessed at regular intervals for the necessity of continued hormone replacement.

Empty Sella Syndrome

Definition/Overview

Empty sella syndrome is often a radiologic diagnosis and is manifest by a sella that may appear to be empty to varying degrees (i.e., partial to complete) (Figures 5.17 and 5.18).

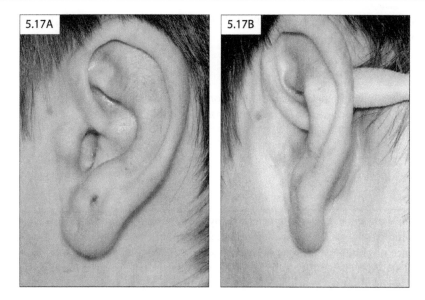

FIGURE 5.17 (A and B) Images depicting auricular calcification. This clinical finding may be seen with acromegaly, hyperparathyroidism, and adrenal insufficiency. This particular subject had secondary adrenal insufficiency secondary to an empty sella syndrome.

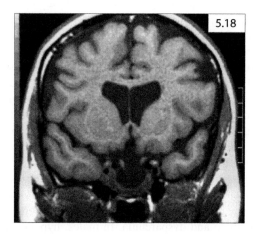

FIGURE 5.18 Coronal image demonstrating an enlarged empty sella. Note that the intrasellar content is the same density as CSF in the lateral ventricles.

Etiology

Whereas the primary empty sella is the result of a congenital diaphragmatic defect, the secondary empty sella may result from previous surgery, irradiation, or infarction of a preexisting tumor.

Diagnosis

The diagnosis of empty sella syndrome is increasingly made owing to the prevalence of CT and MRI. Pituitary fossa enlargement is secondary to communication between the pituitary fossa and subarachnoid space, which causes remodeling and enlargement of the sella. Most patients have no pituitary dysfunction, but a wide spectrum of pituitary deficiencies have been described, especially in those with secondary empty sella. Coexisting tumors may occur.

Management/Treatment

Management is usually with reassurance and hormone replacement, if necessary. Surgery is only necessary if visual field defects occur or if there is cerebrospinal fluid rhinorrhea.

Hypopituitarism

Etiology

Pituitary adenomas are the most common cause of hypopituitarism, but other causes including parasellar diseases, following pituitary surgery or radiation therapy, and head injury must also be considered. The usual consequence of pituitary hormone deficiency secondary to a mass effect is in the following order: GH, LH, FSH, TSH, ACTH, and PRL. PRL deficiency is uncommon except in those with pituitary infarction. Isolated deficiencies of various anterior pituitary hormones have also been described.

Clinical Presentation, Management, and Treatment of Hormone Deficiencies

GH deficiency is now recognized as a pathologic state in adults as well as children and more patients with GH deficiency undergo GH replacement. GH deficiency may contribute to increased mortality in patients with hypopituitarism, with cardiovascular disease being the most common cause of mortality. The symptoms of GH deficiency in adults are more subtle including decreased muscle strength and exercise tolerance, and reduced sense of well-being (e.g., diminished libido, social isolation). Patients with GH deficiency have increased body fat, particularly intra-abdominally, and decreased lean body mass in comparison to normal adults. Some patients have decreased bone mineral density, which may improve with GH replacement. A trial of GH replacement in adults with documented GH deficiency and symptoms or metabolic abnormalities suggestive of GH deficiency is indicated. The most common side effects of GH therapy include fluid retention, carpal tunnel syndrome, and arthralgia. These side effects are usually dose related and improve with dose reduction.

Gonadotropin deficiency may be secondary to a pituitary defect; hypothalamic deficiency of LHRH; or a functional abnormality, such as hyperprolactinemia, anorexia nervosa, and severe disease state. In females, gonadotropin deficiency causes infertility and menstrual disorders including amenorrhea. It is often associated with lack of libido and dyspareunia. In males, hypogonadism is diagnosed less often, since decreased libido and impotence may be considered as a function of aging. Hypogonadism is often diagnosed retrospectively when a patient presents with a mass effect. Osteopenia is a consequence of long-standing hypogonadism and usually responds to hormone replacement therapy.

The symptoms of secondary adrenal insufficiency are similar to primary adrenal insufficiency with one important difference. Mineralocorticoid secretion is mainly regulated by the renin and angiotensin system, and is preserved in patients with pituitary disorders. For this reason, the symptoms are more chronic in nature and commonly include malaise, loss of energy, and anorexia. Hyperkalemia is not a feature of secondary adrenal insufficiency. An acute illness may precipitate vascular collapse, hypoglycemia, and coma.

TSH deficiency is relatively a late finding in patients with pituitary disorders, with symptoms being similar to those with primary hypothyroidism including malaise, leg cramps, lack of energy, and cold intolerance. The degree of hypothyroidism depends on the duration of thyrotropin deficiency.

PITUITARY APOPLEXY

Definition/Overview

Pituitary apoplexy is an endocrine emergency resulting from hemorrhagic infarction of the pituitary, usually associated with a preexisting pituitary tumor.

Etiology

A variety of predisposing conditions, including bleeding disorders, diabetes mellitus, pituitary radiation, pneumoencephalography (of historical interest only), mechanical ventilation, and trauma, have been described.

Diagnosis

Diagnosis is made when a patient presents with classic symptoms of headache, visual disturbance, and an MRI or CT showing hemorrhage within a pituitary adenoma.

Differential Diagnosis

- Aneurysm of the internal carotid
- Basilar artery occlusion
- Hypertensive encephalopathy
- Acute expansion of intrasellar cyst or abscess
- Cavernous sinus thrombosis

Clinical Presentation

The clinical manifestations of this syndrome are related to rapid expansion and compression of the pituitary gland and the perisellar structures, leading to severe headaches, hypopituitarism, visual field defects, and cranial nerve palsies. Extravasation of blood or necrotic tissue into the subarachnoid space may cause clouding of consciousness, meningismus, autonomic dysfunction, fever, and, rarely, sudden death.

Although secondary hypoadrenalism does not usually result in hypotension, acute loss of ACTH in pituitary hemorrhage can result in shock. Other deficiencies of anterior pituitary hormones may be present, but diabetes insipidus is seen only transiently in 4% of cases.

Management/Treatment

If pituitary apoplexy is suspected, anterior pituitary insufficiency should be presumed and the patient must be treated accordingly. The glucocorticoid dose must be adequate for the degree of stress and presumptive cerebral edema. Any evidence of sudden visual field defects, oculomotor palsies, hypothalamic compression, or coma should lead to immediate surgical decompression. The recovery of a variety of pituitary hormone deficiencies following surgery has been documented, and all patients should be reevaluated for possible recovery of their pituitary hormone axes. The choice between initial medical versus surgical management is debated, and more research on prognostic variables and clinical outcomes is needed.

Sheehan's syndrome is the result of ischemic infarction of a normal pituitary gland leading to hypopituitarism secondary to postpartum hemorrhage and hypotension. Patients have a history of failure to lactate postpartum, failure to resume menses, cold intolerance, or fatigue. Some women may have an acute crisis mimicking apoplexy within 30 days postpartum. There is often subclinical central diabetes insipidus (DI).

A patient with untreated hypopituitarism may decompensate acutely with stress, resulting in a coma. This acute decompensation may mimic acute myocardial infarction, overwhelming sepsis, a cerebrovascular accident (CVA), or meningitis. Symptoms may be a blend of acute thyroid and adrenal insufficiency. Clinical clues might consist of a myxedematous or acromegalic appearance and/or decreased body hair.

POSTERIOR PITUITARY

Introduction

The posterior pituitary is a storage site for antidiuretic hormone (ADH, vasopressin) and oxytocin. Clinically, disorders of ADH are the most relevant (Table 5.5). ADH secretion is regulated by changes in serum osmolality and/or plasma volume. Small increments in serum osmolality greater than 290 mOsm/kg lead to prompt secretion of ADH. However, more than a 10% reduction in plasma volume will override any osmolar stimulus. Pain, nicotine, and caffeine can increase ADH secretion. Native ADH is a potent vasoconstrictor, but desmopressin (DDAVP), an ADH analogue, has pure antidiuretic action with little vasoconstriction.

TABLE 5.5   Common ADH-Related Syndromes

CLINICAL PRESENTATION	THIRST	ADH SECRETION	ADH ACTION	DIAGNOSIS
Polyuria/polydipsia	N	⇓	N	Central DI
Polyuria/polydipsia	N	N	⇓	Nephrogenic DI
Polyuria/polydipsia	⇑	N	N	Primary polydipsia
⇑ Na+	⇓	N	N	Hypodipsia
⇓ Na+	⇓	⇑	N	SIADH

DI, diabetes insipidus; SIADH, syndrome of inappropriate antidiuretic hormone secretion.

CENTRAL DIABETES INSIPIDUS

Definition/Overview

Central DI (pituitary origin) is a polyuric syndrome secondary to inadequate ADH secretion and the inability to concentrate urine. Patients have a normal response to administration of vasopressin. Maximum urine output due to complete ADH deficiency is about 18 liters per day, and urine volume over this indicates excess fluid intake.

Etiology

- Familial
- Idiopathic
- Trauma/postsurgical
- Granulomatous disease
- Tumors
- Craniopharyngioma (Figure 5.19)
- Pituitary tumors
- Metastatic cancer
- Infectious
- Vascular
- Aneurysms
- Sheehan's syndrome
- Autoimmune

Diagnosis

Patients with DI who are conscious usually have sufficient thirst to maintain a normal serum sodium in spite of polyuria. In this situation, a standard water deprivation test should be performed, during which patients are allowed no fluid to drink and are closely monitored. When two consecutive voided urine osmolalities differ by less than 30 mmol/L or when 5% of body weight is lost, 5 U of aqueous vasopressin

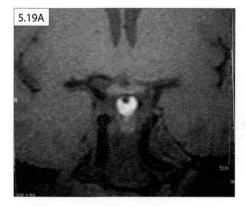
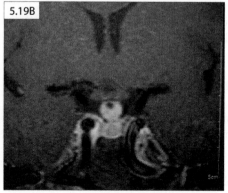

FIGURE 5.19 Craniopharyngioma with suprasellar mass. (A) Precoronal and (B) postcoronal T1-weighted images. (Courtesy of Dr. Amir Hamrahian.)

(approximately 5 µg of DDAVP) is given intravenously with repeating urine osmolality measurements at 30 and 60 minutes.

Desmopressin administration following dehydration will elicit the following responses:

- Less than 9% increase in urine osmolality with maximal urine concentration during the test – normal
- Greater than 50% rise in urine osmolality with inadequate urine concentration during the test – central DI
- No rise in urine osmolality with inadequate urine concentration during the test – nephrogenic DI

The serum ADH level at the end of fast and before administration of vasopressin helps to differentiate between partial central and nephrogenic DI, since both may have modest concentrations of urine with dehydration and a more than 10% increase in urine osmolality in response to vasopressin.

Differential Diagnosis

Patients with psychogenic polydipsia have a diluted medullary concentrating gradient and partial nephrogenic DI may develop. Some of the conditions associated with nephrogenic DI include familial, tubulointerstitial renal disease, electrolytes disorder (hypokalemia and hypercalcemia), drugs (e.g., lithium, demeclocycline), and pregnancy.

Management/Treatment

The posterior pituitary enhances on MRI with gadolinium and is a 'good assay' of ADH reserve, keeping in mind that up to 20% of normal individuals do not have a bright spot. Partial central DI may be treated with chlorpropamide or thiazides, while complete central DI needs to be treated with desmopressin. The drug is available via subcutaneous, oral, and nasal spray administration. The exact dosing and timing have to be individualized.

COVID-19 and Pituitary Disease

Definition/Overview

Since 2020, the COVID-19 pandemic has dominated medicine. With the finding of ACE2 in hypothalamic and pituitary tissue, these organs may be susceptible to direct COVID-19 infection and resulting symptoms. Cases of pituitary apoplexy secondary to COVID-19, have also been described in those with preexisting pituitary disease.

Diagnosis

Diagnosis will require a high index of suspicion in a patient with proven COVID-19 who is presenting with symptoms that could be due to pituitary dysfunction. Very rarely, posterior pituitary dysfunction may occur.

Management/Treatment

Management is the same as for any other pituitary dysfunction. Special attention should be given to steroid courses given for the actual COVID-19 infection. With regard to COVID-19 vaccinations for those with hypopituitarism, most would not recommend stress-dosing of glucocorticoids at the time of vaccination.

Adrenal Disorders

6

Sarah Kanbour, Reza Pishdad,
Ezra Baraban, and Amir H. Hamrahian

ANATOMY AND PHYSIOLOGY OF THE ADRENAL GLAND

The adrenal glands are paired retroperitoneal organs that lie within the perinephric fat, at the kidneys' anterior, superior, and medial aspects. They weigh about 5 grams. The right adrenal gland is located posterior to the inferior vena cava (Figure 6.1). The adrenal glands are pyramidal in shape with a narrow apex and a broader base. In cross-section, they resemble an inverted Y with an anteromedial limb and two posterolateral limbs (Figure 6.1). Each gland consists of an outer cortex and inner medulla, with distinct embryologic origins, and produces different hormones.

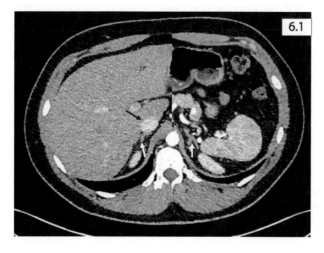

FIGURE 6.1 Normal adrenal gland. The right adrenal gland is located posterior to the inferior vena cava (blue arrow). In cross-section, they resemble an inverted Y with an anteromedial limb and two posterolateral limbs (white arrows).

DOI: 10.1201/9781003100669-6

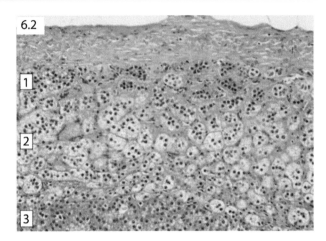

FIGURE 6.2   Normal adrenal cortex is arranged into three discrete layers. The periphery of the gland abutting the retroperitoneum is at the top of the image. The glomerulosa (1), fasciculata (2), and reticularis (3) layers are composed of blue, clear, and pink cells respectively, with the medulla (not pictured) situated deep to the reticularis layer at the bottom. H&E, 200×.

The cortex mainly produces steroid hormones and is composed of three zones (Figure 6.2):

- The outer zona glomerulosa synthesizes aldosterone under the principal control of the renin–angiotensin system and serum potassium concentration. The adrenocorticotropic hormone (ACTH) has a minor effect on aldosterone secretion.
- The middle zona fasciculata secretes cortisol under the influence of ACTH.
- The inner zona reticularis is primarily involved in the synthesis of androgens (dehydroepiandrosterone [DHEA], dehydroepiandrosterone sulfate [DHEAS], and androstenedione).

The adrenal medulla, located in the central portion of the gland, is part of the sympathetic nervous system and produces catecholamines, mostly epinephrine.

ADRENAL INSUFFICIENCY

Definition

Adrenal insufficiency (AI) is a failure of the adrenal cortex to secrete enough glucocorticoids, mineralocorticoids, or both. It can be caused by a primary adrenal disorder or secondary to the pituitary and hypothalamic diseases, or from adrenocorticotropic hormone suppression by drugs such as glucocorticoids and opioids.

TABLE 6.1 Causes of Primary Adrenal Insufficiency

Anatomic Destruction of the Gland (Acute or Chronic)
- Autoimmune adrenalitis (Addison's disease); autoimmune polyendocrine syndromes (APS) type 1 and 2
- Infections (tuberculosis, fungi, HIV, CMV, syphilis)
- Metastatic cancer
- Infiltration (e.g., amyloid)
- Hemorrhage/infarction

Metabolic Failure in Hormone Production
- Congenital adrenal hyperplasia
- Medications (ketoconazole, metyrapone, megestrol, mitotane, etomidate, immune checkpoint inhibitors)

Others
- Adrenoleukodystrophy/adrenomyeloneuropathy
- Congenital adrenal hypoplasia
- ACTH-resistant syndromes

Epidemiology/Etiology

Primary Adrenal Insufficiency

Primary adrenal insufficiency is a rare condition with the highest prevalence of 6–14 individuals per 100,000. It is less common than secondary and tertiary AI. It is caused by an intrinsic adrenal gland pathology such as autoimmune destruction of the adrenal cortex, infections, hemorrhage, metastases, or genetic defects (Table 6.1).

Glucocorticoid deficiency due to autoimmune disease accounts for up to 70% of the cases of primary adrenal failure. Antibodies targeting the 21-hydroxylase enzyme lead to the destruction of the adrenal cortex. Adrenal insufficiency can occur in combination with other autoimmune conditions such as thyroid disease, type 1 diabetes, premature ovarian insufficiency, hypoparathyroidism, autoimmune gastritis, celiac disease, vitiligo, alopecia, hepatitis, or pneumonitis (autoimmune polyglandular syndrome 1 and 2). Adrenoleukodystrophy (ALD) and adrenomyeloneuropathy (AMN) are two phenotypes of an X-linked recessive disorder caused by peroxisomal abnormalities and affect 1 in 20,000 males. The diagnosis may be evaluated by measurement of very long-chain fatty acids and then confirmed by genetic testing. This disorder accounts for up to 10% of all cases of primary adrenal insufficiency.

Secondary Adrenal Insufficiency

Secondary adrenal insufficiency is reported in about 14–28 individuals per 100,000, although the true prevalence is likely underestimated. It presents in two major forms: either as a deficiency of ACTH and other pituitary hormones (pituitary tumors, surgery, or radiation therapy), or less commonly as an isolated ACTH insufficiency (hypophysitis, or hereditary disorders). Hypophysitis is often related to pregnancy or as an adverse event of immune checkpoint inhibitors. Hypopituitarism secondary to trauma, pituitary apoplexy in an adenoma, or pituitary infarction, are less common.

Nearly 1% of the general population is treated with long-term regimens of glucocorticoids for inflammatory diseases. Adrenal insufficiency secondary to exogenous glucocorticoid may occur using 5 mg or more of prednisone for longer than 3 weeks. Concomitant use of drugs that inhibit glucocorticoid metabolism, such as itraconazole and ritonavir, can lead to adrenal suppression, even with local and topical glucocorticoids. In addition, opiates can suppress ACTH release and lead to the impairment of the hypothalamic–pituitary–adrenal (HPA) axis. Adrenal insufficiency should be suspected in any individual taking more than 20 mg morphine-equivalent dose. It occurs in 10%–20% of individuals using daily morphine-equivalent doses of 100 mg or more.

Clinical Presentation

Hallmark clinical features of primary AI are unintentional weight loss, anorexia, and profound fatigue. The patients may also complain of postural hypotension, muscle/abdominal pain, and hyponatremia (Table 6.2). Primary adrenal insufficiency may be associated with skin hyperpigmentation (Figures 6.3–6.7), orthostatic hypotension, and salt craving due to both glucocorticoid and mineralocorticoid deficiency.

TABLE 6.2 Manifestations of Primary Adrenal Insufficiency

SYMPTOM	FREQUENCY (%)	SIGNS	FREQUENCY (%)
Weakness, fatigue	100	Weight loss	100
Anorexia	100	Hyperpigmentation	95
Nausea and/or vomiting	90	Hypotension (systolic BP <100) mmHg)	85–90
Constipation	20–30	Vitiligo	10–15
Diarrhea	15–20	**Laboratory Abnormalities**	
Abdominal pain	30–35	Hyponatremia	80–90
Salt craving	15–20	Hyperkalemia	60–65
Dizziness and/or syncope	12–15	Hypercalcemia	10–20
		Azotemia	50–60
		Anemia and eosinophilia	20–40

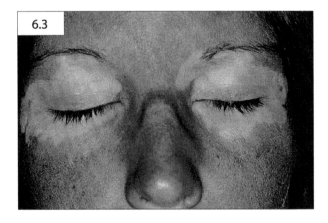

FIGURE 6.3 Vitiligo of the face. (Courtesy of Dr. Leann Olansky.)

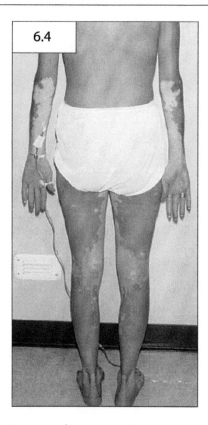

FIGURE 6.4   Vitiligo of the body. (Courtesy of Dr. Leann Olansky.)

Secondary adrenal insufficiency is usually milder than primary adrenal insufficiency because mineralocorticoid production is intact and adrenal insufficiency is more likely to be partial in nature. All patients with unexplained hyponatremia should undergo evaluation for adrenal insufficiency. Hypoglycemia is more common in patients with secondary adrenal insufficiency, which is due to the more chronic nature of secondary adrenal insufficiency.

Diagnosis

Confirmation of the clinical diagnosis of adrenal insufficiency involves the following three steps (Figure 6.8):

- Establishing the presence of adrenal insufficiency
- Measuring the ACTH level to differentiate between primary and secondary causes
- Investigating the underlying etiology

Establishing the Presence of Adrenal Insufficiency

Morning Serum Cortisol
In normal subjects, serum cortisol concentrations are highest about 1 hour before awakening and range from 275 to 550 nmol/L (10–20 μg/dL). An early morning cortisol level <80 nmol/l (3 μg/dL) is usually

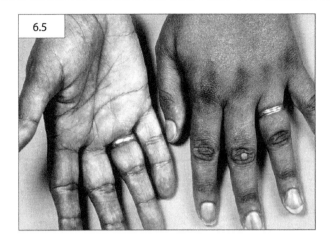

FIGURE 6.5 Hyperpigmentation of palmar creases. (Courtesy of Dr. Charles Faiman.)

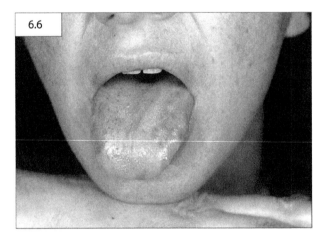

FIGURE 6.6 Hyperpigmentation of tongue. (Courtesy of Dr. Charles Faiman.)

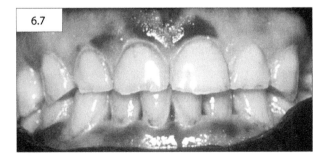

FIGURE 6.7 Hyperpigmentation of gingival mucosa. (Courtesy of Dr. Charles Faiman.)

consistent with adrenal insufficiency, while a value >276 nmol/L (10 µg/dL) makes the diagnosis highly unlikely. Patients with cortisol levels between 80 and 276 nmol/L (3–10 µg/dL) should be further evaluated by the cosyntropin stimulation test (CST). Due to the diurnal variation of cortisol, random serum cortisol levels are only of value during stress.

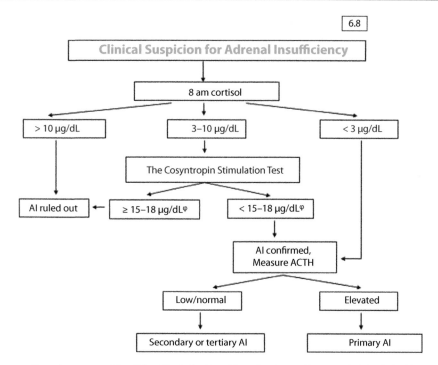

6.8

φ Normal response ≥15 µg/dL at 30 min & ≥18 µg/dL at 60 min post Cosyntropin Stimulation Test

FIGURE 6.8 Algorithm for the diagnosis of adrenal insufficiency (AI). The standard cosyntropin stimulation test (CST) may be used as the first-line test for evaluation of adrenal function, especially in patients who are seen in the clinic later during the day.

The Cosyntropin Stimulation Test
During the standard or high-dose CST (250 µg cosyntropin), plasma cortisol is measured before and at 30 and 60 minutes after intramuscular injection of 250 µg cosyntropin (ACTH analogue). Using the cortisol II assay, a normal response is a serum cortisol concentration >400–414 nmol/L (14.5–15 µg/dL) at 30 minutes and 485 nmol/L (18 µg/dL) at 60 minutes.

The standard dose CST is an excellent test to exclude primary adrenal insufficiency. However, patients with recent-onset pituitary ACTH deficiency (e.g., within 2–4 weeks after pituitary surgery) may have a normal response since the adrenal glands have not undergone sufficient atrophy and still respond to high concentrations of cosyntropin.

Another pitfall is pregnancy and oral estrogen, increasing corticosteroid-binding globulin (CBG) concentrations leading to elevated total cortisol levels. Conversely, critically ill patients and those with cirrhosis can have low levels of CBG and albumin leading to low total cortisol levels.

Differentiation between Primary and Secondary Adrenal Insufficiency

In a patient with a low serum cortisol level, an elevated ACTH level (usually double the upper limit of normal) is consistent with primary AI. Furthermore, low aldosterone and high renin concentrations may be additional clues to the diagnosis of primary adrenal insufficiency. A low or normal range ACTH level in the same setting confirms the diagnosis of secondary AI.

Investigating the Underlying Etiology

The diagnosis of autoimmune adrenal insufficiency is supported by the presence of other autoimmune disorders and adrenal autoantibodies, which may be present in up to 80%–90% of patients. Patients should be screened for other autoimmune conditions, such as autoimmune thyroid disease, type 1 diabetes, celiac disease, and autoimmune gastritis. In patients younger than 20 years old with primary adrenal insufficiency, autoimmune polyendocrine syndrome type 1 should always be considered. The presence of steroid side-chain cleavage enzyme autoantibodies indicates a potential risk of developing ovarian insufficiency.

All male patients with negative autoantibodies against 21-hydroxylase should have their serum very long-chain fatty acid tested to avoid missing an underlying adrenoleukodystrophy (ALD) or adrenomyeloneuropathy. Primary AI can be the initial manifestation in 30%-40% of these patients. Early diagnosis of ALD may improve outcomes of hematopoietic cell transplantation before the development of irreversible cerebral injury.

Patients with primary adrenal insufficiency should undergo an abdominal computed tomography (CT) scan if they have negative adrenal antibodies and normal very long-chain fatty acids (Figure 6.9). Abdominal CT may detect enlarged adrenal glands or adrenal calcification, suggesting an infectious, hemorrhagic, or metastatic cause. In patients with secondary AI, a thorough evaluation of other pituitary hormones and an MRI of the pituitary gland is indicated.

Adrenal Insufficiency in the Critically Ill Patient

More than 90% of measured total cortisol is bound to CBG and albumin. The remaining is free cortisol, which is responsible for its action. Since there is decreased CBG and albumin level in critically ill patients, the total serum cortisol may be a poor indicator of glucocorticoid activity and can be misleading. In critically ill patients without sepsis or septic shock, hypoalbuminemia (<25 μ/L) is usually an indirect marker of low CBG. In such patients, measurement of serum free cortisol may provide a better assessment of adrenal function. However, there is a need for establishing the reference range of serum free cortisol in critically ill patients.

A random cortisol level of <15 and <10 μg/dL may be used as evidence of AI in patients with near-normal (albumin >2.5 g/dL) or hypoalbuminemia, respectively. In patients with equivocal biochemical results or those with volume-resistant hypotension on vasopressors, a trial of glucocorticoids is appropriate. The benefit of a short course of glucocorticoids in patients with sepsis or septic shock may be related to the underlying inflammatory condition and not an underlying adrenal insufficiency. Relative adrenal insufficiency or critical illness-related corticosteroid insufficiency defined by the CST has multiple potential flaws. Therefore, it should not be used as a guide for glucocorticoid therapy in critically ill patients.

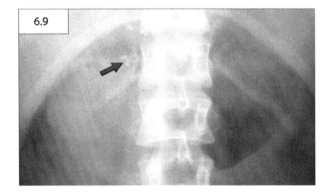

6.9

FIGURE 6.9 Plain X-ray of the abdomen demonstrating adrenal calcification on the right side (arrow) in a patient with a history of adrenal insufficiency secondary to tuberculosis. (Courtesy of Dr. Charles Faiman.)

Management/Treatment

Treatment of Adrenal Insufficiency

Patients with primary AI require lifelong replacement with both glucocorticoids and mineralocorticoids. The minimum dose to treat symptoms should be used, starting with hydrocortisone 10–15 mg in the morning as soon as the patient wakes and 5 mg in midafternoon to avoid sleep disturbances. Some patients may have improved energy by taking hydrocortisone three times per day. Treatment of adrenal insufficiency with steroids with long half-lives, such as prednisolone and dexamethasone, might result in increased adverse events including hyperlipidemia and reduced bone mineral density, and is usually avoided. Plasma ACTH and serum cortisol are not useful parameters to assess the adequacy of glucocorticoid replacement.

Patients require fludrocortisone 0.05–0.2 mg for mineralocorticoid replacement. Physically active people frequently need higher doses than sedentary older people and should be advised to increase their salt intake as needed. The adequacy of treatment is assessed clinically. However, the measurement of plasma renin activity may provide additional information about the adequacy of mineralocorticoid intake. Patients with secondary adrenal insufficiency do not need mineralocorticoid replacement.

During minor illnesses (e.g., flu or fever greater than 38°C), the hydrocortisone dose should be doubled for 2–3 days. Patients must be educated to self-administer hydrocortisone 100 mg intramuscularly if they cannot keep down their oral glucocorticoids. All patients should carry some form of medical alert.

Hydrocortisone 50–75 mg/day orally (or parenterally if the patient is nil by mouth) provides adequate glucocorticoid coverage for outpatient surgeries. Parenteral hydrocortisone 100–150 mg/day (in three to four divided doses) is usually sufficient for moderate to major surgeries with a taper to normal replacement dose during the recovery period.

Adrenal Crisis

Adrenal crisis is a life-threatening condition and refers to the vasomotor collapse associated with infection, stress, or trauma in a patient with adrenal insufficiency. The clinical features include worsening of the initial symptoms of fatigue, anorexia, nausea, vomiting, and abdominal pain, followed by sudden deterioration characterized by refractory hypotension leading to death in untreated patients. Glucocorticoid deficiency should be treated by intravenous administration of 100 mg hydrocortisone. In patients without a history of AI, a random serum cortisol level should ideally be drawn before the administration of hydrocortisone. Large volumes (2–3 L) of 0.9% saline solution with dextrose are initially needed to support blood pressure and hypoglycemia. Hydrocortisone 50 mg every 6–8 hours should be continued until the patient is hemodynamically stable and then gradually tapered to physiologic replacement doses. Possible precipitating causes should be actively searched for and treated. Mineralocorticoid replacement is not needed in patients receiving 100 mg or more of hydrocortisone per day.

PRIMARY ALDOSTERONISM

Definition

Primary aldosteronism (PA), also known as Conn's syndrome, is characterized by hypertension, inappropriately elevated levels of plasma aldosterone, and low levels of plasma renin. PA is the most common curable cause of secondary hypertension. The prevalence of PA is about 20% in patients with resistant hypertension and 6% with uncomplicated hypertension. PA is associated with higher cardiovascular and cerebrovascular morbidity and mortality compared to patients with essential hypertension. Early diagnosis may cure hypertension or provide targeted therapy to prevent irreversible cardiovascular damage and renal disease. However, the screening rate remains extremely low because screening entails follow-up (confirmation, imaging, adrenal venous sampling, and surgery when indicated), and these procedures are time-consuming and costly.

Aldosterone Secretion: Physiology and Pathophysiology

Aldosterone, a mineralocorticoid hormone produced in the zona glomerulosa of the adrenal cortex, binds to mineralocorticoid receptors and regulates the final stages of sodium reabsorption in the distal renal tubules and collecting ducts. Mineralocorticoid receptors are also expressed in cardiomyocytes and neurons in the hippocampus, hypothalamus, and brainstem. The secretion of aldosterone is stimulated by high serum potassium concentration and the renin–angiotensin system and to a much lesser degree by the ACTH stimulation.

In primary aldosteronism, the aldosterone level is inappropriately high and autonomous of the major regulators of its secretion. Aldosterone-producing adenoma (APA) and bilateral idiopathic hyperaldosteronism (IHA) are the two most common subtypes of PA (Table 6.3). IHA may be associated with bilateral micronodular or macronodular adrenal hyperplasia. APAs are generally small (<2 cm in diameter), benign tumors and have a golden yellow color on their cut surface (Figures 6.10–6.12). Unilateral

TABLE 6.3   Causes of Primary Aldosteronism

- Bilateral idiopathic hyperplasia (60-70%)
- Aldosterone-producing adenoma (30-40%)
- Unilateral (primary) adrenal hyperplasia (2%)
- Adrenal carcinoma (<1%)
- Ectopic aldosterone-producing tumors (<1%)
- Familial hyperaldosteronism (FH, types I–IV) (1–5%)
  - ○ FH type I (glucocorticoid-remediable aldosteronism)
  - ○ FH type II (APA or IHA)
  - ○ FH type III (germline KCNJ5 mutations)
  - ○ FH type IV (germline CACNA mutations)

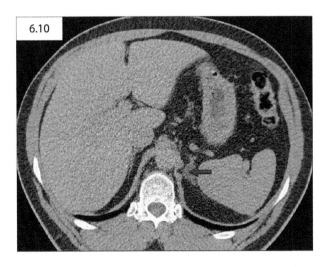

6.10

FIGURE 6.10   Noncontrast CT scan of adrenal glands in a patient with primary aldosteronism showing a 2 cm nodule in the left adrenal gland with Hounsfield units <10, suggesting a benign adenoma (arrow).

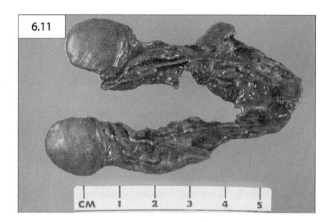

FIGURE 6.11 The cut surface of a resected aldosterone-producing adenoma showing a 1.8 cm discrete golden nodule within the cortex of a bivalve adrenal gland. (Courtesy of Dr. Howard Levin.)

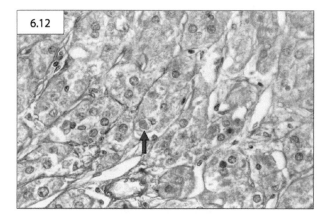

FIGURE 6.12 Microscopic appearance of an aldosterone-producing adenoma showing uniform cells with round nuclei and abundant cytoplasm. A spironolactone body is present in the center (arrow). (Courtesy of Dr. Howard Levin.)

hyperplasia is uncommon and caused by micronodular or macronodular hyperplasia of the zona glomerulosa of one adrenal gland. Familial hyperaldosteronism (FH) is a rare cause of PA (see the section 'Familial Hyperaldosteronism').

Clinical Presentation

PA usually occurs between 20 and 60 years of age. Patients may experience symptoms related to hypertension (headaches), hypokalemia (polyuria and nocturia related to the hypokalemia-induced renal concentrating defect, paresthesia, or muscle cramps), or both. Hypertension is usually moderate to severe and may be resistant to usual pharmacologic treatment. Hypokalemia is encountered in less than half of the cases. Compared to those with essential hypertension, patients with PA experience a fourfold increased risk of strokes, sixfold increase of myocardial infarction, and twelvefold increase of atrial fibrillation.

Diagnosis

Screening Tests

According to the Endocrine Society 2016 guidelines, patients should be screened for PA if they have:

1. Sustained BP above 150/100 mmHg on three occasions measured on different days
2. BP above 140/90 mmHg despite taking three antihypertensive drugs (including a diuretic) at optimal doses
3. Controlled BP (< 140/90 mm Hg) on at least four antihypertensive drugs, including a diuretic
4. Hypertension and unprovoked or diuretic-induced hypokalemia
5. Hypertension or hypokalemia with adrenal incidentalomas
6. Hypertension and sleep apnea
7. Hypertension and a family history of early-onset (before 40 years) hypertension or cerebrovascular accident
8. Hypertension and a first-degree relative with PA

Screening requires the measurement of paired plasma aldosterone concentration (PAC), plasma renin activity (PRA; or direct renin concentration), and a basic metabolic panel (Figure 6.13). These measurements can be conducted while patients are on their antihypertensive medications such as beta-blockers, diuretics, ACE inhibitors, angiotensin receptor blockers, and calcium channel blockers except for mineralocorticoid antagonists, which should be stopped for at least 4 weeks before testing. However, patients with hypokalemia, an aldosterone level >20 ng/dL, and a suppressed plasma renin activity can be assumed to have primary aldosterone without a need for confirmatory tests. In such patients, discontinuing mineralocorticoid antagonists may not be safe. Potassium should be corrected, as hypokalemia may suppress aldosterone secretion in primary aldosteronism.

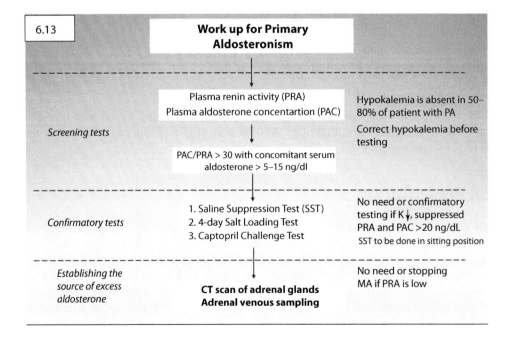

FIGURE 6.13   Algorithm for the workup of patients with suspected primary hyperaldosteronism.

The aldosterone-to-renin ratio (ARR) >20–30 (PAC in ng/dL and PRA in ng/mL per h) may be used for further confirmatory testing. Sensitivity improves when samples are collected in the morning after patients have been out of bed for at least 2 hours, and after they have been seated for 5–15 minutes. A major pitfall of ARR is that some laboratories report PRA values to a lower limit of 0.1 ng mL^{-1} h^{-1}. In such cases, an ARR of 20 can be achieved even when aldosterone is as low as 2 ng dL^{-1}, leading to false-positive results. Therefore, caution should be used in interpreting ARR when PRA is less than 0.6 ng mL^{-1} h^{-1}. There is no consensus on an aldosterone level below which a diagnosis of PA should not be pursued. In the absence of hypokalemia, the authors use an aldosterone cutoff value of 7 ng/dL as the threshold for further testing. Aldosterone levels between 5 and 15 ng/dL have been suggested by experts in the literature.

Confirmatory Tests

Patients with an ARR >20 who have a PRA <1 ng mL^{-1} h^{-1} and PAC >7 ng dL^{-1} should undergo one or more confirmatory tests. Patients should be on pharmacological agents with no effects on the renin–angiotensin–aldosterone system during confirmatory testing, including nondihydropyridine calcium channel blockers, alpha-1 blockers, and hydralazine.

In most centers, one of the following three tests is used for confirmatory testing:

1. Oral salt loading test (4 days)
2. Saline suppression test
3. Captopril challenge test

During the oral sodium loading test, a urinary sodium level of more than 200 mmol/24 h confirms an adequate salt load. An aldosterone excretion of >12 mcg/24 h is consistent with autonomous aldosterone secretion.

In the saline infusion test, serum aldosterone is collected after a saline infusion of 2 L over 4 hours. PAC >7 ng dL^{-1}, measured by mass spectrometry, is consistent with PA. In the captopril challenge test, blood samples are drawn for measurement of PRA, plasma aldosterone, and cortisol at time 0 and at 1 or 2 hours after 25–50 mg captopril intake. Normal suppression is defined as a PAC less than 11 ng/dL and a PAC:PRA ratio less than 50 ng/dl per ng/ml per hour. This test is recommended when salt loading is contraindicated (for patients with heart failure or uncontrolled hypertension).

Lateralizing Studies

Lateralization of the source of the excessive aldosterone secretion is critical to guide the management of PA. Unilateral adrenalectomy of aldosterone-producing adenoma or unilateral adrenal hyperplasia results in the normalization of hypokalemia, improvement of hypertension in all patients, and cure of hypertension in about half of affected patients.

The adrenals in IHA may be normal on CT or show thickening or nodular changes. Adrenal CT is inferior to adrenal venous sampling in distinguishing between APA and IHA. When the adrenal venous sampling is performed by an experienced radiologist, it has 95% sensitivity and nearly 100% specificity for detecting unilateral aldosterone excess (Figure 6.14). Adequate training and experience are essential, especially in terms of successfully cannulating the smaller right adrenal vein. In most centers, the adrenal venous sampling is performed under cosyntropin infusion. An aldosterone lateralization ratio (ratio of PAC/cortisol from the dominant side to that of the nondominant side) >4 indicates unilateral aldosterone excess. A ratio of <2 suggests bilateral aldosterone hypersecretion. A ratio between 2 and 4 is indeterminate. In young patients (<35 years of age) with a discrete adrenal nodule, and a normal contralateral adrenal gland, unilateral adrenalectomy may be considered without a need for adrenal venous sampling.

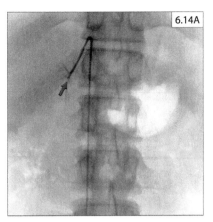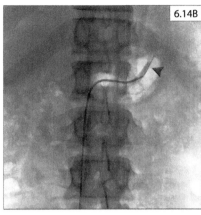

FIGURE 6.14   Abdominal radiographs that show adrenal venous sampling for identifying the source of hyper-aldosteronism. A catheter is placed in the (A) right adrenal (arrow) and (B) left adrenal (arrowhead).

Familial Hyperaldosteronism

FH accounts for 1%–5% of PA cases (Table 6.3). Genetic testing for FH is indicated in patients with PA diagnosed at <20 years, particularly if they have a family history of PA and/or stroke at an early age (<40 years). To date, there are four forms of FH characterized by their germline mutations.

FH type I (also known as glucocorticoid-remediable aldosteronism) is autosomal dominant and results from the expression of a chimeric gene, which fuses the promoter region of the 11β-hydroxylase gene (CYP11B1) with the aldosterone synthase gene (CYP11B2). The enzyme encoded by this hybrid gene produces aldosterone under the regulation of adrenocorticotropic hormone (ACTH) in the zona fasciculata, where cortisol is normally made. Most patients have a normal potassium level.

FH type II is clinically indistinguishable from sporadic PA except for the early-onset hypertension and familial occurrence. The underlying mutation is in the voltage-gated chloride channel in adrenal glomerulosa cells.

FH type III results from a mutation in the gene encoding the potassium channel leading to changes in sodium conductance, zona glomerulosa cell depolarization, calcium entry, and aldosterone production. Although the clinical features are variable, FHA type III patients often present with an early onset of severe hyperaldosteronism that is resistant to pharmacological therapy, associated with hypokalemia and diabetes insipidus-like symptoms. Bilateral adrenalectomy is often required.

FH type IV is caused by a mutation in a gene encoding L-type voltage-gated calcium channels. Patients may have mild mental retardation and social skill alterations.

Management/Treatment

The optimal treatment of APA or unilateral hyperplasia is curative surgery. Medical management with mineralocorticoid receptor antagonists (MRAs) is the treatment of choice for IHA and glucocorticoid-remediable aldosteronism. Spironolactone treatment in men may result in gynecomastia. Therefore, treatment with eplerenone in men who require long-term MRAs is preferred.

In patients with FH type I (glucocorticoid-remediable aldosteronism), hypertension is usually controlled by treatment with glucocorticoids in low doses. Spironolactone and amiloride are alternative treatments. Genetic counseling is advisable for patients with this autosomal dominant disorder.

PHEOCHROMOCYTOMA

Definition

Pheochromocytomas and paraganglioma are rare neuroendocrine tumors of catecholamines hypersecretion (norepinephrine, epinephrine, and dopamine) that arise from chromaffin cells of the adrenal medulla (pheochromocytomas) or ganglia of the autonomic nervous system (paragangliomas). Paragangliomas can occur in any region from the base of the skull to the pelvic floor. Their incidence is about 0.6 cases per 100,000 person-years. Functional pheochromocytomas and paragangliomas can be lethal if untreated (Figures 6.15–6.17).

Clinical Features

Catecholamine-secreting tumors affect men and women equally and occur primarily in the third to fifth decades. They are rare in children, and when discovered, are associated with hereditary syndromes. Presenting symptoms are nonspecific and may include the classic triad of headaches, palpitations, and profuse sweating, often triggered by stressful situations, which occur in less than half of the patients. Patients may present with resistant hypertension or hypertensive spells. Blood pressure lability is attributed to the episodic release of catecholamines, volume depletion, and altered sympathetic vascular tone regulation.

Head and neck paragangliomas are rarely hypersecreting and manifest as painless, slowly growing masses (carotid-body tumors and vagal paragangliomas), conductive hearing loss, or pulsatile tinnitus (jugulotympanic paragangliomas).

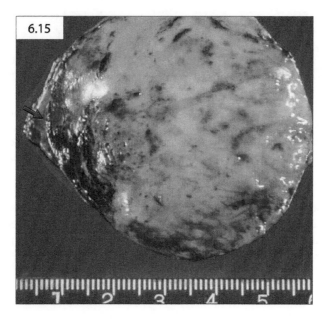

FIGURE 6.15 Gross appearance of pheochromocytoma. A 6 cm predominantly gray-tan mass with some areas of hemorrhage is seen within the substance of the adrenal gland. A small remnant of the normal adrenal cortex is visible (arrow). (Courtesy of Dr. Howard Levin.)

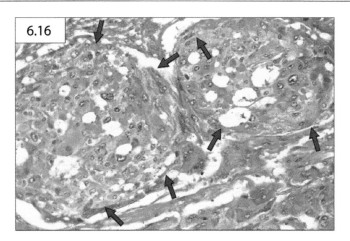

FIGURE 6.16   Microscopic appearance of pheochromocytoma. Cell balls ('zellballen'; arrows) are demarcated by connective tissue containing capillaries. Nuclei are round to oval. The cytoplasm is pink, somewhat granular, and focally vacuolated. (Courtesy of Dr. Howard Levin.)

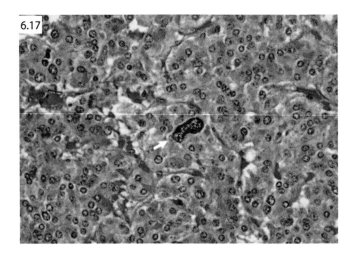

FIGURE 6.17   In pheochromocytoma, the tumor cells are characteristically arranged in tightly packed nests separated by a delicate branching vasculature. Tumor cells have strikingly purple cytoplasm due to their dense complement of cytoplasmic chromaffin granules containing catecholamines. Scattered markedly enlarged cells (arrow) are not uncommon. These are regarded as degenerative in nature and have no prognostic significance. H&E, 400×.

Asymptomatic cases of pheochromocytoma and paraganglioma are increasingly being discovered with the widespread use of imaging and germline-mutation testing of family members of affected individuals or those with the associated syndrome. The indications for screening patients with suspected pheochromocytoma are listed in Table 6.4.

Diagnosis

Metanephrine is the metabolite of epinephrine, and normetanephrine is the metabolite of norepinephrine. Elevated plasma-fractionated metanephrines (metanephrine and normetanephrine) have a 97% sensitivity and 93% specificity for diagnosing pheochromocytoma and paraganglioma. Plasma-fractionated

TABLE 6.4 Indications for Screening of Patients Suspected of Having Pheochromocytoma

- Episodic symptoms of headaches, tachycardia, and diaphoresis (with or without hypertension)
- Family history of pheochromocytoma or predisposing familial syndromes pheochromocytoma
- Lipid-poor adrenal incidentaloma
- Unexplained paroxysms of tachy-bradyarrhythmia or hypertension during anesthesia, surgery, parturition or prolonged and unexplained postoperative hypotension
- Adverse cardiovascular reactions to certain drugs including anesthetic agents, beta-blockers, glucagon, glucocorticoids, tricyclic antidepressants, metoclopramide, phenothiazine, and tyramine-containing foods
- Spells or attacks during exertion, movements of torso, straining, coitus, or micturition
- Refractory or labile hypertension

metanephrines have a similar specificity and more sensitivity than urinary metanephrines when compared to the same control groups (normotensive versus hypertensive). Fractionated catecholamines (epinephrine, norepinephrine, and dopamine) are less sensitive, and their measurement is not routinely indicated. Although sympathetic paragangliomas can secrete norepinephrine, they do not synthesize epinephrine since they lack the enzyme for converting norepinephrine to epinephrine, which requires a high level of cortisol for its expression. Head and neck paragangliomas may only display increased excretion of the dopamine metabolite 3-methoxytyramine.

Typically, pheochromocytomas and paragangliomas that induce clinical symptoms are associated with metanephrine or normetanephrine levels that are >4 times above the upper limit of the reference range. Less than two times the elevated plasma and urine normetanephrine are commonly attributed to enhanced sympathoadrenergic tone (e.g., stress, illness), the use of catecholamine reuptake inhibitors (e.g., tricyclic antidepressants, antipsychotic agents, serotonin-reuptake or norepinephrine-reuptake inhibitors), and renal insufficiency, causing false-positive test results. Medications that may interfere with biochemical testing should be discontinued (Table 6.5). Patients with plasma normetanephrine levels about two- to fourfold above the upper limit of normal may undergo the clonidine suppression test for further evaluation (Figure 6.18). Any degree of elevated plasma or urinary fractionated metanephrines should be further evaluated by repeating the level and, if still elevated, pursued with adrenal imaging (Figures 6.19–6.21).

Management/Treatment

Preoperative Management

Surgical resection of pheochromocytoma or paraganglioma is the mainstay of therapy. To control blood pressure and prevent hypertensive crises intraoperatively, combined α- and β-adrenergic blockade is usually started at least two weeks before surgery.

The adrenergic blockade is accomplished with either a nonselective (phenoxybenzamine) or a selective α-adrenergic receptor antagonist (doxazosin) with a blood pressure goal of <140/90 mmHg and tolerable adverse events. β-adrenergic antagonists (e.g., extended-release metoprolol for a heart rate goal of 80 beats per minute) should be administered to control tachycardia only after α-adrenergic blockade has been initiated since β-adrenergic blockade alone can cause a hypertensive crisis because of unopposed α-adrenergic stimulation. Postoperative sustained hypotension can be a complication of the preoperative adrenergic blockade and the downregulation of the alpha receptors; therefore, close monitoring is needed. When blood pressure control is inadequate with combined α- and β-adrenergic blockade or when patients develop intolerable side effects, calcium channel blockers (nicardipine and amlodipine) may be used with adequate efficacy.

TABLE 6.5   Medications and Stimulants to Avoid before Measuring Plasma and Urinary Catecholamines and Metanephrines

Tricyclic antidepressants

  Beta-blockers: labetalol and sotalol

  Acetaminophen

  Phenoxybenzamine

  Monoamine oxidase inhibitors

  Antipsychotics

  Sympathomimetics: ephedrine, pseudoephedrine, amphetamines, albuterol

  Stimulants: caffeine, nicotine, theophylline

  Miscellaneous: levodopa, carbidopa, alcohol, cocaine

Imaging studies

The imaging modality of choice to assess those neuroendocrine tumors depends on three clinical scenarios.

  1. Patients with typical symptoms and significantly elevated metanephrines: In this group, contrast-enhanced computed tomography (CT) or magnetic resonance imaging (MRI) of the abdomen and pelvis is recommended since nearly 95% of the pheochromocytomas and paragangliomas are in the abdomen and pelvis (Figures 6.18–6.20). Those tumors demonstrate high contrast avidity (often with heterogeneous enhancement) on CT imaging with intravenous contrast. The CT washout characteristics of pheochromocytomas are not reliable to confirm or exclude the diagnosis. On MRI, pheochromocytomas usually display hyperintensity on T2-weighted imaging and have features suggestive of low lipid content (no loss of signal intensity on out-of-phase T1 images).

  2. Patients with incidental adrenal mass: CT without contrast is recommended in this second group, because low attenuation on unenhanced CT imaging (<10 Hounsfield units) of a lipid-rich mass rules out the diagnosis of pheochromocytoma and biochemical testing is not necessary.

  3. Carriers of asymptomatic germline mutation of a susceptible gene: The specific gene guides the tailoring of imaging studies as the anatomical locations of pheochromocytomas and paragangliomas differ among the syndromes.

Once a pheochromocytoma or paraganglioma has been identified, additional testing including functional imaging (123I-labeled metaiodobenzylguanidine [MIBG] or Gallium Dotatate scan) may be performed to assess the extent of the disease or further evaluation of patients with positive biochemical testing and negative CT or MR imaging studies (Figure 6.21).

Surgical Management and Follow-Up

Endoscopic resection of pheochromocytomas with transabdominal or retroperitoneal access is the standard practice. This procedure has a shorter operative time and hospital stay as well as fewer intraoperative and postoperative complications compared to open laparotomy. For bilateral pheochromocytomas, cortical sparing adrenalectomy may be considered to avoid lifelong glucocorticoid and mineralocorticoid replacement.

For patients with a head and neck paraganglioma, treatment options include surgery, stereotactic radiosurgery, external radiation therapy, and a watchful waiting strategy depending on the location, presence of tumor extension, symptoms, and staging. With advanced cervical and jugular paragangliomas, deficits of the lower cranial nerves are frequently seen after surgery and therefore nonsurgical treatment options including radiotherapy may be considered. Long-term follow-up is necessary for all patients.

Pheochromocytoma-Associated Syndromes

About 40%–50 % of patients have an identifiable mutation, and this number is expected to grow. A brief description of paraganglioma-associated familial syndromes is discussed here. A more detailed description of them may be found in Chapter 9. Genetic screening is recommended for almost all patients with pheochromocytoma.

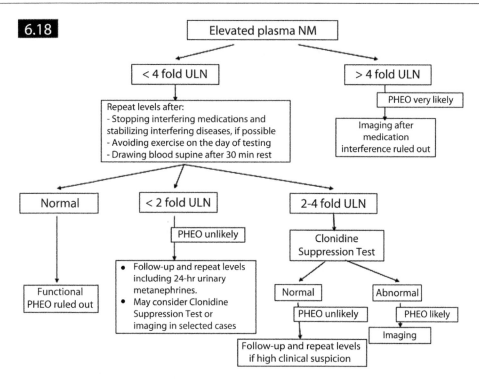

FIGURE 6.18   Algorithm for the biochemical evaluation of patients suspected of having pheochromocytoma.

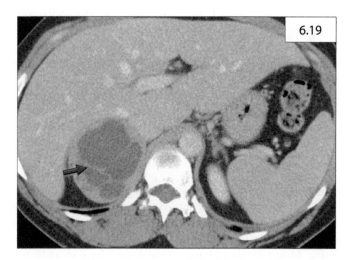

FIGURE 6.19   Pheochromocytoma. CT scan of adrenal glands showing an 8 cm right adrenal mass, with central necrosis (arrow). The mass deforms the contour of the liver without evidence of invasion.

- Multiple endocrine neoplasia, type 2 (MEN-2) is caused by germline mutations of the RET protooncogene. Pheochromocytomas occur in about 50% of individuals with MEN-2. MEN-2 is subclassified into two distinct syndromes: type 2A (MEN-2A) and type 2B (MEN-2B). The classic MEN-2A is composed of medullary thyroid cancer, pheochromocytoma, and primary hyperparathyroidism. The latter is not part of the MEN-2B syndrome. They are diagnosed at an earlier age and are more likely to be bilateral than sporadic tumors. Malignant transformation occurs in only about 4% of cases.

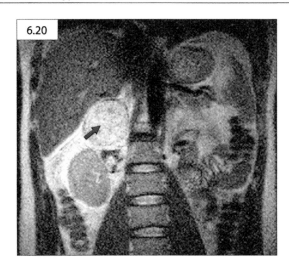

FIGURE 6.20 Coronal MRI image showing a heterogeneous 6 cm right adrenal mass exhibiting a bright T2 signal intensity suggestive of pheochromocytoma (arrow).

Von Hippel–Lindau disease is caused by mutations in the VHL tumor-suppressor gene. Pheochromocytomas associated with VHL predominantly make norepinephrine due to a lack of expression of phenylethanolamine N-methyltransferase enzyme. They are often benign but may metastasize if left untreated. About 40% are bilateral. Other features of the disease include renal cell carcinoma, retinal and central nervous system (CNS) hemangioblastomas, and pancreatic neuroendocrine tumors.

Neurofibromatosis type 1 is caused by mutations in the NF1 tumor-suppressor gene. Pheochromocytomas and paragangliomas are present in only 1% to 3%. The risk of malignancy is higher than MEN-2 and is about 10%–12%. It is characterized by neurofibromas, café-au-lait spots, axillary freckling, iris hamartomas, bony abnormalities, CNS gliomas, macrocephaly, and cognitive deficits.

Paraganglioma syndromes 1 through 5 are caused by mutations of the succinate dehydrogenase genes. They are all characterized by an autosomal dominant inheritance pattern with varying penetrance. Tumor risk and malignancy rates vary by mutation type.

SDHB carries a greater risk for malignancy and metastatic pheochromocytoma (10%–40%).

Metastatic Pheochromocytoma

The diagnosis of malignant pheochromocytoma and paraganglioma is problematic. It remains difficult to predict the clinical behavior of individual tumors based on clinical, biochemical, and histologic features, and accordingly, only metastases are proof of underlying malignancy. The most frequent locations for metastasis include bones, lymph nodes, liver, lung, and brain. The extent of the disease may be best documented on nuclear imaging. Most patients with metastatic disease have sporadic tumors, whereas, among patients with heritable pheochromocytoma in whom metastatic disease develops, tumors caused by *SDHB* mutations account for most cases. Treatment options include surgical resection, targeted radiolabeled therapies (e.g., ^{131}I-MIBG, ^{90}Y-DOTATATE, and ^{177}Lu-DOTATATE), thermal ablation, chemotherapy, and external irradiation.

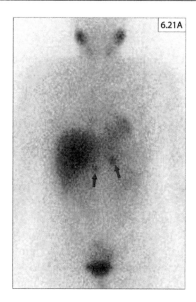

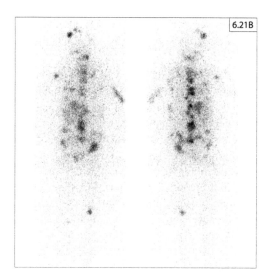

FIGURE 6.21 ^{123}I-metaiodobenzylguanidine (MIBG) scan of patients with (A) bilateral pheochromocytoma and (B) metastatic pheochromocytoma. In panel A, arrows indicate abnormal uptake in the region of adrenals. (Courtesy of Dr. Donald Neumann.)

CUSHING SYNDROME

Definition

Cushing syndrome (CS) comprises signs and symptoms associated with prolonged exposure to inappropriately elevated levels of plasma glucocorticoids. Untreated, it has significant morbidity and mortality. Despite the progress in biochemical evaluation and imaging, diagnosing and managing CS in some patients continues to be a challenge.

Etiology/Pathophysiology

The most common cause of CS is the use of supraphysiologic amounts of exogenous glucocorticoids. Here, we will discuss endogenous CS.

Approximately one-third of the US population is obese, and the chance that a person with obesity, hypertension, hirsutism, type 2 diabetes, and dyslipidemia has endogenous CS is about 1 in 500. In those with poorly controlled diabetes and hypertension, the reported prevalence of CS is ~2%–5%, although there may be some referral bias in such estimates. In addition, some of these rates are based on biochemical evaluation and not the final pathology.

The etiology of CS can be classified into ACTH-dependent and ACTH-independent. Excluding patients with mild autonomous excess cortisol secondary to an adrenal nodule or hyperplasia, the ACTH-dependent CS is responsible for 80%–85% of endogenous CS. Pituitary adenomas make about 80% of ACTH-dependent CS, and the rest are secondary to ectopic ACTH syndrome (EAS). Up to half of ectopic ACTH syndrome cases are due to small-cell lung carcinoma. Other etiologies may include bronchial carcinoids, pheochromocytoma, pancreatic neuroendocrine tumors, and gut carcinoids.

ACTH-independent CS accounts for the remaining 15%–20% of cases. About half of those patients have a benign adrenal adenoma. The remaining are secondary to unilateral adrenal hyperplasia, adrenal carcinoma, primary pigmented nodular adrenal disease, bilateral macronodular, and micronodular adrenal hyperplasia (Table 6.6 and Figures 6.22–6.25).

Primary Pigmented Nodular Adrenocortical Disease and Carney Complex

Primary pigmented nodular adrenal disease (PPNAD) is usually associated with adrenal nodules that may be too small to be visualized on imaging (Figure 6.26). In addition, clinical features might be mild and cyclical, making the diagnosis challenging. The disease can be sporadic or part of the Carney complex (an autosomal dominant multiple neoplasia syndrome), which may present with blue nevi; atrial myxomas; spotty skin pigmentation; peripheral nerve tumors; and various tumors including breast, testicular, and growth hormone-secreting pituitary adenomas. Most cases present in late childhood or young adults. The Carney complex is the most common form of familial CS and requires lifelong surveillance for cardiac myxomas and other potentially fatal tumors. Germline mutations of the regulatory subunit R1A of protein kinase A (PRKAR1A) are present in about half of the patients with Carney complex and in sporadic primary pigmented nodular adrenal disease. Dexamethasone stimulates cortisol release through a glucocorticoid receptor-mediated effect on protein kinase A catalytic subunits. Therefore, these patients usually show a paradoxical rise in cortisol secretion in response to dexamethasone, which sometimes may be mistaken for misplaced blood samples.

McCune–Albright Syndrome

McCune–Albright syndrome is a rare disorder defined as the triad of peripheral precocious puberty, irregular café-au-lait skin pigmentation, and fibrous dysplasia of bone. It is due to activating mutations of the G_{sa} receptor in adrenal cells. This mutation leads to constitutive activation of the cyclic AMP pathway and continued stimulation of endocrine function, leading to precocious puberty, thyrotoxicosis, growth hormone excess, CS, and renal phosphate wasting (rickets) in several combinations.

TABLE 6.6 Causes of Adrenal Cushing Syndrome

UNILATERAL	BILATERAL
Benign adrenal adenoma	Primary pigmented nodular adrenocortical disease
Adrenocortical carcinoma	Bilateral macronodular hyperplasia
Unilateral adrenocortical hyperplasia	Bilateral micronodular adrenal hyperplasia

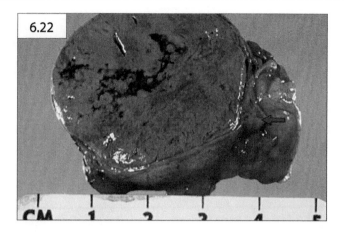

FIGURE 6.22 Adrenal cortical adenoma associated with Cushing syndrome: a well-encapsulated 3.6 cm yellow-tan intra-adrenal mass with focal hemorrhage. Normal adrenal tissue is seen to the right (arrow). (Courtesy of Dr. Howard Levin.)

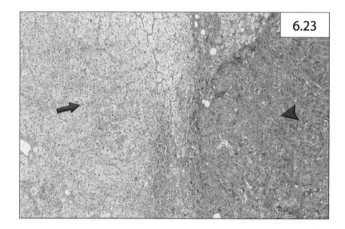

FIGURE 6.23 Nodular hyperplasia associated with Cushing syndrome. Coalescing large nodules are seen, which are comprised of cells with clear cytoplasm (arrow) and eosinophilic cytoplasm (arrowhead). (Courtesy of Dr. Howard Levin.)

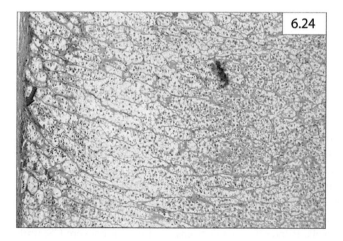

FIGURE 6.24 Diffuse cortical hyperplasia in a patient with pituitary Cushing syndrome. There is a marked expansion of the zona fasciculata and reticularis. The zona glomerulosa is not visible. The normal capsule is seen to the left (arrow). (Courtesy of Dr. Howard Levin.)

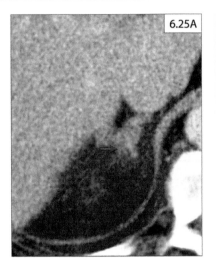
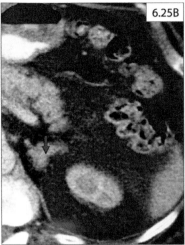

FIGURE 6.25   CT scan of the abdomen in a patient with pituitary Cushing syndrome showing bilateral hyperplastic (thickened) adrenal glands (arrows). The adrenals tend to maintain their shape.

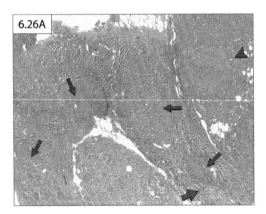
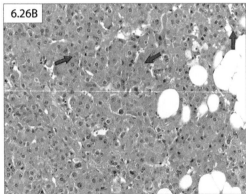

FIGURE 6.26   Primary pigmented nodular adrenocortical disease. (A) In low power magnification, four discrete intracortical eosinophilic nodules are seen (arrows). A larger nodule extends into periadrenal fat (arrowhead). A strip of normal medullary tissue is present in the lower center-right (large arrow). (B) High-power magnification of an eosinophilic nodule present within periadrenal fat. There is a mild variation in nuclear size. Many adrenal cortical cells contain abundant fine brown lipochrome pigment (arrows), accounting for the black color of nodules in the gross specimen. (Courtesy of Dr. Howard Levin.)

Bilateral Macronodular Adrenal Hyperplasia (BMAH)

Recent evidence shows that cortisol production by some adrenal tumors is triggered by aberrant expression and pathologic activation of several G-protein-coupled receptors, such as vasopressin, gastric inhibitory peptide (GIP), vasoactive intestinal polypeptide (VIP), LH/hCG, and catecholamines. Different stimuli, such as posture, food, and pregnancy, may result in the excessive release of cortisol from the adrenal tumor, resulting in clinical manifestations of CS. Patients with GIP-dependent CS have a 'food-dependent' pattern of cortisol hypersecretion. The diagnosis is made in patients with bilaterally enlarged nodular adrenals (Figure 6.27). Hypercortisolemia may range from mild disease to overt CS with suppressed ACTH and DHEAS levels. Bilateral adrenalectomy is offered for severe CS; unilateral adrenalectomy to remove the larger adrenal gland may be considered when there is a significant asymmetry in adrenal sizes.

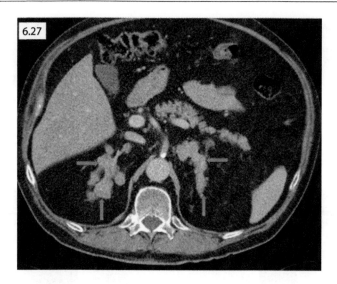

FIGURE 6.27 Noncontrast CT scan of the abdomen in a patient with bilateral macronodular adrenal hyperplasia showing bilateral nodules in the adrenals (arrows).

Clinical Presentation

Some of the clinical features of CS are listed in Table 6.7. Among these, skin manifestations and serial photographs warrant special attention (Figure 6.28). The pathological striae in CS are red-purple and usually greater than 1 cm in width (Figure 6.29). They are uncommon in older patients. Skin is thinned and wrinkled (Liddle's sign – 'cigarette paper' – on the dorsum of the hands), and minimal trauma results in easy bruising. The patients usually have a round face (moon facies) and plethoric appearance, and acne may be present. Patients may have myopathy involving the proximal muscles of the lower limb and the shoulder girdle. Supraclavicular and dorsocervical fat pads (buffalo hump) are less specific findings and may be seen in most patients presenting to obesity clinics. Both sexes complain of decreased libido, and women may present with irregular menstruation and hirsutism.

Hypertension and hypokalemia may be seen in patients with CS and are mainly due to the binding of excess cortisol to the nonspecific type 1 aldosterone receptors. The onset of clinical features is usually gradual in patients with adrenal adenomas but rapid in adrenocortical carcinomas and ectopic CS. Virilization and feminization may be part of the clinical picture in patients with adrenocortical carcinoma cosecreting androgens and estrogen, respectively.

Diagnosis

Once CS due to exogenous administration of glucocorticoids is excluded, the evaluation of a patient with suspected CS should take place in two stages (Figure 6.30):

1. Establishing hypercortisolemia (confirm presence of CS)
2. Establishing the etiology of CS

TABLE 6.7 Clinical Features Suggestive of Cushing Syndrome

• Central obesity	• Wide purplish striae (>1 cm)
• Proximal myopathy	• Changes in serial photographs
• Spontaneous bruising	• Hypokalemia
• Facial plethora	• Osteoporosis

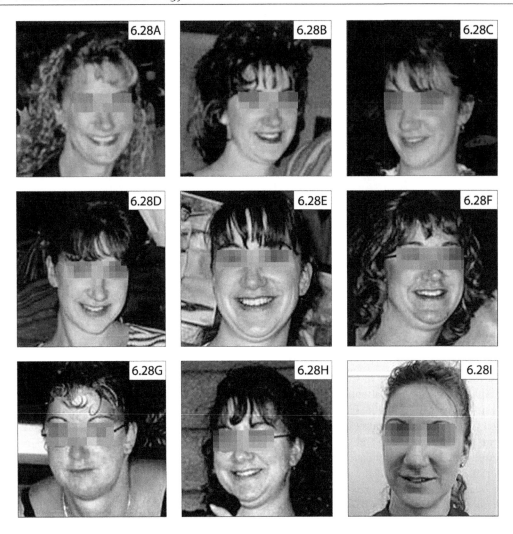

FIGURE 6.28 Serial photographs of a patient with Cushing syndrome demonstrating gradual development of moon face, acne, and facial plethora. The patient underwent surgery in 2003. Note the dramatic improvement in facial appearance 9 months after surgery. (A) 1995; (B) 1996; (C) 1998; (D) 1999; (E) 2000; (F) 2001; (G) 2002; (H) 2003; (I) 2004. (Not taken as clinical pictures.)

The diagnosis of ACTH-dependent CS has been discussed in detail in the section on hypothalamic–pituitary disorders. Plasma ACTH levels should be measured once hypercortisolemia is established. ACTH concentrations below 3.3 pmol/L (15 μg/mL) are consistent with an ACTH-independent CS secondary to an adrenal etiology. ACTH levels >25 pg/mL point toward an underlying ACTH-dependent CS. In patients with ACTH levels between 15 and 25 pg/mL, repeating ACTH levels in the morning or performing additional dynamic testing such as the corticotropin-releasing hormone (CRH), desmopressin stimulation, and high-dose dexamethasone suppression tests would be indicated.

Once the diagnosis of ACTH-independent CS has been established, the adrenals need to be imaged by a noncontrast CT scan. In patients with unilateral hyperfunctioning adrenal tumors, the contralateral adrenal gland may appear atrophic (Figure 6.31).

In patients with adrenocortical carcinoma, an MRI may provide additional information about the vascular invasion, particularly of the inferior vena cava, and the adrenal and renal veins. In BMAH, the

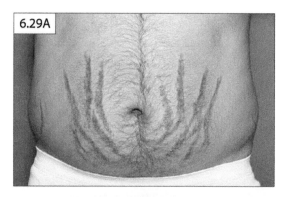

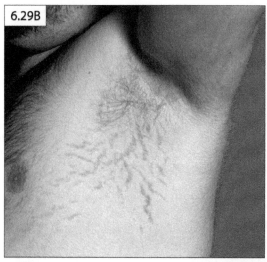

FIGURE 6.29   (A) Abdominal and (B) axillary striae in a patient with Cushing syndrome. The striae are purple and broad (>1 cm in width). (Courtesy of Dr. Charles Faiman.)

adrenal glands can be replaced by the presence of multiple nodules up to 4 cm in diameter (Figure 6.27); in other cases, the adrenal appears diffusely enlarged without macroscopic nodules. In PPNAD, imaging of the adrenal glands may reveal slightly enlarged glands with or without nodules.

Differential Diagnosis

Pseudo-Cushing State

A pseudo-Cushing state can be defined as some or all of the clinical features of CS that may be associated with some degrees of hypercortisolism but lack an identifiable etiology for CS. Several causes have been described including alcoholism, sleep apnea, depression, obesity, uncontrolled type 2 diabetes, and anorexia nervosa. Resolution of the underlying cause results in the disappearance of the cushingoid state. The 24-hour urine free cortisol (UFC) in patients with pseudo-Cushing is usually less than four times the upper limit of normal, although this may vary based on the assay used. It may be necessary to treat the underlying condition and then repeat the biochemical evaluation for CS.

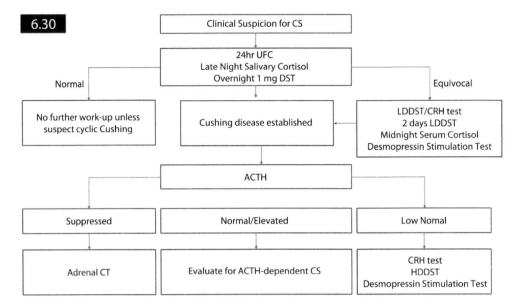

FIGURE 6.30   Algorithm for evaluation of patients suspected of having Cushing syndrome. ACTH, adreno-corticotrophic hormone; CRH, corticotropin-releasing hormone; CS, Cushing syndrome; CT, computed tomography; DST, dexamethasone suppression test; HDDST, high-dose dexamethasone suppression test; LDDST, low-dose dexamethasone suppression test; UFC, urine free cortisol.

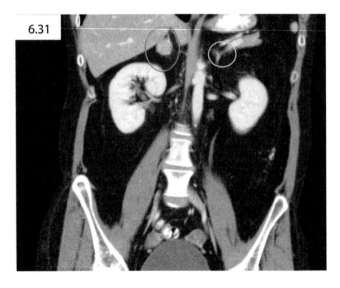

FIGURE 6.31   Patient with left adrenal gland atrophy due to Cushing syndrome from the contralateral adrenal nodule.

Management/Treatment

The treatment goals of CS include normalization of cortisol levels, eradicating the tumor, and avoiding permanent hormonal deficiency, when possible. Hormone-secreting adrenal adenomas should be surgically removed. Compared to the open adrenalectomy, the laparoscopic approach is associated with decreased postoperative pain, reduced time to return of bowel function, and decreased length of hospital stay. Surgical resection of adrenocortical carcinoma at an early stage is the only therapy that may offer a potential cure. Bilateral adrenalectomy is recommended for patients with PPNAD and BMAH with CS.

Medical therapy may be used in patients who are not surgical candidates, have bilateral disease, do not wish to undergo bilateral adrenalectomy, and cannot have a complete tumor resection. Patients with adrenal CS may be treated with steroidogenesis enzyme inhibitors such as osilodrostat, metyrapone, ketoconazole, levoketoconazole, mitotane, or a cortisol receptor blocker (mifepristone). Etomidate, an 11β-hydroxylase inhibitor, is the only parenteral agent used in severe hypercortisolism to achieve normal cortisol levels in a short time. This may be a great option before bilateral adrenalectomy. Chemotherapeutic agents and immune check inhibitors are used for advanced adrenocortical carcinomas.

CONGENITAL ADRENAL HYPERPLASIA

Definition

Congenital adrenal hyperplasia (CAH) is an autosomal recessive disorder of adrenal steroid biosynthesis that can be life-threatening in its classic (severe) form and cause hyperandrogenism and infertility in women in its nonclassic (mild) form. While testicular adrenal rest tumors and infertility are common in men, men with nonclassic CAH are usually asymptomatic. The severity of the disease relates to the degree to which the mutations compromise enzyme activity.

Epidemiology/Etiology

21-Hydroxylase deficiency is the most common cause of CAH, which accounts for >95% of all diagnosed cases. Classic CAH occurs in 1 in 10,000 to 1 in 20,000 live births. Nonclassic CAH occurs in 1 in 200 to 1 in 1,000 persons. 11β-Hydroxylase deficiency is the second most common cause of CAH, with an incidence of 1 in 100,000 live births. Other enzyme deficiencies like 3β-hydroxysteroid dehydrogenase deficiency, 17α-hydroxylase deficiency, and steroidogenic acute regulatory protein deficiency are very rare. This section will focus on the CAH due to 21-hydroxylase deficiency.

Pathogenesis

Deficient cortisol production is the key aberration in all forms of CAH. CYP21A2 is the gene that encodes for 21-hydroxylase, a cytochrome P-450 enzyme required to produce cortisol and aldosterone in the adrenal cortex (Figure 6.32). Reduced cortisol biosynthesis results in the overproduction of corticotropin (ACTH), which stimulates the accumulation of cortisol precursors and their subsequent diversion through the steroid pathways that produce adrenal androgens (Figure 6.33). The classic form is the most common cause of atypical genitalia in 46,XX newborns and primary adrenal insufficiency during childhood.

Clinical Presentation and Diagnosis

The clinical presentation of CAH is classified as classic versus nonclassic. The terms 'salt-wasting' and 'simple virilizing' have fallen out of favor because all patients lose salt to some degree.

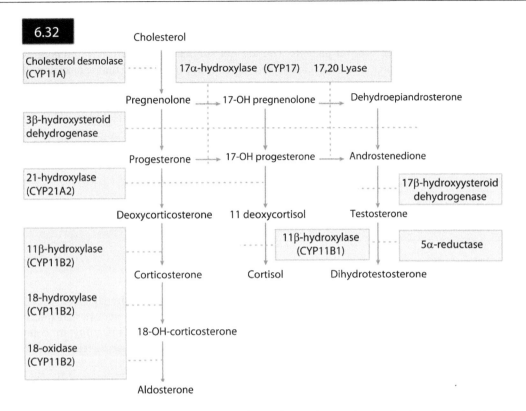

FIGURE 6.32 Pathways of steroid biosynthesis. The pathways for synthesis of mineralocorticoids (aldosterone), glucocorticoids (cortisol), and androgens (testosterone and dihydrotestosterone) are arranged from left to right. The enzymes coded by a single gene catalyzing each bioconversion are shown in boxes.

Infancy

Most cases of CAH are first detected by newborn screening, which has reduced morbidity and mortality. Detection is based on the presence of elevated 17-hydroxyprogesterone levels. 17-Hydroxyprogesterone levels can be elevated in healthy neonates during the first 1 to 2 days of life and in premature or ill newborns. Adjusting for age and weight, using second-tier screening by liquid chromatography and tandem mass spectrometry, measurement of 21-deoxycortisol, or genetic testing improves accuracy. 21-Deoxycortisol is a more specific biomarker of 21-hydroxylase deficiency because this cortisol precursor is not produced in the gonads and is uniquely adrenal-derived.

Elevation of 17-hydroxyprogesterone levels may also occur with 11β-hydroxylase and 3β-hydroxysteroid dehydrogenase (3βHSD) deficiency. They are distinguished by measuring several steroids with ACTH stimulation testing. In 3βHSD, the elevated 17-hydroxyprogesterone level in the face of defective steroidogenesis from 17-hydroxypregnenolone is related to the intact activity of the type-1 3βHSD in peripheral tissues and liver rather than the type-2 3βHSD enzyme that is expressed in adrenal glands.

The clinical presentation differs according to sex. In classic CAH, high levels of androgens affect the development of external genitalia in 46,XX fetuses, beginning in the first trimester. Clitoral enlargement (Figure 6.34), partially fused labia majora, and a urogenital sinus in place of separate urethral and vaginal openings are common. The uterus, fallopian tubes, and ovaries are formed normally. Correctional surgery for ambiguous genitalia is often performed between 2 and 6 months of age. Excess adrenal androgens do not affect 46,XY sexual differentiation.

About 75% of infants with classic CAH have a salt-wasting adrenal crisis within the first 3 weeks after birth if not treated. The diagnosis of classic CAH should be suspected in infants with poor weight gain or feeding, and dehydration with hyponatremia and hyperkalemia.

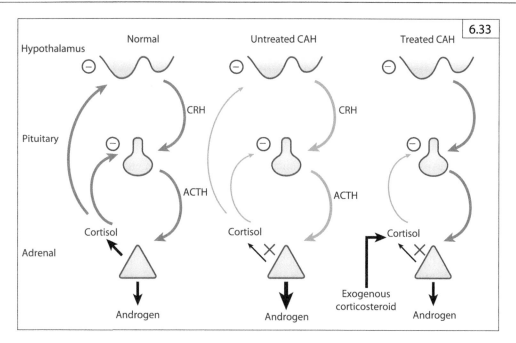

FIGURE 6.33 Pathogenesis of CAH. In a patient with normal adrenal function, the adrenals produce both cortisol and androgens, and the HPA axis is controlled by negative feedback. In the untreated patient with CAH, the block in cortisol synthesis leads to a lack of negative feedback and increased secretion of CRH and ACTH, leading to adrenal hyperplasia and oversecretion of androgens. In the patient with treated CAH, the exogenous corticosteroid replacement leads to suppression of excess androgen secretion.

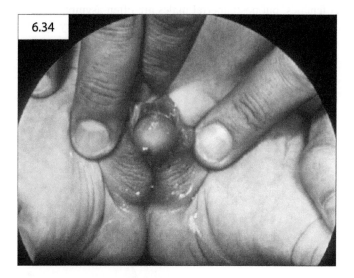

FIGURE 6.34 Female infant with classic 21-hydroxylase deficiency presenting with ambiguous genitalia as a result of in utero exposure to excess androgens. (Courtesy of Dr. Charles Faiman.)

Childhood

In approximately 25% of classic CAH, aldosterone production is sufficient to maintain sodium balance in early childhood. Without newborn screening, affected children present with signs of androgen excess (pubic hair) typically before the age of 4 years, and girls may have clitoromegaly or a urogenital sinus. The diagnostic criterion for classic CAH in childhood is the same as that in infancy. Patients who are inadequately treated show rapid somatic growth leading to premature epiphyseal fusion and subsequent short stature. Children with nonclassic CAH may have hyperandrogenism and often are diagnosed during adulthood.

Adolescence and Adulthood

Women with Classic CAH

Women may present with clinical manifestations secondary to excess androgen (irregular menses, acne, hirsutism, deep voice) due to inadequate treatment or noncompliance. In contrast, women treated with excess glucocorticoids may present with clinical manifestations of hypercortisolism, such as excess weight gain, easy bruising, and myopathy. During the transition of care from childhood into adulthood, women should be assessed for vaginal stenosis. Women with CAH are at increased risk for infertility.

Men with Classic CAH

Men with classic CAH might develop testicular adrenal rest tumors (TARTs), which can masquerade as testicular tumors. TARTs develop in 30% to 50% of adolescent boys and men with classic CAH, particularly after periods of poor control. TARTs are usually bilateral and arise from the rete testis. The tumors are identified with ultrasonography, which should be performed on completion of puberty in boys with classic CAH. The pathogenesis of TARTs is unknown but thought to be related to ectopic adrenal cortex remnants in the testis or from reprogrammed Leydig stem cells that grow under the influence of chronically elevated ACTH. The mass effect impairs blood flow to the testis and hinders the outflow of semen leading to irreversible damage. The presence of a TART and elevated follicle-stimulating hormone levels are poor prognostic factors for male fertility.

Nonclassic CAH

Mild hyperandrogenism (hirsutism, acne, menstrual dysfunction, and subfertility) associated with nonclassic CAH can affect females, but postpubertal males are often asymptomatic. Those clinical features may be difficult to differentiate from the more common polycystic ovary syndrome (Figure 6.35), and

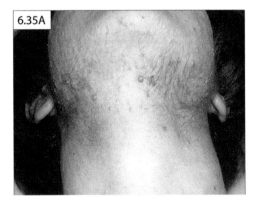
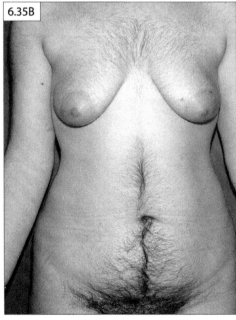

FIGURE 6.35 Adult female with nonclassic congenital adrenal hyperplasia presenting with (A) facial acne and hirsutism and (B) body hirsutism. (Courtesy of Dr. Charles Faiman.)

measurement of corticotropin-stimulated 17-hydroxyprogesterone levels by liquid chromatography-tandem mass spectrometry helps establish the diagnosis.

A level greater than 1500 ng/dL, when measured before 8 a.m. and during the early follicular phase, is usually diagnostic. Levels between 200 and 1500 ng/dL are suggestive and can be confirmed with a CST. An increase in 17-hydroxyprogesterone to greater than 1500 ng/dL is confirmatory. A level less than 200 ng/dL rules out CAH in almost all patients. Genetic testing may be done for family planning and in patients with inconclusive biochemical testing.

Genetics

The diagnosis of CAH can be confirmed by genotyping and is part of newborn screening programs in some countries. Mutations in the CYP21A2 gene located on chromosome 6p21.3 is responsible for causing 21-hydroxylase deficiency. 11β-Hydroxylase deficiency is caused by mutations of the CYP11B1 gene located on chromosome 8q21-q22, whereas 17α-hydroxylase deficiency is caused by mutations in the CYP17 gene, which is located on chromosome 10. 3-β-Hydroxysteroid dehydrogenase deficiency is related to mutations in the HSD3B2 gene that impairs both adrenal and gonadal steroid production.

Differential Diagnosis

Nonclassic CAH is the cause of hirsutism in about 4% of cases worldwide, and it is commonly misdiagnosed as polycystic ovary syndrome. Therefore, screening for nonclassic CAH is appropriate in the evaluation of hirsutism or polycystic ovary syndrome. Other differential diagnoses include virilizing adrenal and ovarian tumors.

Management/Treatment

The treatment goals for CAH include:

1. Treatment of adrenal insufficiency by replacing cortisol deficiency without causing cushingoid features and aldosterone deficiency with fludrocortisone (if there is a lack of adequate mineralocorticoid activity)
2. Addressing excess ACTH secretion that leads to hyperandrogenism in females and increased risk for TARTs in males

Classic CAH

Management of adrenal insufficiency was addressed in the section 'Adrenal Insufficiency'.

In children with CAH, an additional major goal of therapy is to sufficiently suppress adrenal-derived androgen production to allow for the achievement of normal adult height. Hydrocortisone is preferred in doses of 10–20 mg/m² of body surface area per day in three divided doses. During the transition to care in adulthood, after linear growth has stopped, control of adrenal-derived androgen excess is often relaxed to limit exposure to prolonged glucocorticoid excess. Androstenedione and 17-hydroxyprogesterone levels are usually used to guide the intensity of glucocorticoid treatment. Nocturnal glucocorticoids are especially effective at lowering morning rises in ACTH and adrenal androgen production but impart a greater risk for CS and mood disorders.

In women who desire pregnancy, the goal is to suppress adrenal-derived progesterone to less than 0.6 ng/mL during the follicular phase. Dexamethasone is not inactivated by placental 11β-hydroxysteroid dehydrogenase type 2 and will expose the fetus. Accordingly, hydrocortisone, prednisone, or prednisolone are preferred for women who desire fertility. Preconception genetic counseling is advised for all patients with classic or nonclassic CAH to assess the risk of fetuses for CAH.

In pregnancies where the fetus is at risk for classic CAH, maternal dexamethasone treatment instituted early in the first trimester can successfully suppress the fetal HPA axis and prevent the genital ambiguity of affected female infants. Chorionic villus sampling or amniocentesis should be performed for the determination of fetal sex and genotyping for the CYP21A2 gene. The treatment with dexamethasone can be safely discontinued if the fetus is male or the female is unaffected.

Men with TARTs require glucocorticoid intensification to achieve corticotropin suppression and tumor shrinkage; however, TARTs develop fibrotic elements over time, which do not regress in response to glucocorticoids. Large TARTs can be surgically removed, but testicular testosterone and sperm production rarely return to normal levels.

Nonclassic CAH

In symptomatic patients with nonclassic CAH, the combined oral contraceptive pill is the most effective treatment for hyperandrogenism and oligomenorrhea. It would normalize estrogen and menses, increase SHBG, and decrease free androgen bioavailability. Spironolactone can be added to the oral contraceptive pill if there is insufficient improvement of hyperandrogenism. If undesired clinical signs of hyperandrogenism persist after 6 to 12 months of treatment with an oral contraceptive and spironolactone, a discussion regarding a low-dosage glucocorticoid can be considered. To improve fertility, a low-dosage glucocorticoid therapy could also be considered.

ADRENOCORTICAL CARCINOMA

Incidence/Epidemiology

Adrenocortical carcinoma (ACC) is a rare and aggressive malignancy, with an annual incidence of 1 to 2 cases per million. Although ACC can occur at any age, there is a bimodal age distribution, with disease peaks before 5 and between 40 and 50 years. The incidence is almost tenfold higher in children in southern Brazil, due to the high prevalence of a TP53 germline mutation. In an adrenal incidentaloma, the risk of ACC is less than 2% with tumors smaller than 4 cm, 6% with tumors between 4 to 6 cm, and >25% with tumors measuring at least 6 cm.

Molecular Pathogenesis

Most cases of ACC appear to be sporadic, and some present as a component of hereditary cancer syndromes, such as Li–Fraumeni syndrome, Beckwith–Wiedemann syndrome, Lynch syndrome, and MEN-1. Li–Fraumeni syndrome is an autosomal dominant disorder associated with inactivating mutations of the TP53 tumor-suppressor gene at the 17p13 locus. Beckwith–Wiedemann syndrome is associated with abnormalities in 11p15 leading to IGF-2 overexpression. MEN-1 is associated with inactivating mutations of the MEN-1 gene on chromosome 11q. Lynch syndrome is an autosomal dominant disease and is associated with mutations in the *MLH1, MSH2, MSH6, PMS2,* and *EPCAM* genes.

Clinical Presentation

There are three main clinical scenarios in which ACC patients present. Approximately half of the patients have signs and symptoms of hormone excess (commonly hypercortisolism and/or hyperandrogenism). A third presents with nonspecific symptoms from local tumor growth (abdominal/flank pain or fullness, early satiety) since the tumors are generally large, measuring on average 10 to 13 cm. The remaining cases are incidental.

Hypercortisolism presents with plethora, muscle weakness, hypertension, diabetes mellitus, hypokalemia, and osteoporosis. Hyperandrogenism presents with rapid-onset male pattern baldness, hirsutism, virilization, and irregular periods (Figure 6.36). Concurrent androgen and cortisol production is evident in about half of all ACC patients with hormone excess. Isolated hyperandrogenism in men is often challenging to recognize; however, some patients present with gynecomastia and testicular atrophy related to estrogen excess. Autonomous aldosterone secretion is rare in ACC. Paraneoplastic syndromes are uncommon and include IGF-2–mediated hypoglycemia, hyperreninemic hyperaldosteronism, and erythropoietin-associated polycythemia.

Diagnosis

Imaging

Available imaging techniques for suspected ACC include CT, MRI, and 18FDG-PET. The initial evaluation is usually an unenhanced CT of the abdomen (Figure 6.37). Large tumors commonly demonstrate necrosis or hemorrhage and may contain calcifications. Masses with a density of 10 HU or more should be evaluated with a dedicated adrenal contrast-enhanced CT scan. Almost all ACCs have a noncontrast CT density >20 HU. Lesions with >60% absolute contrast washout at 15 minutes are likely benign.

If initial CT imaging is highly suspicious for malignancy, additional chest and pelvic CT is needed to determine the extent of the disease. Although CT imaging is the study of choice, MRI (Figure 6.38) may provide better resolution on venous tumor thrombus, venous invasion, and small hepatic metastasis. 18F-Fluorodeoxyglucose (FDG)–positron emission tomography (PET)/CT may help to assess disease extent.

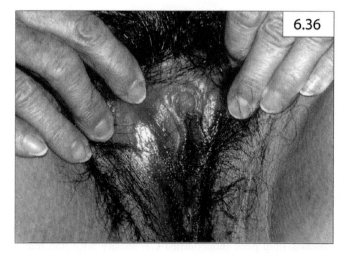

FIGURE 6.36   Clitoromegaly in a woman with adrenocortical carcinoma secondary to excess androgen secretion. (Courtesy of Dr. Charles Faiman.)

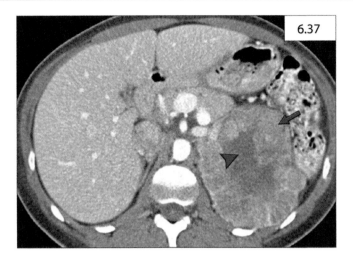

FIGURE 6.37 CT scan of the abdomen with intravenous contrast in a patient with adrenocortical carcinoma showing a 12.6 cm heterogeneous lobulated mass occupying the left renal fossa (arrow). An area of necrosis is seen in the center (arrowhead).

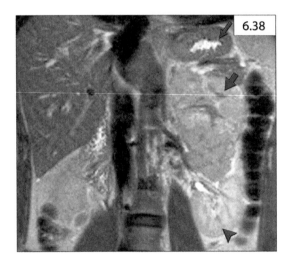

FIGURE 6.38 Coronal view of T1-weighted gadolinium-enhanced abdominal MRI of the same patient in Figure 6.37 showing a large lobulated mass in the left upper quadrant of the abdomen (large arrow) displacing the left kidney inferiorly (arrowhead) and the stomach superiorly (arrow). There is heterogeneous enhancement after giving contrast.

Hormonal Workup

The biochemical workup of an adrenal mass suspicious for ACC should include basal cortisol, ACTH, DHEAS, and testosterone levels; a 1 mg dexamethasone suppression test; and/or 24-hour urine free cortisol, aldosterone, and plasma renin activity, as well as plasma metanephrines to rule out an underlying pheochromocytoma. It is important to note that imaging studies cannot reliably distinguish ACC from pheochromocytoma, which is lipid poor (noncontrast CT density >10) and may appear heterogeneous. The measurement of other adrenal steroidogenesis intermediary hormones such as 17-hydroxyprogesterone, androstenedione, and 11-deoxycortisol may serve as a tumor marker and is recommended by some experts. In addition, urine steroid profiling may reveal increased steroid precursors and metabolites even in clinically nonfunctioning ACC. Hormonal evaluation is essential in guiding the postoperative need for hormone replacement and may be a potential tumor marker for surveillance.

Pathology and Staging

Patients with ACC without evidence of extensive multiorgan involvement or widespread distant metastases should undergo open surgical resection (Figure 6.39), providing a potential cure.

The pathology is used to confirm the diagnosis and determine the grade and stage of the cancer. The Weiss scoring system relies on microscopic features to make the pathologic diagnosis (Figure 6.40). The scoring includes the nuclear grade, mitotic rate, presence of atypical mitosis, necrosis, clear cells, venous invasion, sinusoidal invasion, and capsular invasion. A Weiss score of 3 or more confirms ACC diagnosis. Adrenal cortical tumors with a Weiss score of 2 are considered to have uncertain malignant potential. It is worth noting that the Weiss score may overestimate the malignant potential of adrenal cortical tumors in pediatric patients and in tumors with predominantly oncocytic morphology. In such cases, the Wieneke and Lin–Weiss–Bisceglia criteria, which have modified criteria for malignancy tailored to these subsets of tumors, are recommended.

The histologic appearance of adrenal cortical carcinoma is often nonspecific and can overlap with carcinomas from other sites, such as the liver, kidney, and thyroid, in addition to a variety of mesenchymal tumors. Correlation with clinical history, hormone levels, and imaging studies, as well as confirming adrenal cortical origin with immunohistochemistry are critical (Figure 6.41). SF1 is the most reliable immunohistochemical marker to confirm the adrenocortical origin and is useful to exclude metastasis and pheochromocytoma. Inhibin, Melan-A, chromogranin, and GATA3 are other markers of adrenal cortical origin, although less sensitive and specific than SF1. Synaptophysin expression can be seen in both adrenal cortical tumors and pheochromocytoma; therefore, it cannot differentiate these entities. After the diagnosis of ACC is made, the grade of the tumor is determined by the Ki67 proliferation index, where greater than 10% is considered high-grade. High-grade tumors have a poor prognosis.

Management/Treatment

The most effective therapy is surgical resection. Surgery often needs to be extensive with en bloc resection of involved organs. The presence of a tumor thrombus in the inferior vena cava or the renal vein does

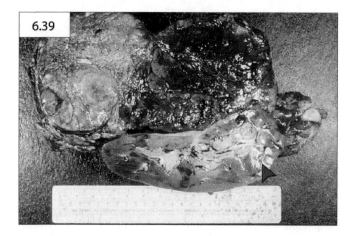

FIGURE 6.39 Gross appearance of adrenocortical carcinoma: 15 cm gray-tan and hemorrhagic, variegated tumor totally replacing the adrenal gland (arrow). The normal kidney is seen inferior to the mass (arrowhead). (Courtesy of Dr. Howard Levin.)

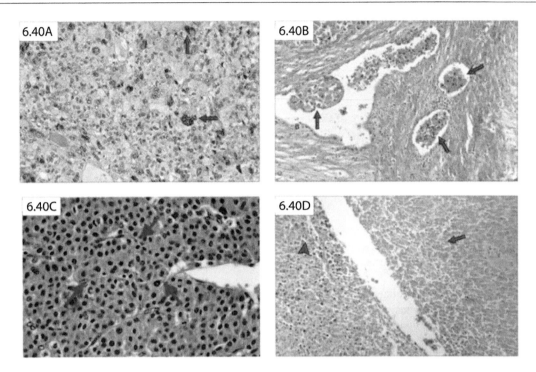

FIGURE 6.40   Microscopic appearance of an adrenal cortical carcinoma. (A) Marked hypercellularity with loss of sinusoidal architecture and marked nuclear pleomorphism (arrows). (B) Vascular invasion. Arrows show the presence of carcinomatous cells within three blood vessels. (C) Nests and sheets of pink cells, with readily identifiable mitotic activity (arrows). (D) Extensive necrosis (arrow) and focal residual viable adrenal cortical carcinoma cells (arrowhead). (Courtesy of Dr. Howard Levin.)

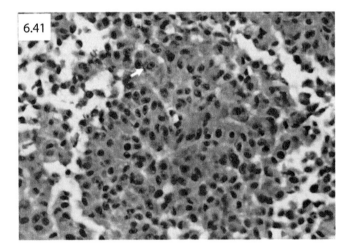

FIGURE 6.41   Metastatic melanoma to the adrenal. Malignant neoplasm is composed of pink cells with prominent nucleoli (arrow), which could be mistaken for an adrenal cortical neoplasm out of context. This case illustrates the critical importance of correlation with clinical history and imaging studies in diagnosing adrenal tumors. If metastasis is suspected, the diagnosis can readily be confirmed with immunohistochemistry. Lack of expression of adrenal cortical markers such as SF1 along with expression of melanocyte-specific markers was confirmatory in this case. H&E, 400×.

not preclude complete tumor resection but occasionally necessitates cardiac bypass technique. An open adrenalectomy is advised, since the laparoscopic technique may be associated with a higher risk for local recurrence. Tumor debulking does not improve survival but may help control the symptoms of hormonal excess. Surgery for local recurrences or metastatic disease may be associated with improved survival.

Mitotane is the only adrenal-specific agent available for the treatment of ACC. It has adrenolytic and adrenostatic properties, and it can control symptoms of hormone excess in most patients.

Adjuvant mitotane therapy is recommended for high-grade stage I and II disease, all stages III and IV, and in those with incomplete surgical resection. Progression of the disease while on mitotane should trigger an escalation of therapy, including chemotherapy (etoposide, doxorubicin, cisplatin), immunotherapy, repeated surgery, radiotherapy, and radiofrequency ablation of metastases.

Patients on mitotane should be treated with glucocorticoids with or without mineralocorticoids, as all patients will eventually develop adrenal insufficiency. Patients often need supraphysiologic dosages of glucocorticoids because mitotane increases cortisol-binding globulin and accelerates glucocorticoid metabolism by activating P450 CYP3A4. Patients on mitotane commonly develop central hypothyroidism and should have their free T4 levels monitored. Men may also develop hypogonadism, which is often challenging to treat due to very high levels of sex hormone-binding globulin.

Follow-Up and Prognosis

Hormonal markers and imaging studies are monitored after surgery for early detection of tumor recurrence. CT scan of the abdomen, chest, and pelvis is the preferred imaging modality. ^{18}F-FDG PET may be helpful in selected cases for detecting local recurrence or distant metastasis.

After radical surgery, more than 50% of patients with ACC will develop a recurrence within 5 years. The 5-year survival rate for patients with metastatic disease is less than 15%. The introduction of new therapies, including immune check inhibitors, has provided additional tools to combat this aggressive cancer.

ADRENAL INCIDENTALOMA

Definition

Adrenal incidentaloma is defined as an adrenal lesion measuring 1 cm or more that is detected on imaging in the absence of symptoms or clinical findings suggestive of adrenal disease. This definition excludes patients who are undergoing screening and surveillance because of hereditary syndromes or as part of the staging of an underlying malignancy.

Prevalence/Etiology

The prevalence of adrenal incidentaloma is about 4%–6%. The prevalence increases with age: adrenal incidentaloma occurs less than 1% in patients younger than 30 years old and about 7% in those over 70 years old.

When faced with a patient with an adrenal incidentaloma, the clinician must answer two important questions:

1. Is the lesion functioning?
2. Is there any possibility of a primary or secondary (metastasis) malignant tumor?

These determinations are guided by clinical and radiographic features and biochemical assessments.

Evaluation/Management

Ruling Out an Underlying Malignancy

An adrenal incidentaloma may be a primary malignant tumor of the adrenal cortex (adrenocortical carcinoma) or medulla (pheochromocytoma), or metastases from another primary site such as lung, gastrointestinal tumors, melanoma, and renal cell carcinoma (Table 6.8). Tumor size and imaging characteristics help determine the likelihood of cancer and guide treatment. Since benign incidentalomas are uncommon in patients younger than 40 years of age, close monitoring is important in this age group, even for masses smaller than 4 cm. Suspicious imaging features include irregular tumor margins, heterogeneity, necrosis, increased vascularity, and calcification. A low noncontrast CT attenuation <10 Hounsfield units excludes malignant lesions (Figures 6.42–6.45). Attenuations of more than 10 Hounsfield units require follow-up imaging with contrast-enhanced CT to calculate washout characteristics. An absolute washout of more than 60% and a relative washout of more than 40% are suggestive of an adenoma, but the sensitivities and specificities of these cutoff values vary across studies owing to variations in technique and timing of measurement of the washout.

In patients with borderline imaging characteristics, monitoring the tumor size would be a reasonable approach. A change in tumor size of 0.5–1 cm has been used as a threshold for surgical intervention. While a change in adrenal mass is a significant predictor of a malignant tumor, it should be used in conjunction with other imaging and clinical characteristics when surgical resection is considered.

MRI with chemical-shift analysis may also help differentiate between benign and malignant adrenal masses. On T1-weighted images, a drop in signal intensity during the opposed phase (out-of-phase) compared to in-phase images is consistent with the high fat content seen in benign adrenal masses (Figure 6.46). It has 94% sensitivity and 95% specificity for identifying adenomas.

During the 18F-FDG PET-CT adrenal imaging, using the ratio of maximum standardized uptake in the adrenal tumor compared with the spleen or liver may be used to distinguish benign from malignant tumors with inconclusive CT or MR images (sensitivities and specificities of 85% to 91% and 89% to 91%, respectively).

TABLE 6.8   Causes and Prevalence of Adrenal Incidentalomas

ETIOLOGY	PREVALENCE (%)
Adrenal cortical tumors	
Adenoma	80–90
Nodular hyperplasia	7–17
Carcinoma	0.1–2
Adrenal medullary tumors	
Pheochromocytoma	1.5–5
Other adrenal tumors	
Myelolipoma	7–15
Lipoma	0–11
Cysts and pseudocysts	4–22
Hematoma and hemorrhage	0–4
Infections and granulomas	Rare
Metastases	0–21

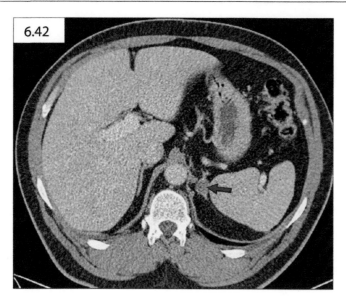

FIGURE 6.42 A left adrenal mass with noncontrast CT scan HU of –5, which is consistent with a benign adenoma (arrow).

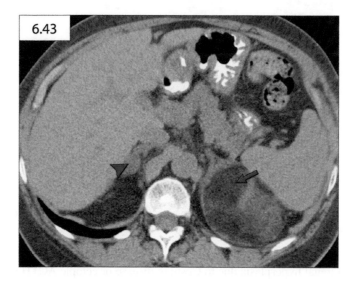

FIGURE 6.43 Adrenal myelolipoma. Noncontrast CT scan image of a left adrenal myelolipoma. The lesion appears heterogeneous, with areas of very low Hounsfield units (<–30) due to the high fat content (arrow). A right adrenal adenoma is also seen (arrowhead).

Adrenal Biopsy
Biopsy of an adrenal mass may not distinguish between benign adenoma and ACC and may lead to tumor seeding of an underlying adrenocortical carcinoma. It should only be considered if an adrenal metastasis is highly suspected, and confirmation of such a diagnosis would change the management. Pheochromocytoma must be excluded before a biopsy or any adrenal surgery to avoid a hyperadrenergic crisis.

Assessment of Bilateral Adrenal Masses
About 15% of adrenal incidentaloma are bilateral. The differential diagnosis of bilateral adrenal masses includes primary macronodular adrenal hyperplasia and adenomas, pheochromocytomas, congenital

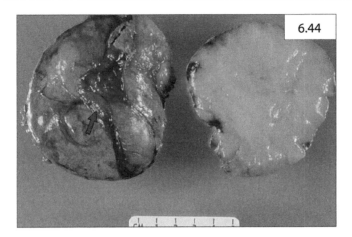

FIGURE 6.44 Gross specimen of an adrenal myelolipoma; 7.5 cm bivalved yellow mass is shown. Normal adrenal cortex is splayed over the surface (arrow). (Courtesy of Dr. Howard Levin.)

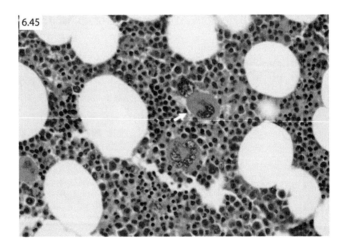

FIGURE 6.45 Microscopic appearance of adrenal myelolipoma. It consists of admixed mature fat and bone marrow elements, including maturing erythroid and myeloid cells and megakaryocytes (arrow).

adrenal hyperplasia, adrenal hyperplasia due to Cushing disease or ectopic ACTH syndrome, metastases or primary cancers, myelolipomas (Figures 6.44 and 6.46), infections, hemorrhage, and partial glucocorticoid resistance. Hormonal assessments should also include measurement of the serum 17-hydroxyprogesterone level to rule out congenital adrenal hyperplasia. Testing for adrenal insufficiency is indicated if the lesions appear hemorrhagic or infiltrative, or if there is suspicion of bilateral metastasis. Management depends on the underlying etiology.

Hormonal Evaluation

Initial hormonal evaluation in patients with adrenal incidentalomas includes 1 mg DST; in all patients, plasma or urinary metanephrines in lipid-poor lesions and aldosterone; and PRA levels in those with HTN or a history of hypokalemia. The measurement of plasma ACTH and serum DHEAS levels may provide additional information about chronic mild autonomous cortisol excess secretion.

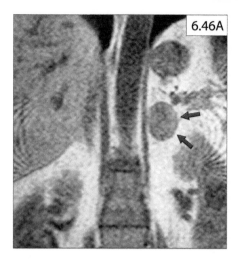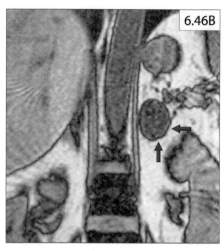

FIGURE 6.46 (A) In-phase and (B) out-of-phase coronal MRI image in a patient with left adrenal mass (arrows). There is a decrease in signal intensity of the mass in the out-of-phase image due to high fat content, which is consistent with adenoma/hyperplasia.

Mild Autonomous Cortisol Excess (MACE)
About 5% to 30% of patients with incidentally detected adrenal masses (adrenal incidentalomas) have mild cortisol hypersecretion in the absence of the typical clinical features of CS such as facial plethora, muscle wasting, or wide purplish striae. The MACE has also been referred to as subclinical CS.

MACE is associated with a higher incidence of coexisting hypertension, obesity, hyperglycemia, dyslipidemia, and low bone density as compared with nonfunctioning adrenal tumors.

The initial workup includes overnight 1 mg DST. A cortisol level <1.8 mcg/dL after overnight DST suggests normal cortisol secretion. In the absence of recent glucocorticoid therapy, low plasma ACTH and serum DHEAS levels support autonomous cortisol secretion. False positives may occur in patients receiving medications such as phenytoin, rifampin, and phenobarbital that accelerate the hepatic metabolism of dexamethasone or in those taking estrogen. Following an abnormal overnight 1 mg DST, a 24-hour urinary free cortisol or late-night salivary cortisol level is reasonable to assess the magnitude of cortisol excess.

Adrenalectomy may improve diabetes mellitus, hypertension, low bone density, and hyperlipidemia compared to patients undergoing active surveillance. Patients with MACE may develop temporary adrenal insufficiency following removal of the adrenal tumor due to chronic suppression of the contralateral adrenal gland.

Evaluation/Management/Follow-Up

An approach to incidentally discovered adrenal masses is shown in Figure 6.47. Homogeneous adrenal masses <4 cm in size with a maximum noncontrast CT <10 HU do not require routine follow-up imaging study. Patients with a normal 1 mg DST do not require continued workup unless they develop new or worsening comorbidities suggestive of autonomous excess cortisol secretion. Adrenal masses >2.4 cm are more likely to develop MACE and a closer follow-up is needed.

Patients with a noncontrast CT ≥10 HU and tumor size >4 cm should be referred for surgery. Those with a noncontrast CT density ≥10 HU and tumor size <4 cm should have their absolute CT washout percentage calculated and referred for surgery if the mass has a poor washout (<60%). In patients with a high washout percentage, a follow-up imaging study in 6–12 months is reasonable. There is no good evidence

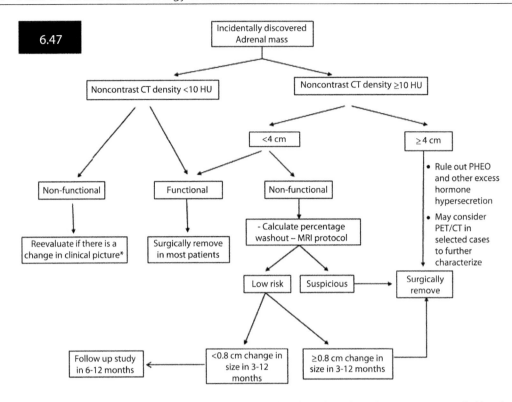

FIGURE 6.47 Algorithm for management of patients with adrenal incidentaloma. HU, Hounsfield unit.

supporting continued radiological surveillance in lipid-poor adrenal masses with no significant change in tumor size beyond 2–3 years.

BIBLIOGRAPHY

Bovio et al., *J Endocrinol Invest* (2006). PMID: 16699294
Young et al., *Endocrinol Metab Clin North Am* (2000). PMID: 10732270
Morelli et al., *JCEM* (2014). PMID: 24423350
Bornstein. *NEJM* (2009). PMID: 19474430
Husebye et al., *Lancet* (2021). PMID: 33484633
Li et al., *JCEM* (2020). PMCID: PMC7470471
Boonen et al., *NEJM* (2013). PMID: 23506003
Hamrahian et al., *Endocr Pract* (2017). PMID: 28332876
Hamrahian et al., *NEJM* (2004). PMID: 15084695
Javorsky et al., *J Endocr Soc* (2021). PMID: 33768189
Funder et al., *JCEM* (2016). PMID: 26934393
Byrd et al., *Circulation* (2018). PMID: 30359120
Rossi. *J Am Coll Cardiol* (2019). PMID: 31779795
Young. J Intern Med (2019). PMID: 30255616
Milliez et al., *J Am Coll Cardiol* (2005). PMID: 15837256
Neumann et al., *NEJM* (2019). PMID: 31693823
Kannan et al., *Clin Endocrinol* (2014). PMID: 24494743
Geroula et al., *Eur J Endocrinol* (2019). PMID: 31370000
Newell-Price et al., *Lancet* (2006). PMID: 16698415

Feelders et al., *Lancet Diabetes Endocrinol* (2019). PMID: 30033041
Loriaux. *NEJM* (2017). PMID: 28402781
Yogi-Morren et al., *Endocr Pract* (2015). PMID: 26121435
Merke et al., *NEJM* (2020). PMID: 32966723
Speiser et al., *JCEM* (2018). PMID: 30272171
Fassnacht et al., *JCEM* (2013). PMID: 24081734
Kiseljak-Vassiliades et al., *Endocr Pract* (2020). PMID: 33875173
Else et al., *Endocr Rev* (2014). PMID: 24423978

Male and Female Reproductive Disorders

7

Rhoda H. Cobin, MD

ABSTRACT

Reproductive disorders in males and females include those which are congenital or aquired, structural or functional and range from the very common to the very rare. Understanding normal development and function as well as basic pathophysiology allows appropriate evaluation and management. This chapter will provide this information and current evidence based treatment recommendations for these disorders.

AMENORRHEA

Normal women experience regular ovulatory menses from an average age of onset (menarche) of 12.4 years (range 10–16 years) until their cessation (menopause) at an average age of 51.5 years (range 45–55 years). 'Normal' menses can be viewed as a sign of normal anatomy, pubertal development, hypothalamic–pituitary–ovarian axis function, and general good health. Although irregular menses can be a sign of failure to ovulate, menses can be regular but anovulatory in anywhere between 4% and 20% of otherwise normal women. In the first 2–3 years after menarche and several years before total cessation of menses (perimenopause; vide infra), anovulatory cycles, which may be regular or irregular, are extremely common. In conditions such as polycystic ovary syndrome (PCOS; vide infra), up to 20% of regular cycles may be anovulatory (1).

Normal

The development of normal female anatomy is dependent on the absence of a functional Y chromosome (codes for the development of testes, male internal genitalia, androgen production, and regression of Müllerian duct structures). In the female, Müllerian duct structures (uterus, fallopian tubes, upper vagina) develop, external genitalia remain female in the absence of androgen, while ovaries secrete estrogen, resulting in female external genitalia and secondary sex characteristics, and ultimately ovulation during 'reproductive years'.

DOI: 10.1201/9781003100669-7

Menses result from cyclic estrogen (and progesterone after ovulation) stimulation of endometrial tissue. Ovarian hormone secretion and ovulation are stimulated by appropriate pulsatile release of pituitary gonadotropins, luteinizing hormone (LH), and follicle-stimulating hormone (FSH) of variable frequency and amplitude during the menstrual cycle, which in turn are controlled by pulsatile hypothalamic kisspeptin–stimulated gonadotropin-releasing hormone (GnRH). Kisspeptin release by hypothalamic KNDy neurons is intricately coordinated by integrating signals via neurokinin and kappa opioid peptide receptors from sex steroid feedback as well as metabolic signals including leptin, ghrelin, adiponectin, insulin, melanocortin, GLP-1, inflammatory signals, and opioids, and neuronal input from POMC/CART and AgRP/NPY hypothalamic neurons. In both the hypothalamus and pituitary, sex steroids and gonadotropin inhibitory protein reduce LH, while inhibin from ovarian granulosa cells inhibits FSH release. Ovarian estrogen production initially causes feedback inhibition in the early phase of the menstrual cycle, which then becomes positive resulting in the LH surge, which causes ovulation. After ovulation, the ovarian corpus luteum secretes progesterone, which inhibits gonadotropin and hence estrogen production, beginning the next cycle. As noted, menses can occur without ovulation, with uterine bleeding being caused by estrogenic stimulation of the endometrium and with subsequent estrogen withdrawal. (Unopposed estrogen can cause endometrial hyperplasia, which can in turn result in endometrial carcinoma; this will be important in evaluation and management to be discussed later.)

For a more detailed description of normal development and reproductive function, see Cobin et al. (2).

Females are born with a full complement of ovarian follicles numbering approximately 2 million, which normally decline over one's lifetime to about 300,000 at puberty and to 100,000 at age 30 with eventual further decline thereafter. In addition to gonadotropin stimulation, intraovarian signaling, including anti-Mullerian hormone (AMH), growth factors, transcription factors, and complex signaling cascades with endocrine, paracrine, and autocrine regulation result in the development of a dominant follicle and ovulation each cycle, with graduation atresia and loss of oocytes during a woman's lifetime (3, 4).

Amenorrhea is the inappropriate absence of menses in women of reproductive age. Oligomenorrhea is a reduced frequency/longer interval between menses, often but not always associated with absent or less frequent ovulation. Pathologic amenorrhea is considered primary if a woman has never menstruated by the average age of 15 (age 14 without signs of puberal development [breast tissue development, axillary/pubic hair] or by age 16 with breast development). Secondary amenorrhea is the absence of menses in a woman who previously had established menstrual function, with the definition being the absence of menses for 3–12 months, according to various authorities. (It should always be remembered that the most common cause of secondary amenorrhea is not pathologic but pregnancy!)

The etiology, impact, and therapy of amenorrhea and oligomenorrhea are influenced by this distinction. Since normal menstrual function requires normal structural development and normal function of the hypothalamic–pituitary–ovarian axis as well as a normal outflow tract (uterus, vagina, hymen), in women with primary amenorrhea, there may be defect(s) at any of these levels, whereas, by definition, women with secondary amenorrhea must have had normal anatomy as well as function.

Table 7.1 summarizes the most common etiology of amenorrhea at each of these levels in both the primary (congenital) and secondary (acquired) settings.

Hormone replacement treatment (HRT) for all forms of amenorrhea in women in the 'reproductive age group' is indicated. Treatment goals include restoration of normal menses, preservation of bone mass, reduced psychological concern, and, when appropriate, treatment for infertility. Therapy should be individualized based on age, goals, expectations, and possible risks. Estrogen is available in multiple formulations, doses, and routes of administration. Progesterone is required with estrogen therapy in the presence of a uterus to avoid endometrial hyperplasia and possible endometrial cancer. Contraindications to estrogen therapy in young women include thrombogenic mutations or a history of venous thromboembolic disease (VTE), pulmonary embolism, and a strong risk of hereditary breast cancer. But it should be emphasized that the potential risks of HRT commonly cited for menopause, especially cardiovascular and brain risk (see 'Menopause' section) do not apply to this group of young women in which benefit almost always outweighs risk.

TABLE 7.1   Etiology of Amenorrhea

LEVEL OF AXIS	CONGENITAL	ACQUIRED*
Hypothalamus	Syndromic[†] Isolated GnRH deficiency	Craniopharyngioma Meningioma Other tumors
Pituitary	Agenesis	Hyperprolactinemia Tumor or other cause Acromegaly Cushing's Nonsecretory tumors
Ovary	Chromosomal ovarian dysgenesis	PCOS[‡] Androgen-secreting tumors Premature ovarian failure
Uterus	Mullerian duct defects	Pregnancy
Outflow tracts	Mullerian duct defects	
Adrenal	Congenital adrenal hyperplasia	Cushing's, androgen- secreting tumors
Thyroid		Hyper-/hypothyroidism
Miscellaneous	Androgen insensitivity syndrome 5α-reductase deficiency	Constitutional delay of puberty

Source: Cobin RH, Goodman NF, Jain S, Reproductive disorders, Chapter 5, in *Evidence-Based Endocrinology*, Camacho, P. et al. ed., 4th edition, pp. 166–265, Wolters Kluwer, Philadelphia, 2020.

*Congenital disorders always present as 'primary amenorrhea', while acquired disorders may present as primary amenorrhea if their onset is before puberty/menarche or as secondary amenorrhea if they develop afterward.

†*Multiple complex genetic syndromes associated with congenital hypogonadotropic hypogonadism have been described with known genetic mutations. A variety of associated nonreproductive anomalies may be present. For more complete details, see https://www.ncbi.nlm.nih.gov/books/NBK1334/table/kms.T.syndromes_associated_with_hypogona/.*

‡While PCOS is thought to be genetically determined, it does not typically present clinically until puberty. Women with this disorder undergo normal development of internal and external genitalia and secondary sexual characteristics.

Primary Amenorrhea

Constitutional Retardation of Puberty

When a young female fails to develop at an expected age, there is often concern for pathology, however, many young women simply have delayed or 'constitutional delay of puberty', a normal variant. Although this is more common in males than females, it does occur. Lab studies are indistinguishable from primary hypothalamic hypogonadism, but there are no associated anosmia or somatic abnormalities. There may be a family history of late menarche and often slight breast development may have started. Both adrenarche and gonadarche are concomitantly delayed, and bone age is appropriate for height age rather than chronologic age. Once puberty eventually starts, it progresses to normal menses, normal body proportions, and family-appropriate height (5).

Imperforate Hymen

The first step in evaluating a woman with normal growth and pubertal development and primary amenorrhea is to determine the patency of the vaginal introitus. Imperforate hymen is readily apparent on thorough examination of the external genitalia. The critical need for full physical examination in any woman presenting with primary amenorrhea cannot be emphasized strongly enough.

This congenital anomaly is present in only about 0.5% of females. It consists of a persistent band of tissue without the usual small aperture of the hymen, thus obstructing the flow of menstrual blood from the vaginal outflow tract. It can sometimes be apparent in newborn females but is often unnoticed until

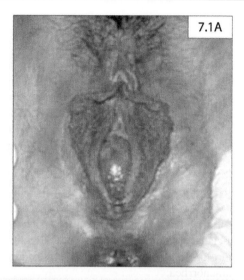

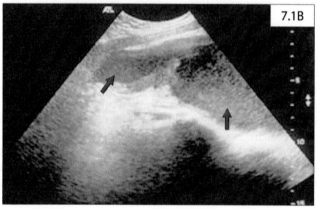

FIGURE 7.1 Imperforate hymen. (From Stone SM, Alexander JL. Images in clinical medicine. Imperforate hymen with hematocolpometra. *N Engl J Med* 2004;351(7):e6.)

the time of menarche when, after fully normal female pubertal development and otherwise normal anatomy and hormone secretion, amenorrhea is reported (or sometimes scant infrequent blood flow). Many girls present with lower abdominal pain and/or distention and sometimes lower back pain. Occasionally, women have urinary tract symptoms. Laboratory studies are completely normal. Sonography will show hematocolpos (distended vaginal and uterus filled with blood). Correction is by a simple hymenotomy or hymenectomy, resulting in a complete, durable cure with normal menses and reproductive function (6).

Mullerian Agenesis (Mayer-Rokitansky-Kuster-Huaser)

Primary amenorrhea results from absent or rudimentary Müllerian-derived structures in a woman with otherwise normal growth, development, hormone secretion, and secondary sexual characteristics. A rudimentary vaginal canal may be present but with an absent uterus and fallopian tubes. Other congenital anomalies may be present including scoliosis, unilateral renal agenesis, and, rarely, cardiac defects. Most cases are sporadic, but autosomal dominant inheritance has been reported in some families. The disorder has been associated with genetic mutations of various transcription factors involved in embryonic development of the reproductive tract including the SHOX, WNT, LHX1, and TBX genes. The diagnosis is made with sonography. Levels of estrogen and gonadotropins are normal. Treatment may include vaginal reconstructive procedures (8, 9).

Turner Syndrome

Turner syndrome is a relatively common cause of primary amenorrhea with failure of normal pubertal development. It results from mitotic error leading to XO or mosaic XX genotypes. Deletion of the short arm of the X chromosome leads to degeneration of ovarian follicles and typical streak gonads. Variable somatic abnormalities are associated. Deletion in the SHOX gene on the short arm of the X chromosome leads to short stature and other abnormalities, while other X chromosome genes may contribute to anomalies that may include micrognathia, a high-arched palate, short fourth metacarpals, genu valgum, Madelung wrist deformities, short limbs, wide-spaced nipples, webbed neck, and low-set hairline. There may be associated hearing loss, renal developmental abnormalities (30%), and autoimmune disease, especially Hashimoto thyroiditis (30%) (10).

Liver disease, type 2 diabetes mellitus (T2DM), and metabolic syndrome (MBS) are also more common in these women.

The presence of Turner syndrome may be diagnosed with prenatal amniotic fluid genetic testing, it may be apparent because of associated somatic abnormalities before puberty; may be found with evaluation of growth retardation, failure of development of secondary sexual characteristics, or may only be diagnosed because of primary amenorrhea.

Laboratory studies in addition to karyotype will show low estrogen. FSH is elevated due to lack of ovarian inhibin in early childhood, falling during prepuberty (as GnRH production normally falls during this time, occasionally causing diagnostic confusion), then rising to high levels at the time of puberty and remaining elevated thereafter (12).

Of great importance, congenital heart disease is present in about 50% of women with Turner's syndrome, with mortality being three times higher than in the general population, with cardiovascular disease the most common cause of death. The most common anomalies are a bicuspid aortic valve, coarctation of the aorta, and thoracic aortic aneurysm. Hypertension, coronary artery disease, myocardial infarction, and stroke risk are exacerbated by the underlying predisposition to MBS and diabetes mellitus. Thus, it is strongly advised to regularly screen all women with Turner syndrome with initial and regularly followed noninvasive imaging combining echocardiography, cardiovascular MRI, and sometimes cardiac computed tomography, because of the high incidence of serious lesions that often remain subclinical. A recent statement on cardiovascular health in Turner syndrome from the American Heart Association outlines the details of these lesions and suggests guidelines for appropriate screening and management (13).

Some mosaic genotypes include all or portions of a Y chromosome, increasing the risk of gonadoblastomas and therefore requiring a gonadectomy at the time of diagnosis (14).

Growth hormone treatment may significantly improve final adult height and should be considered early in childhood if growth velocity (determined with Turner-specific growth curves) predicts final height less than the fifth percentile. Estrogen is added at the time of predicted puberty. Because it will cause epiphyseal fusion and limit further growth, the timing of growth hormone and estrogen administration is important (15).

Progesterone in estrogen-treated women is necessary because of the presence of a uterus to prevent endometrial hyperplasia.

Bone density testing should be performed in adulthood and periodically thereafter. HRT in these women has been shown to significantly improve bone density and reduce fractures, compared with no treatment (16, 17).

It should be noted that in this and other conditions with amenorrhea in young women, the possible concerns of menopausal HRT are not relevant.

Occasional spontaneous ovulation and pregnancy have been reported in women with mosaic Turner syndrome, but outcomes are usually poor. The presence of a uterus, however, allows assisted reproduction with donor ova, resulting in better outcomes (18).

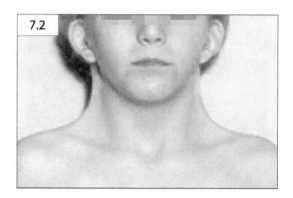

FIGURE 7.2   Turner syndrome with neck webbing and shield chest (11). (Courtesy of Dr. Donald Gordon.)

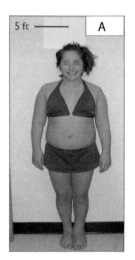 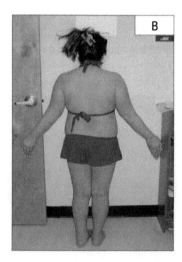 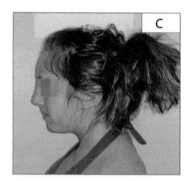

FIGURE 7.3   Turner syndrome. (A) Short stature, (B) increased carrying angle in the upper extremities, (C) low set ears. (Courtesy of Dr. Rhoda Cobin.)

Pure Ovarian Dysgenesis

Women presenting with female phenotype, failure of pubertal development, and primary amenorrhea may have a normal XX karyotype (and occasionally XY). Although ovarian dysgenesis with low estrogen and elevated FSH is present, unlike Turner syndrome, there are no somatic anomalies. Müllerian duct–derived organs (uterus, vagina) are normal. The condition is inherited as an autosomal recessive trait. Some women with familial ovarian dysgenesis have been found to have mutations in the nucleoporin and/or BRCA2 genes, both of which have been associated with ovarian dysgenesis in drosophila (19–21).

Androgen Insensitivity Syndrome (Testicular Feminization Syndrome; Complete Variant)

Phenotypic females with primary amenorrhea may be found to have XY karyotype and normal testes that secrete bioactive testosterone and AMH but have mutations in the androgen receptor gene causing structural abnormalities in the receptor that result in abnormal binding. Occasionally no gene mutation is found, but there is epigenetic repression of androgen receptor transcription. Male range circulating

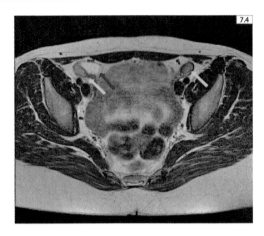

FIGURE 7.4   Axial T2-weighted images revealing the testes (green arrows) with adjoining cysts on both sides (red arrows). 3T Magnetic Resonance Imaging. Axial 4 mm fast T2-weighted image, TR/TE 5030/119. (From Nezzo M, De Visschere P, T'Sjoen G, Weyers S, Villeirs G. Role of imaging in the diagnosis and management of complete androgen insensitivity syndrome in adults. *Case Rep Radiol* 2013:Article ID 158484, 6 pages, 2013.)

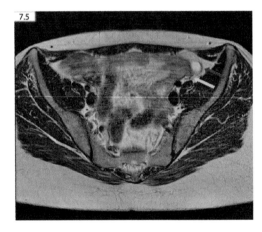

FIGURE 7.5   Coronal T2-weighted images revealing the testes (green arrows) with adjoining cysts on both sides (red arrows). (From Nezzo M, De Visschere P, T'Sjoen G, Weyers S, Villeirs G. Role of imaging in the diagnosis and management of complete androgen insensitivity syndrome in adults. *Case Rep Radiol* 2013:Article ID 158484, 6 pages, 2013.)

testosterone and dihydrotestosterone (DHT) are found, with the former being aromatized to estrogen. Clinically normal growth and development of breast tissue occur with minimal to modest axillary and pubic hair and absent Müllerian duct structures. The testes may be intra-abdominal or inguinal and may be visualized on sonography or MRI. Because of the presence of a Y chromosome, there is a risk of gonadoblastoma; therefore, a gonadectomy must be performed but can be deferred until around the time of puberty, as these tumors do not occur earlier. After removal, estrogen replacement is required to maintain breast development and bone density. Since no uterus is present, progesterone is not required and menses do not occur (22–24). (Note: Incomplete androgen insensitivity results in male phenotype with incomplete virilization; see 'Male Hypogonadism' section.)

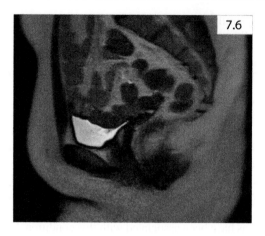

FIGURE 7.6   Sagittal image showing the absence of the Müllerian structures and the presence of the lower vagina (yellow arrowheads). 3T Magnetic Resonance Imaging. Sagittal 5 mm HASTE-sequence, TR/TE 6500/89. (From Nezzo M, De Visschere P, T'Sjoen G, Weyers S, Villeirs G. Role of imaging in the diagnosis and management of complete androgen insensitivity syndrome in adults. *Case Rep Radiol* 2013:Article ID 158484, 6 pages, 2013.)

5-Alpha Reductase Deficiency

This autosomal recessive trait, clinically expressed in XY males, is caused by mutation of the SRD5A2 gene, which codes for the 5-alpha reductase enzyme, whose function is to catalyze the conversion of testosterone to DHT, thus reducing the active hormone that binds to the androgen receptor in androgen-sensitive tissues. Male internal genitalia, adult male muscle mass, voice, and other signs of virilization are responsive to testosterone, while intrauterine development of external genitalia, adult prostate tissue, and male pattern baldness require DHT. XY males are not virilized in utero or in prepuberal life even though normal testes are present and produce AMH, which causes regression of Müllerian structures. Wolffian duct male internal genitalia develop normally.

Thus in the newborn, external genitalia may appear to be female with mild clitoromegaly, may show ambiguous genitalia, or may appear male with a micropenis or hypospadias (26, 27).

At the time of puberty, however, the testosterone level becomes high enough to cause virilization (and/or to result in overcoming a partial defect and cause some DHT production) to cause enlargement of the phallus and normal virilization. Because the prostate and hair follicles are dependent upon relatively high DHT concentrations, in the adult male, prostate enlargement and male pattern baldness do not occur and there is a variable beard and male pattern body hair (28).

Mature men may be fertile but often have abnormal spermatogenesis with low sperm counts and thick ejaculate, requiring assisted fertilization (29).

In areas where this mutation is common, it is often recognized by the family and people are raised as males, awaiting 'penis at 13' development (30).

XX females with this mutation may be completely normal or may have delayed menarche, minimal acne, and minimal body hair, with normal fertility.

If XY subjects are raised as girls, when puberty and masculinization occur, gonadectomy and estrogen replacement are performed. Since no uterus is present, pregnancy is not possible (31).

Autoimmune Oophoritis

Although this usually presents as secondary amenorrhea, occasionally ovarian destruction occurs before the onset of first menses and would prevent normal pubertal development as well as amenorrhea. Elevated

LH and FSH and low estrogen similar to other ovarian failure disorders are present; antiovarian antibodies would distinguish this condition from the others.

Primary Hypogonadotropic Hypogonadism

Although this condition is more common in males than females, it may present with failure of pubertal development and primary amenorrhea in females. Very rarely, spontaneous thelarche and menarche that fail to progress may occur. Normal female phenotype, normal ovaries, and normal internal and external genitalia are present. Anosmia is present in 50% of cases, which are labeled Kallmann syndrome. Other variants may present with midline facial defects, cleft lip/palate, hearing loss, or syndactyly. The diagnosis may be suggested because of the presence of these features and/or family history.

Laboratory studies show low estrogen, inappropriately low gonadotropins, normal androgens, and normal prolactin.

Multiple hereditary patterns have been associated with this condition. Some cases are part of complex genetic syndromes, including Prader–Willi syndrome and Laurence–Moon–Bardet Biedl syndrome (32).

In classic Kallmann syndrome, various mutations of the KAL gene, inherited in an X-linked recessive manner, have been shown to cause failure of normal migration of GnRH-producing cells from the olfactory area to the hypothalamus. Other gene mutations presenting as hypogonadotropic hypogonadism with anosmia and many associated nonreproductive developmental anomalies include autosomal dominant inherited SOX10, SEM3A, and IL17RD, and autosomal recessive inherited FEZF1. Hypogonadotropic hypogonadism without anosmia has been linked to various mutations of either kisspeptin or the kisspeptin receptor, which play important roles in the regulation of GnRH and subsequent gonadotropin release. Additional mutations in the GNRH1 (prepro-GnRH production), GNRHR (receptor), and TAC3 and TAC3R genes encoding neurokinin B and its receptor in KNDy neurons have been described. Oligogenic complex inheritance has also been described. Some of these disorders are associated with nonreproductive abnormalities (2).

Treatment of hypogonadotropic hypogonadism in females with estrogen and progesterone should be initiated after full height is attained, to stimulate and maintain secondary sex characteristics and bone health. In appropriate clinical settings, pulsatile GnRH therapy delivered by pump has restored sex steroid production and fertility, though this is cumbersome and rarely used.

Pituitary and Hypothalamic Tumors

Most pituitary adenomas present as secondary amenorrhea but can occasionally present earlier. Craniopharyngiomas and other pituitary–hypothalamic tumors (gliomas, meningiomas, etc.) may present prepuberally. Infiltrative diseases of the pituitary–hypothalamic area rarely begin in childhood and more commonly cause secondary amenorrhea.

Hypothalamic Amenorrhea

This disorder is described in greater detail later. Although it generally presents with secondary amenorrhea, if the underlying predisposing factors are present early enough in life, primary amenorrhea may be the presenting feature, usually in young girls who may have had otherwise normal growth and development but fail to menstruate. In this situation, it must be differentiated from hypothalamic hypogonadism and constitutional retardation of puberty, and thus requires full investigation being a diagnosis of exclusion, with all other causes of primary amenorrhea fully ruled out.

Secondary Amenorrhea

Uterine Dysfunction (Asherman's Syndrome)

Destruction of the endometrium is most commonly caused by overly aggressive D&C performed for termination of pregnancy or incomplete or missed abortion, retaining the placenta after delivery, for removal of uterine polyps, testing for endometrial cancer, or surgery to remove uterine polyps. These women have no other symptoms or physical findings, and laboratory studies are normal, with normal estrogen, gonadotropins, prolactin, androgens, and otherwise general good health. The diagnosis is suggested by the failure to bleed after a progesterone challenge (a positive test would indicate adequate estrogen) but also after priming with estrogen, indicating an inadequate endometrium. Saline sonography or hysterosalpingography may be suggestive, but a definitive diagnosis may require a hysteroscopy. Since these women are hormonally normal, no treatment is indicated, but pregnancy cannot be achieved (33).

Premature Ovarian Failure

Women with previously normal menses that end before the expected age of menopause (usually <40 years old) are said to have premature ovarian failure. They may present with amenorrhea and may experience hot flashes, vaginal dryness, and other typical menopausal symptoms. Since estrogen levels are low, a progesterone challenge will fail to produce bleeding, but estrogen priming will result in a positive progesterone challenge since the uterus is normal. Because of primary ovarian failure with loss of follicles, serum AMH, estrogen, and inhibin are low, and LH and FSH are elevated. Some genetic causes of premature ovarian failure have been identified (34).

There is a strong association with other autoimmune disorders, including Hashimoto's disease, autoimmune adrenal insufficiency, autoimmune polyglandular syndrome, and vitiligo. Circulating antiovarian antibodies are found in up to 67% of women with this disorder. A candidate antigen (MATER) has been identified. Antibodies to adrenocortical and thyroid may sometimes be found.

Often an alerting, easily detected physical finding suggestive of autoimmune disease is the presence of vitiligo.

Treatment with estrogen and progesterone is indicated to preserve bone density, treat menopausal vasomotor symptoms, and possibly have cardioprotective effects (see 'Menopause' section) unless there are specific contraindications to HRT. Fertility with assisted reproductive technology with donor ova has been achieved (35).

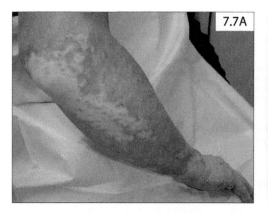 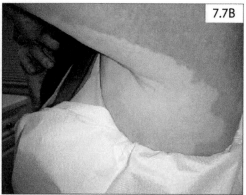

FIGURE 7.7 Vitiligo of the (A) arm and (B) abdomen in a patient with premature ovarian failure and Hashimoto's thyroiditis. (Courtesy of Dr. Rhoda Cobin.)

Fragile X Syndrome

All women with premature ovarian failure should be screened for fragile X syndrome, an X-linked dominant disorder in which 20% of female carriers have premature ovarian failure. They are at risk of tremor/ataxia syndrome, neuropathy, dizygotic twinning, and musculoskeletal problems. Their offspring suffer cognitive impairment, worse in males than females. Genetic studies can identify the condition to avoid its transmission. Preimplantation genetic testing is available (36).

PCOS

This disorder is extensively discussed in its own section. Although it is congenital and may present with primary amenorrhea, it usually presents as oligomenorrhea first noticed at the time of puberty.

Hyperprolactinemia

This disorder is discussed in its own section.

Pituitary and Hypothalamic Tumors and Infiltrative Disease

Any space-occupying lesion, infiltrative disease, or destruction of the hypothalamic/pituitary region may produce amenorrhea, either by destroying the production of normal regulatory peptides or by producing hyperprolactinemia by direction secretion or by 'stalk section', which causes hyperprolactinemia by lack of dopaminergic inhibition of pituitary prolactin production. Sheehan's syndrome, or postpartum pituitary necrosis, generally occurs in the setting of obstetrical bleeding in a physiologically hypertrophic gland, often with preexistent anemia. Fortunately, it is increasingly rare in developed countries.

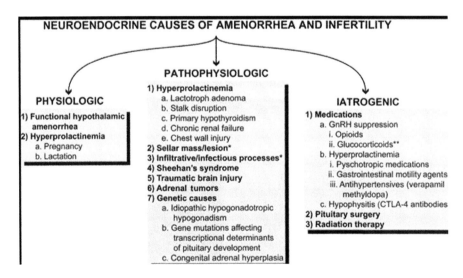

FIGURE 7.8   Neuroendocrine Causes of Amenorrhea and Infertility. (Image from Fourman, LT, Fazeli PK. Neuroendocrine causes of amenorrhea—An update. *J Clin Endocrinol Metab* 2015;100(3):812–824.)

Functional Hypothalamic Amenorrhea (HA)

In clinical practice, functional hypothalamic amenorrhea is a diagnosis of exclusion. It is important to take a full history and perform a full physical examination to exclude all other conditions listed earlier.

HA is often termed 'diet-stress amenorrhea', as it is thought to be caused by perturbations that disturb the complex regulatory mechanisms in the hypothalamus involving the KNDy neuron system. This system integrates multiple intrinsic and extrinsic signals, as described earlier.

The typical history is one of regular menses that become irregular, anovulatory, and/or cease altogether. A physical exam reveals normal growth and development, normal secondary sex characteristics, lack of galactorrhea, and lack of hyperandrogenism. There may be evidence of weight loss and or anorexia/bulimia, but this is not always present. Excessive exercise, nutritional deficiency, and emotional stress may play a role, but this is not always apparent or forthcoming in an initial history.

Laboratory studies include normal to low estrogen, inappropriately low/'normal' gonadotropins, normal thyroid, adrenal hormones, normal prolactin, and normal androgens. Because of the inappropriate low gonadotropin levels, it is critical to exclude structural pathology in the hypothalamic–pituitary area with imaging (38).

Treatment goals include restoring menses (and fertility when indicated) and, importantly, restoring normal nutrition, body weight, and fat mass. Bone loss is a serious issue in these women, and often when bone accretion in adolescence is inadequate, it is very difficult to restore and may result in fracture risk even later in life.

Sometimes, counseling to address underlying psychosocial issues and to advise appropriately beneficial but not excessive exercise will result in restoration of menses, normal body weight, better nutrition, improved bone mass, and improved psychological status. If not adequate, HRT is indicated.

Although estrogen/progesterone therapy will restore normal menses (and often psychological reassurance), it is not always successful in restoring bone mass. Lack of IGF-1 may also contribute to bone loss caused by undernutrition. Treatment with antiresorptive and/or bone anabolic agents, although helpful in adults, has not been as useful in adolescents. Novel treatments, including IGF and DHEA, have been tried (39, 40).

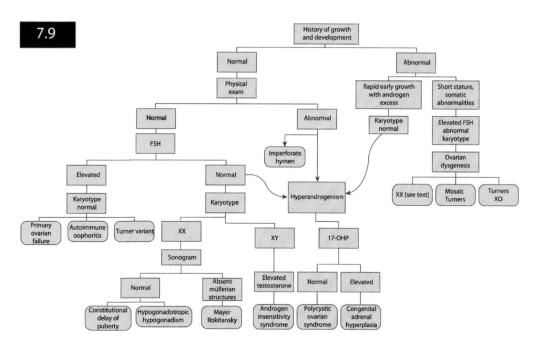

FIGURE 7.9 Clinical algorithm for amenorrhea evolution. (Algorithm from Cobin RH, Goodman NF, Jain S, Reproductive disorders. Chapter 5, in *Evidence-Based Endocrinology*, Camacho, P. et al. ed., 4th edition, pp. 166–265, Wolters Kluwer, Philadelphia, 2020.)

Algorithm for Evaluation of Amenorrhea

Polycystic Ovarian Syndrome (PCOS)

PCOS is the most common endocrine disorder of women in the reproductive age group, affecting as many as 8% of women. It is the most common cause of anovulatory infertility and hyperandrogenism. Its metabolic consequences have profound medical consequences that persist beyond menopause (41, 42).

Confusion regarding the diagnosis, incidence, and consequences of PCOS occurs because of different sets of criteria. Specifically, under the original Rotterdam classification, women may have only menstrual/ovulatory irregularity along with polycystic ovarian morphology (PCOM) (which in itself is a major issue, both because of the need for precise dedicated sonography equipment and experienced readers, and because of the clinical overlap with hypothalamic amenorrhea, especially in adolescents, who may have polycystic ovarian morphology without having the syndrome).

Authorities emphasize the need for caution in interpreting sonography in adolescence, often deferring this to 8 years after menarche. The International PCOS Network guidelines published in 2018 (see later) recently endorsed modified Rotterdam criteria in adolescence to require both hyperandrogenism and menstrual/ovulatory dysfunction without considering PCOM, i.e., making them the same as the National Institutes of Health (NIH) criteria, reducing prevalence in the group from 29% to 16% of women in one study, reducing overdiagnosis. One study found that women with the updated criteria had a higher body mass index (BMI) and greater risk of long-term weight gain. This fits with a long series of observations of the strong connection between insulin resistance and androgen levels (see later) (43).

Since acne and insulin resistance may be part of normal adolescence, and rising testosterone and falling sex steroid-binding globulin (SSBG) (within range) are typical in this age group, a diagnosis of PCOS by these criteria in adolescence should be made with caution; excessive hirsutism and age-inappropriate chemical hyperandrogenism, however, may allow an earlier diagnosis

Women may have regular menses yet be anovulatory. It is estimated that about 90% of diagnosed PCOS adult women have PCOM, suggesting that 10% do not.

Conversely, many normal adult ovulatory women may have PCOM on sonography, rarely progressing to PCOS and frequently normalizing over time (44).

TABLE 7.2   Definitions of PCOS

All sets of criteria, other causes of hyperandrogenism and menstrual irregularities including congenital adrenal....(content in notes)

- NIH (need all)
  - Clinical and/or biochemical hyperandrogenism
  - Menstrual dysfunction
- Rotterdam (ES) (2 of following)
  - Clinical and/or biochemical hyperandrogenism
  - Oligoovulation or anovulation
  - Polycystic ovaries
- AES-PCOSA (AACE) (need all)
  - Clinical and/or biochemical hyperandrogenism
  - Ovarian dysfunction and/or polycystic ovaries
- Consequence of which criteria used:
  - Rotterdam may include women with amenorrhea/PCOM only; not PCOS
  - Requirement of hyperandrogenism increases likelihood of MBS, etc
  - Influences diagnosis and management

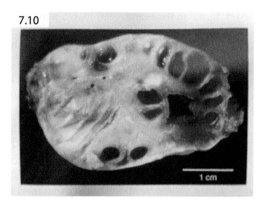

FIGURE 7.10 Gross pathology, cut section polycystic ovary. (From Kurman RJ, Ellenson LH, Ronnett BM, *Blaustein's Pathology of the Female Genital Tract*, Springer. doi: 10.1007/978-3-319-46334-6.)

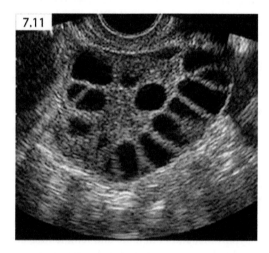

FIGURE 7.11 Ultrasound appearance of polycystic ovary. (From Giménez-Peralta I, Lilue M, Mendoza N, Tesarik J, Mazheika M. Application of a new ultrasound criterion for the diagnosis of polycystic ovary syndrome. *Front Endocrinol* 2 September 2022, Sec. Developmental Endocrinology.)

Pathophysiology

Insulin resistance is present in the majority of patients with PCOS and provides a plausible explanation for many of the abnormalities seen. Impaired insulin-mediated glucose uptake in fibroblasts of PCOS women, compared with controls, independent of but exacerbated by obesity and greater than that seen in T2DM, led to the hypothesis that downstream pathways of insulin action are affected, with excess phosphorylation of serine over tyrosine leading to resistance in insulin's metabolic effects and to increased ovarian 17,20-lyase, resulting in excess ovarian androgen production. This action is exacerbated by a direct effect of compensatory hyperinsulinism in multiple sites: in the ovary, causing stimulation of androgen production, in the hypothalamus where persistent rapid GnRH release with increased frequency and amplitude of LH pulses increased LH secretory burst mass, disorderly LH release, and elevated in vitro LH bioactivity all are affected, indirectly leading to greater stimulation ovarian androgen production and in the liver where SSBG production is decreased, leading to higher levels of circulating free testosterone.

Genetic variants in DDEN1A, which is involved with regulating androgen production have been found in a significant number of families with PCOS (45).

Increased production of AMH, found in the majority of PCOS patients, is produced by ovarian granulosa cells, reflects a larger pool of preantral and small antral follicles, and not only affects follicular development but decreases aromatase activity in the ovary increasing relative androgen/estrogen levels in a paracrine manner.

Hypothalamic dysfunction may be intrinsic to the disorder and also affected by hyperinsulinism and hyperandrogenism, as suggested by improvement with insulin sensitizers and anti-androgens.

Genetic variants in AMH or its receptor have been found to affect AMH signaling in 7% of Caucasian women with PCOS (46).

AMH and its receptor have been found in hypothalamic neurons, GnRH neurons, and the pituitary. It is unclear whether AMH can act in neurons that control the GnRH pulse generator in the arcuate nucleus, in kisspeptin neurons, and in other neuronal afferents that control GnRH/LH secretion. In animal studies, complex interactions between AMH, either produced locally in neural tissue or derived from ovarian sources in the circulation, may play a role in both the normal development and functioning of this system, There is a positive correlation between AMH and LH, with AMH likely stimulating the GnRH pulse generator, and LH increasing AMH production in the ovary (47–49).

SHBG (sex hormone-binding globulin), which binds testosterone and estradiol, a product of the liver, is reduced in insulin resistance, metabolic syndrome (MBS), nonalcoholic fatty liver disease (NAFLD), and PCOS. Androgens and insulin reduce SSBG production, and lower SHBG results in higher levels of bioavailable testosterone. Studies now suggest a possible etiologic role of SHBG in the pathogenesis of PCOS, as in vitro studies suggest that it may be a signal transduction factor itself. Using cellular models of human insulin resistance, decreased expression of SHBG protein and mRNA may downregulate the PI3K/AKT pathway, leading to insulin resistance and hence to hyperandrogenism (50).

Although discrepant results have previously been reported, a recent meta-analysis has revealed the presence of eight or more SHBG-specific polymorphisms associated with low SHBG levels and an increased risk of PCOS (51).

Familial Clustering

A complex genetic etiology is clear from strong familial clustering with mothers of PCOS women having a greater likelihood of the syndrome, and both male and female first-degree relatives having a higher incidence of MBS, HBP (high blood pressure), and DM. Despite this, no specific genotype/phenotype correlation has yet been found.

Prenatal exposure to androgens may also play a role in hypothalamic dysfunction in adult offspring. In animal models, prenatal exposure to high levels of AMH results in hyperandrogenism in female fetuses, in part due to the effect of AMH in reducing placental aromatase of androgens to estrogen. In a small portion of PCOS patients, genetic alterations leading to altered AMH function have been found. Epigenetic alterations may also explain transgenerational effects on AMH regulation in both male and female offspring (52–55).

Recent advances in the genetics of various subtypes of PCOS may eventually clarify more fundamental genomic physiologic explanations for the heterogeneity seen within the broader definition of PCOS, possibly revealing separate genotypes producing distinct or overlapping phenotypes.

Genome-wide association studies (GWAS) of PCOS have suggested genetic association with gonadotropin secretion and action, androgen biosynthesis, metabolic regulation, and ovarian aging. Only 1 of 14 PCOS susceptibility loci identified seemed to differentiate between the various clinical phenotypes, being significantly more strongly associated with the NIH phenotype compared to non-NIH Rotterdam phenotypes or to self-reported PCOS. Therefore, the current phenotypic diagnostic criteria do not correlate with genetically distinct disease subtypes.

Using an unsupervised clustering approach of reproductive and metabolic quantitative traits from a large cohort of women with PCOS, a new study characterized phenotypic subtypes of PCOS. Subjects were 13–45 years old and fulfilled the NIH criteria of hyperandrogenism and chronic anovulation, after

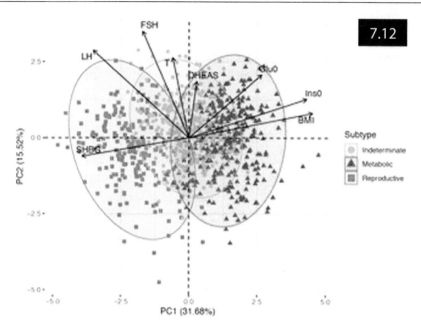

FIGURE 7.12 Subtypes of PCOS by genetic analysis. (From Dapas M, et al. Distinct subtypes of polycystic ovary syndrome with novel genetic associations: An unsupervised, phenotypic clustering analysis. *PLOS Med* 2020;17(6):e1003132.)

excluding other etiologies. Clustering was performed in PCOS cases on eight adjusted quantitative traits: BMI, T, dehydroepiandrosterone sulfate (DHEAS), insulin, glucose, SHBG, LH, and FSH. There were 893 genotyped cases from the GWAS samples with complete quantitative trait data available for clustering. Clustering analysis revealed two distinct phenotypic subtypes: (1) a group (23%) characterized by higher LH and SHBG levels with relatively low BMI and insulin levels, which were designated 'reproductive'; and (2) a group (37%) characterized by higher BMI and glucose and insulin levels with relatively low SHBG and LH levels, which were designated 'metabolic'. The key traits distinguishing the reproductive and metabolic subtypes were BMI, insulin, SHBG, glucose, LH, and FSH, in order of importance, while the remaining cases (40%) were designated 'indeterminate'. The reproductive and metabolic subtypes clustered along opposite ends of the SHBG versus the insulin/BMI axis.

The clustering procedure was then repeated in an independent, nongenotyped cohort of 263 NIH PCOS cases diagnosed according to the same criteria as the genotyped clustering cohort. The clustering yielded similar results, with a comparable distribution of reproductive (26%), metabolic (39%), and indeterminate clusters (35%).

This important study will allow further work to help determine the genetic basis for the pathophysiology of what we now label PCOS, but which may represent several different genetic entities with similar phenotypes.

Clinical Presentation

The clinical presentation of PCOS, as well as its treatment, depends upon the time in a woman's life when it becomes an issue. Precocious pubarche may be an early clue in some women. The most common presentation is oligomenorrhea/amenorrhea beginning at the time of puberty with slowly progressive signs of hyperandrogenism (hirsutism, acne, alopecia) and insulin resistance (acanthosis nigricans, skin tags). Often, infertility may bring the woman to seek medical attention. Although obesity is often present and may exacerbate the metabolic consequences of PCOS, it is not considered a necessary part of the definition of the syndrome. Because of the effect of 'unopposed estrogen' (i.e., anovulation resulting in loss of progesterone secretion), endometrial hyperplasia and ultimately endometrial carcinoma may occur but can be prevented by regular exogenous progesterone.

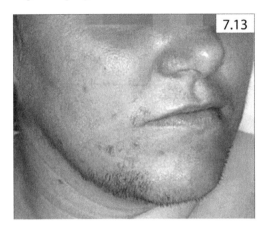

FIGURE 7.13 Acne and hirsutism in a PCOS female. (From Cobin RH, Fenichel R, Chapter 6, in *Clinical Endocrinology and Metabolism*, Camacho, P. ed., p. 151, Manson Publishing Ltd, London, 2011.)

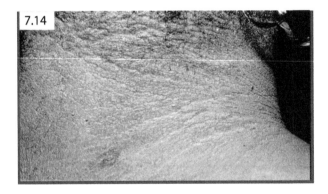

FIGURE 7.14 Acanthosis at nape of neck. (Courtesy Dr. Rhoda H. Cobin.)

Diagnosis

A full history should be taken, including growth, development, menarche, menstrual frequency, presence of molimina, and family history including reproductive, and cardiometabolic factors.

Physical examination should include height, weight, BMI, blood pressure, waist circumference, skin evaluation for acanthosis, careful evaluation of the type, quantity (vellus or terminal) and distribution of facial and body hair, voice, muscle development, presence and severity of acne and alopecia, as well as a complete physical examination, including external genitalia. Gynecologists usually are the providers who perform full pelvic examinations.

Laboratory studies should be done both to rule out other causes of menstrual disturbances and/or hyperandrogenism (cortisol, prolactin, 17 OH progesterone, TFT). In very young women, androgen levels may not be especially elevated but progress with age. LH, FSH, testosterone, SSBG, free testosterone, DHEAS, and androstenedione should be measured. It is important to use accurate testosterone measurements by LC/MS and free testosterone preferably by equilibrium dialysis, or if not available, by correcting total testosterone by SSBG. Testing should be done in the follicular phase of women who are menstruating. In women who are having either regular or irregular menses, evidence of ovulation may be sought (progesterone level, cervical mucus) for those who are seeking fertility and to exclude the need for supplemental progesterone.

Very high levels (usually T >150–200), rapid progression of symptoms, and severe hyperandrogenic signs (virilization: increased musculature, deepening of the voice, clitoromegaly, and severe male pattern baldness) should lead to suspicion of etiology other than PCOS. Although DHEAS is commonly thought of as a purely adrenal precursor, it is often mildly elevated in PCOS. Likewise, mild elevations of prolactin may be noted.

The level of AMH is higher in PCOS women than in normal controls or women with other forms of amenorrhea. AMH levels correlate with the number of large preantral and early antral follicles. It has been suggested as a surrogate marker for PCOS, especially when sonography is not possible. AMH levels in relation to the diagnostic criteria for PCOS have been examined. The highest AMH levels were found in cases where all three main diagnostic criteria existed. AMH has been shown to play a role in intraovarian signaling in the recruitment and survival of follicular cells. New evidence (see earlier) has suggested that it also plays a role in the neuroendocrine regulation of menses and may have a role in the pathogenesis of PCOS. As yet, however, there is not enough evidence to allow AMH levels to become part of the diagnostic criteria for PCOS (60).

If the diagnosis is suspected or confirmed, FBS, lipids, and Hb1ac should be done (guidelines differ on screening for MBS and frequency of follow-up; see later).

Management

Treatment of PCOS depends upon the time of diagnosis, the goal of therapy, and patient preference.

In young women, acne and hirsutism are often the most significant issue. Androgen suppression using oral contraceptive pills (OCPs) may be the most effective therapy, often combined with androgen receptor blockers including spironolactone in the USA, while in other countries, finasteride and glutamine are often added to estrogen. Progestational agents with antiandrogenic properties in OCPs may be helpful. Of note, drospirenone has been linked to a higher risk of VTE. Cyproterone, used outside the USA, is effective but is not approved by the US Food and Drug Administration (FDA). A topical ornithine decarboxylase inhibitor of hair growth, eflornithine, is approved but is costly and of variable success. Electrolysis may be helpful.

Menstrual irregularity may be treated by OCPs, with or without metformin, providing suppression of androgen production and action, improving menstrual regularity and providing contraception.

If OCPs are not used, cyclic progestins to create a secretory endometrium will eliminate the risk of endometrial hyperplasia and carcinoma.

Anovulatory infertility may be treated with antiestrogen letrozole, clomiphene, and/or with metformin, in descending order of effectiveness. If these measures fail, gonadotropin stimulation may be required, with special attention to the risk of hyperstimulation syndrome.

There is a greater risk of gestational diabetes, hypertension, preeclampsia, early miscarriage, and preterm delivery. Prepregnancy counseling, early and regular screening, and treatment are advised. There is conflicting data regarding the efficacy of metformin prior to or during pregnancy.

Weight loss, exercise, and bariatric surgery, when necessary, result in improvement in ovulatory function, menses, and metabolic consequences by reducing insulin resistance. Lifestyle interventions to promote healthy eating and adequate exercise are always the cornerstone of therapy.

Treatment of individual cardiometabolic risk factors (i.e., DM, HBP, hyperlipidemia, obesity) should be treated 'to target'.

Metformin reduces hepatic glucose output and has other less well-understood actions that lead to a reduction in insulin resistance/hyperinsulinism. It is often the first therapy tried. It is moderately successful in ovulation induction, helpful in regularizing menses, and in preventing or improving dysglycemia and its complications (61).

Thiazolidinediones (PPAR gamma agonists) may improve ovulation but are not approved for PCOS, are Class C in pregnancy, and may cause weight gain and fluid retention, as well as potentially reducing bone density, thus limiting their use in PCOS.

Newer drugs, including SGLT 2 inhibitors and GLP1 agonists, already approved for DM, although not specifically approved for PCOS per se, are quite effective in producing weight loss, improving glycemic control, and reducing the risk of cardiovascular disease (CVD) and kidney disease, while GLP1, especially semaglutide, already approved for weight loss in very obese patients, has significant benefit in NAFLD. Thus some patients may already meet the criteria for their use, while many practitioners are already using them off-label. Formal studies of SGLT2 specifically in PCOS are ongoing (https://clinicaltrials.gov/ct2/show/NCT04700839 (62).

Both exenatide and liraglutide in obese/overweight women resulted in improvements in reproductive function, body weight, insulin action, and psychological health; increases in the remission rate of prediabetes; decreases in free testosterone and free androgen index; amelioration of dyslipidemia and ectopic fat accumulation leading to improved glucoregulation, inflammatory markers, and cardiovascular parameters; and reduced body weight, total fat, HOMA-IR, menstrual frequency, and rate of natural pregnancy. Studies with semaglutide in this population are ongoing (63).

Cardiometabolic Consequences

PCOS, especially but not exclusively, using the NIH/AES criteria is strongly associated with insulin resistance, often appearing at an early age, with metabolic syndrome (glycemic dysregulation, hypertension, dyslipidemia [high Tg/low HDL], large waist circumference, and elevated inflammatory markers). There is a strong association with T2DM, often beginning at a younger age, independent of BMI but exacerbated by obesity. Several studies confirm this risk. In a meta-analysis of 40 studies, impaired glucose tolerance (IGT) was 3.26 and for T2DM was 2.87 for PCOS women compared with controls. Ethnicity and location contributed significantly to IGT risk: fivefold greater for Asians, fourfold for Americans, and threefold for Europeans. Obesity increased the risk further, but the difference among groups persisted when BMI was adjusted (64).

However, in nonobese Nordic PCOS women aged 14 to 57, only 3% had T2DM and 23% had IGT. The prevalence of BMI over 25 was 66% in this population. Although dysglycemia was related to BMI and waist circumference, no diabetes was detected in women with a BMI less than 25, and 91% of subjects with T2DM had a BMI of over 30. In contrast to other studies, neither the PCOS phenotype nor testosterone level was related to the presence of dysglycemia (65).

Additional consequences of insulin resistance, including NAFLD and obstructive sleep apnea (OSA), exacerbated by obesity, are more prevalent in PCOS, as is depression, the latter both as a consequence of poor body image and perhaps more intrinsic dysregulation. Even after menopause, these disorders persist. Thus there is theoretically a high risk of coronary artery disease and stroke.

The clinical impact of the metabolic derangements seen in PCOS has been shown to include a greater frequency of abnormal surrogate markers of cardiovascular disease. Carotid intima-media thickness (CIMT), a well-validated surrogate for coronary artery disease, is higher in PCOS lean women than in age- and BMI-matched controls as early as in the third decade of life, especially in those women with the highest androgen levels. CIMT was also correlated with subcutaneous and visceral fat mass and insulin resistance.

Obese, sedentary PCOS teenagers have also been shown to have high CIMT, increased arterial wall stiffness, and more atherogenic lipids than obese, sedentary non-PCOS girls despite normal blood pressure and lipids.

Coronary artery calcification, likewise, is nearly twice as high (40% vs. 20%) in young women with mean age 38 as compared with age- and BMI-matched controls. In a 10-year prospective study in middle-aged women with PCOS, coronary artery calcification was greater than in controls, related to MBS, insulin resistance, and HDL cholesterol, and worsened by obesity.

Despite the high prevalence of CVD risk factors, the demonstration of early-onset dysglycemia, and worse surrogate markers for CVD, an excess of clinical major adverse cardiovascular events (MACE) is not universally reported, because of a lack of high-quality studies using strict criteria, but this is strongly suspected (see later). Some of the disparities in clinical studies and resulting guideline recommendations are due to the actual ascertainment of disease; the age of patients studied; the nature, methodology, duration, and statistical power of the study; and the differences in geography and ethnicity of subjects (2). Indirect but compelling evidence of this association comes from longitudinal cohort studies As PCOS is the most common cause of oligomenorrhea in reproductive-age women, irregular menses have been thought to likely be a surrogate marker of PCOS.

In a community-based longitudinal cohort study of women born between 1946 and 1951 (N = 13,714) over a 20-year follow-up period, women with irregular menstrual cycles had a 20% higher risk of developing heart disease and a 17% higher risk of diabetes than women who had regular menstrual cycles (66).

This study confirms similar data described 2 decades ago in the landmark Nurses' Health Study, where a 14-year cohort prospective questionnaire-based study of 82,439 female nurses who provided information on prior menstrual regularity at ages 20–35 years, followed for incident reports of nonfatal myocardial infarction, fatal coronary heart disease (CHD), and nonfatal and fatal stroke were made. Medical records were reviewed for confirmation. Compared with women reporting a history of very regular menstrual cycles, women reporting usually irregular or very irregular cycles had an increased risk for nonfatal or fatal CHD (age-adjusted relative risks [RR], 1.25 and 1.67, respectively), remaining significant after adjustment for BMI but slightly attenuated when adjusted for hypertension, diabetes, and hyperlipidemia, as these markers of CVD risk themselves were more frequent in women with less regular cycles. Adjustments for confounding variables, including smoking, physical activity, alcohol, and menopausal status, did not change outcomes (67).

Clinical Cardiovascular Disease Events

A systematic review and meta-analysis of controlled observational showed a twofold risk of macrovascular disease for patients with PCOS, including all major definitions of the condition, relative to women without PCOS. This result was unaffected by controlling for BMI. The study concluded that PCOS doubles the risk of CHD and stroke independent of obesity. Another meta-analysis showed that in five studies where the average age was more than 45 years old, the risk of nonfatal stroke was significantly increased, while in six studies, the risk of CHD was insignificantly increased in PCOS compared with controls. In three studies with BMI-matched subjects over age 45, both stroke and CHD risks were greater in PCOS women, though not reaching statistical significance. An additional meta-analysis of five case–control studies and five cohort studies was performed involving a total of 104,392 subjects. PCOS was significantly associated with the increased risk of CVD in both case–control and prospective cohort studies. In this analysis, PCOS was significantly associated with CHD but not with myocardial infarction. A recent study demonstrated a clear-cut increase in stroke risk in PCOS women. A meta-analysis of nine cohort studies found a statistically increased risk of stroke in PCOS patients not entirely explained by higher BMI. There was no increase in all-cause mortality (68–71).

In contrast, an extensive review of studies published from 1990 to 2021, including participants with or without PCOS diagnosed according to the 2003 Rotterdam (without specifying phenotype) or the 1990 NIH criteria, with data on cardiometabolic outcomes, consisted of 31 longitudinal studies with 28,316 participants from four continents. Women were 19 to 49 years old at onset with a follow-up period ranging from 2 to 32 years. Changes in BMI and the risk of coronary heart disease were similar in adult women with and without PCOS. Women with PCOS had a higher risk of type 2 diabetes than their non-PCOS counterparts. It was noted, however, that "evidence for the majority of all other outcomes was conflicting and with inadequate data".

Commenting on the current state of knowledge, the authors note the inadequate information on cardio-vascular morbidity and mortality and focus on women of reproductive age (with the oldest being 69 years), a cohort in whom the absolute rates of CVD events are low regardless of risk factor profiles. Therefore, event rates are low and longer follow-up periods are necessary to determine if there is a true increase in actual CVD risk. CVD risk may be higher if women are menopausal or have had premature menopause.

The heterogeneity of the studies precluded meta-analyses. A substantial number of included studies had no control group. Further, given the role played by phenotypic differences such as the hyperandrogenemic phenotype in cardiometabolic outcomes, longitudinal findings that are PCOS phenotype-specific will clarify true cardiometabolic risk. Homogeneous long-term longitudinal cohort studies reporting key metabolic features of PCOS over time are lacking in the current literature and suggest the need for further investigation (72).

Guidelines for PCOS Diagnosis and Management have been Published by a Number of Organizations

- Androgen Excess/PCOS Society (AES) (73, 74)
- Endocrine Society (ES) (75)
- American Association of Clinical Endocrinologists, American College of Endocrinology, Androgen Excess and PCOS Society (41, 42)
- American College of Obstetrics and Gynecology (ACOG) (76)
- Pediatric Endocrine Society (77)
- American Association of Family Physicians (AAFP) (78)
- International PCOS Network (79, 80)

Given the heterogeneity of presentation and frequency of DM and MBS in background populations, it is not surprising that guidelines and recommendations from different bodies may be somewhat different, depending on their perspective.

The AES, which considers hyperandrogenism a sine qua non for the diagnosis, emphasizes the critical link between it and lipid and glycemic risk and the importance of screening for these risk factors.

The ACOG, not surprisingly, focuses its guidelines on reproductive consequences and their management, most recently endorsing letrozole as a first-line treatment.

AACE/PCOSA guidelines are comprehensive, emphasizing pathophysiology as a determinant of clinical and therapeutic issues.

AAFP guidelines outline findings in other guidelines and provide practical advice for clinicians. The international guidelines of the International PCOS Network, authored by a consortium of 3,000 people from 37 countries, including experts in various fields, multiple societies as well as consumers, are somewhat more flexible in accommodating differences in regional or ethnic likelihood of various components, e.g., hirsutism, hyperglycemia, and hypertension. These comprehensive guidelines are divided into sections regarding all aspects of the syndrome and transparency in evidence used to support the recommendations, which are very specific.

Unlike the AES, ES, and AACE/PCOSA guidelines, the international guidelines recommend screening for metabolic syndrome and dysglycemia in young women only if obese, with follow-up determined by risk. They also state assessment of biochemical hyperandrogenism is recommended only when signs of clinical hyperandrogenism are missing or unclear. They emphasize the need for more accurate standardized laboratory testing of androgen levels in women. They do not recommend routine testing of 17-OHP to rule out CAH.

Despite these differences, there is now consensus regarding diagnostic criteria, recognizing the pitfalls of sonography, especially in adolescents, and recommending against its use in that age group for diagnosis. The link between PCOS and insulin resistance and its consequences is recognized by all groups, with the understanding that not all women fit in this category and that further genomic information as well as more accurate measurements will be helpful in the future in determining recommendations for screening, diagnosis, and treatment.

Evaluation of Guidelines

A review of the recommended PCOS assessment criteria from the 2018 international evidence-based guidelines highlights the need to optimize the diagnosis of PCOS. In particular, it notes the need to standardize terms including the definition of oligomenorrhea, the clinical evaluation of hirsutism (as opposed to hypertrichosis), and its variation by ethnicity, variability in measurement of androgen level by age and laboratory methods, and sonographic features (especially during the first 8 postmenarchal years (81).

Two semiquantitative analyses of guidelines have been published.

The guidelines were evaluated by mapping clinical recommendations in each guideline and assigning them to prespecified domains: diagnosis in adolescents and adults; lifestyle interventions; management of menstrual irregularity, hirsutism, acne, and infertility; and risk assessment for metabolic disease, cardiovascular disease, mental health, and cancer.

The methodological quality of 23 guidelines organized into six domains (scope and purpose, stakeholder involvement, rigor of development, clarity and presentation, applicability, and editorial independence) were scored according to set formulas.

Guidelines were mostly focused on screening for and managing metabolic disease (12/13, 92%), followed by cardiovascular risk assessment (10/13, 77%). Mental health (8/13, 62%) and diagnosis in adolescents (7/13, 54%) were the least reported domains. Most clinical practice guidelines (CPGs) had a high quality for scope and purpose description (12/13, 92%), while stakeholder involvement and applicability of recommendations to clinical practice were appropriate in only two CPGs (2/13, 15%). Inconsistency was found in recommendations on PCOS diagnosis in adolescents, optimal lifestyle interventions, hirsutism and acne treatments, interventions to reduce the risk of ovarian hyperstimulation syndrome, the frequency and screening criteria for metabolic and cardiovascular disease, and optimal screening tools for mental health illness in women with PCOS (82).

Another analysis from China used an assessment tool, the RIGHT checklist, which contains 22 requirements organized into 7 sections with a total of 35 items: basic information (6 items), background (8 items), evidence (5 items), recommendations (7 items), review and quality assurance (2 items), funding and declaration and management of interest (4 items), and other information (3 items). Two authors independently assessed the adherence of each PCOS clinical guideline with the RIGHT checklist, and a yes indicated full reporting of necessary information, whereas a no indicated partial or no reporting. High quality was determined if the yes responses were >70%, medium quality if they were 40% to 70%, and low quality if they were <40%. Assessment by this method revealed that the reporting quality varied among guidelines. Low-quality items were the processes of evidence decision and the declaration of funding in most included CPGs (83). This novel guideline evaluation approach highlights the overall lack of high-quality evidence to make specific consistent recommendations, as well as the various issues most relevant to specific societies.

Future Investigation

Because of the limited data regarding normative cutoffs for the diagnostic features in different subpopulations, leading to inconsistent study populations affecting diagnostic features and ultimately clinical outcomes, a systematic review is proposed. In an attempt to further quantify and characterize participants in studies to better distinguish PCOS from non-POS patients, by the creation of an international database of de-identified subjects with variables to include directly assessed modified Ferriman–Gallwey scores; menstrual cycle lengths; follicle number per ovary, ovarian volume, and AMH; and circulating androgens, including total testosterone (TT), free testosterone, bioavailable testosterone, free androgen index (FAI), androstenedione (A4), and DHEAS. Normative ranges and cutoffs will be defined using cluster analysis. It is hoped that this will provide much-needed differentiation among subjects and lead to further clarity in subsequent studies (84).

MENOPAUSE

Menopause is defined as a period of amenorrhea lasting 12 months or longer in women with previous menses. Laboratory studies show FSH and low AMH, reflecting a lack of ovarian inhibin and low follicular reserve, respectively. The average age of natural or spontaneous menopause is 51 years (range 45–55). If menses cease at an appropriate time, with no other extenuating signs or symptoms, no further investigation is required.

Premature menopause is defined as ovarian failure before the age of 40. This may be caused by hysterectomy, although without oophorectomy, menses are absent but ovarian function may remain normal for years afterward. (The distinction may be made by measuring estrogen, FSH, AMH, and inhibin.) There may be a family history of early menopause and early menarche. In addition to surgical menopause, premature ovarian failure commonly is produced by chemotherapy and/or radiation for cancer. Conditions such as chromosomal abnormalities, fragile X syndrome, autoimmune oophoritis, mumps, thyroid, or chronic inflammatory disorders may contribute to early menopause.

Spontaneous menopause is preceded by a transition period – perimenopause – in which estrogen production is declining and erratic, ovulation is less regular or absent, menses may become irregular, and bleeding may be heavier or lighter. This period may last for 2 to as long as 14 years in some women, and 'menopausal symptoms' may be present for many years before final menses. Some women experience few or no symptoms, while in others, the symptoms may be so severe as to be life-altering. The timing and duration of perimenopause may be influenced by lifestyle factors such as smoking, age of onset, race, and ethnicity.

Menopausal vasomotor symptoms include hot flashes, flushing, night sweats, and insomnia. These vasomotor symptoms are caused by cutaneous vasodilation, a result of the lack of negative inhibition of estrogen on hypothalamic infundibular thermoregulatory neurons that are innervated by the KNDy system. Within the KNDy complex, neurokinin binds to the NK3R receptor, dynorphin to kappa opioid receptors, and kisspeptin to its receptors, integrating multiple signals to regulate menstrual function. Estrogen is inhibitory at NK3 receptors and with its decline at menopause, KNDy neurons exhibit hypertrophy and there is dysregulation of the thermoregulatory neurons, leading to increased heat dissipation. Understanding this system has led to the development of novel NK3 receptor antagonists, which may be useful in treatment.

Modifiable risk factors for hot flashes include smoking, a BMI greater than 30, and sedentary behavior. Nonmodifiable risks include maternal history; menopause earlier than age 32; and abrupt menopause from surgery, radiation, or chemotherapy.

Estrogen deprivation causes urogenital atrophy with resulting dyspareunia, dysuria, and more frequent urinary tract infections.

Estrogen deprivation is a well-known cause of bone loss, osteoporosis, and fragility fractures.

Sexual dysfunction, mood disorders, and cognitive issues are often considered menopausal symptoms, though they may be multifactorial in origin and secondary to previously mentioned primary symptoms.

Other asymptomatic pathology in menopause may not be a direct effect of estrogen loss alone but rather that of aging or other disorders, perhaps compounded by estrogen deprivation; this includes cardiovascular disease and cognitive impairment.

It has also been noted that the age of menopause or duration of reproductive years may be related to the risk of T2DM, CVD, all-cause mortality, and cognitive dysfunction, with longer reproductive years having a beneficial effect. This data comes from cross-sectional epidemiologic studies that may suggest association rather than causation (85–88).

Treatment of menopausal symptoms may include estrogen (with progesterone in the presence of a uterus), in various chemical formulations, doses, and routes of administration. Estrogen is nearly always effective in treating estrogen-deficiency symptoms. It has salutary effects on bone. Its benefit in other aspects of menopause (i.e., less clearly estrogen withdrawal symptoms) is more controversial.

The FDA has approved the use of menopausal hormone therapy for the following applications:

1. Treatment of moderate to severe vasomotor such as hot flashes and night sweats associated with menopause.
2. Treatment of moderate to severe symptoms of vulvar and vaginal atrophy such as dryness, itching, and burning associated with menopause. Topical estrogen may be effective for this purpose.
3. Prevention of postmenopausal osteoporosis.

The FDA notes:

(When menopausal hormone therapy is being prescribed solely for the prevention of postmenopausal osteoporosis, approved non-estrogen treatments should be carefully considered. Estrogens and combined estrogen/progestin products should be considered only in women with a substantial risk of osteoporosis that outweighs the potential drug-related risks.)

The FDA has recommended that menopausal hormone therapy should generally not be prescribed to women with the following conditions (89):

1. Current, past, or suspected breast cancer
2. Known or suspected estrogen-sensitive malignant conditions
3. Undiagnosed genital bleeding
4. Untreated endometrial hyperplasia
5. Previous idiopathic or current venous thromboembolism (deep vein thrombosis, pulmonary embolism)
6. Active or recent arterial thromboembolic disease (angina, myocardial infarction)
7. Untreated hypertension
8. Active liver disease
9. Known hypersensitivity to the active substances of menopausal hormone therapy or any of the excipients
10. Porphyria cutanea tarda (absolute contraindication)

Hormone replacement therapy may be administered orally, transdermally, intravaginally, or, less commonly, parenterally. Therapy may consist of estrogen only, either as conjugated equine estrogen (CEE), estradiol, or various synthetic estrogens. Progesterone, either separately or in combination with estrogen, may be synthetic (medroxyprogesterone acetate [MPA]), various steroid congeners, or micronized progesterone. Evidence suggests that transdermal estrogen may produce less risk of thromboembolic disease by bypassing the liver where it can induce thrombogenic proteins. Likewise, intravaginal progesterone might be considered when women have a risk of breast cancer (see later) but still have a uterus and need to have protection from 'unopposed estrogen' to avoid endometrial hyperplasia. Available formulations are listed in reference (90).

Consumers have been told by some sources that compounded 'bioidentical hormones' are superior to pharmaceutical hormone products, despite the lack of any scientific evidence.

The FDA has warned consumers regarding these claims (91):

The FDA is also not aware of sound evidence showing the superiority of compounded BHRT [bioidentical hormone replacement therapy] products over FDA-approved drugs. Likewise, FDA has no information indicating that the side effects and risks of compounded BHRT products are dissimilar to those of FDA-approved drugs. Thus, claims regarding the safety, efficacy, and superiority of compounded BHRT products have not been substantiated by FDA and may mislead patients and practitioners ... The absence of warnings and risk information may be viewed by patients as implicit evidence that compounded BHRT products are safer than FDA-approved drugs, when there is no data to support this conclusion.

The FDA approved a formulation of a pharmaceutically produced estradiol/micronized progesterone oral capsule, which is being termed a bioidentical product. But, unlike compounded products, it must meet FDA standards and oversight (92).

Risks and Benefits of HRT

In addition to being the most effective treatment for vasomotor symptoms and urogenital atrophy, HRT is associated with a lesser risk of colon cancer, although it is not recommended for its prevention. HRT improves bone density and quality, but other non-hormonal therapies are as or more effective and are first line treatment.
HRT benefit in improving libido and sexual performance is controversial, as other factors, including improving dyspareunia and a significant placebo effect may play a role.
In line with current evidence, the US Preventive Services Task Force does not recommend HRT for the prevention of chronic disorders including CVD, colon cancer, cognitive impairment, and osteoporosis (93).

Known risks of HRT include venous thromboembolic disease, gallbladder disease, and endometrial hyperplasia/carcinoma (the latter when estrogen is used without progesterone).
The relative risk of stroke is higher in women taking HRT compared with nonusers, particularly in older age groups, where the absolute risk of stroke is greatest. Multiple studies of various designs suggest that later initiation of HRT, older age, and use of oral as compared with transdermal estrogen increase the risk (94–97).

Breast Cancer

In the Women's Health Initiative (WHI), the most robust long-term prospective randomized controlled trial (RCT), the use of estrogen alone (CEE 0.625 mg) in the 7.2-year intervention phase was associated with a lower risk of breast cancer and breast cancer death (hazard ratio [HR] 0.55 compared with placebo), even in the long-term 18-year follow-up period. Although the number of users was smaller in this study, using different doses of CEE or using oral estradiol or transdermal estradiol there was no difference in this comparative risk.

The addition of progestin (MPA 2.5 mg) to (CEE) estrogen increases the risk of breast cancer, even in the prolonged 18-year follow-up after the 5.6-year intervention phase, with an HR 1.44 for death from breast cancer compared with placebo (98).

The use of progestins other than MPA (used in WHI) has been associated with a lesser risk of breast cancer in some observational studies of lower power than the WHI. The use of combined estrogen–progestin conferred a greater risk than sequential regimens. Some studies have noted an amplification of risk related to older age and duration of therapy (99–102).

For a more detailed description of these studies, see Cobin et al. (2).

Cognitive Function

The use of HRT in the development of cognitive decline has shown conflicting results. Cumulative knowledge from multiple studies of various design suggest that HRT is likely not deleterious to cognitive function in younger recently postmenopausal women with low inherent cardiovascular risk. However, for older women, those with diabetes, or those with inherent cardiovascular risk, long-term use of HRT or those already developing early dementia may be more adversely affected (103).

A recent study confirmed earlier findings that early menopause itself is associated with greater dementia risk, with greater tau deposits on PET scans, but only if elevated beta-amyloid deposits were already present. Younger initiation of HRT use did not affect tau levels, while delayed initiation was associated with greater risk (104).

A promising strategy was reported in 2023. A longitudinal study featured 1,906 healthy persons in 10 European countries with no demonstrable dementia, categorized by APOE4 and non-E4 genotypes and HRT use, type, and duration. The study measured brain volumes in areas significant for cognition, as well as the performance of standardized cognitive testing. The study found that HRT introduction is associated with improved delayed memory and larger entorhinal and amygdala volumes in APOE4 homozygotes only (who are at higher risk of dementia at baseline), especially when introduced early. The authors postulated that some of the discrepant findings of HRT effect on cognition in previous studies may be ascribed to different APOE genotypes and the age of HRT initiation, and suggested that APOE genotype testing may present an opportunity for more selective personalized targeted therapy (105).

Since these recent studies require further investigation, prudent guidance would suggest against HRT use in at-risk individuals, but reassurance in younger, low-risk individuals who require HRT for symptom relief in early menopausal years.

Diabetes

Estrogen deficiency itself is not associated with an increased risk of diabetes. As women age, however, insulin resistance, metabolic syndrome, and diabetes become more prevalent. The use of HRT, by any route and any formulation, has yielded overall neutral results with respect to glucose intolerance in many trials, despite a small increase or decrease in risk in some subpopulations, which did not persist with longer follow-up (106, 107).

Cardiovascular Disease

Although HRT has been shown to lower LDL, raise HDL, and raise triglycerides, the overall effect on CVD and mortality has now been explored in multiple significant clinical trials, the most robust of which has been the ongoing WHI.

In the WHI, a series of prospective double-blind placebo-controlled trials, the effect of HRT on cardiovascular health is beneficial or at least neutral if given to women within 10 years of menopause onset or less than 60 years old, while in older women further removed from menopause onset, there is an increased risk, at least in the intervention phase of the trial. Over a longer observation period, however, the risk of CVD equalized between HRT-treated and placebo groups, likely the result of aging.

Over an 18-year follow-up of women, in the WHI trial, age 50–79 treated with CEE/MPA or CEE alone for a median of 5.6 and 7.2 years, respectively, there was no increase in CVD, cancer, or all-cause mortality (108–110).

The use of HRT in women with MBS is associated with greater CVD risk than in treated women without MBS (111).

Subsequent and ongoing studies examining differences in CVD surrogate outcomes, including cardiovascular disease itself, breast cancer, and other outcomes with the use of formulations of estrogen and progestins other than CEE/MPA, have been smaller non-RCT, epidemiologic, observational, and unlikely to ever be as statistically robust as the large WHI RCT, leading to inconclusive outcomes regarding risk/benefit profiles. Nonetheless, the trend to use pure estradiol and micronized progesterone transdermally has significant advocates among experts (112–114).

Alternatives to HRT

When hormonal therapy to treat menopausal symptoms is medically contraindicated or unacceptable to patients, several nonhormonal treatments are available. Some, such as SSRIs, gabapentin, clonidine, and SERM–estrogen combination, have been formally studied.

In a double-blind RCT with the strategy to minimize the placebo effect, the SSRIs escitalopram and venlafaxine were compared with estradiol and were found to have equal benefit in reducing hot flashes, with all conferring modestly improved sleep. Other SSRIs and SNRIs have also been effective (115).

In breast cancer patients using tamoxifen, fluoxetine and paroxetine should not be used, as they inhibit the effect of tamoxifen (116).

Both gabapentin and pregabalin in relatively high doses have shown benefit in reducing hot flashes, compared with placebo. Their side effect of causing drowsiness may make bedtime administration useful (117).

Clonidine has modest effects in reducing hot flashes compared with placebo in 39 studies reviewed by a literature search, although a significant placebo effect was noted in these studies (118).

Adverse effects of nonhormonal therapy included somnolence, dizziness, hypotension, and dry mouth for clonidine; weight gain, reduced appetite, nausea, sleepiness, and sweating with SSRIs; and constipation, headache, and somnolence with gabapentin (119).

A combination of bazedoxifene, a selective estrogen receptor modulator, and CEE is effective in treating hot flashes and reducing fracture risk. Vaginal dryness is improved. No progestin is necessary, as endometrial hyperplasia does not develop. There is a risk of venous thromboembolic disease and stroke (120).

A new drug, fezolinetant, a nonhormonal selective neurokinin 3 receptor (NK3R) antagonist blocks binding of neurokinin B to the KNDy neurons to restore normal sensitivity of the thermoregulatory center in the hypothalamus. It has been shown to have significant efficacy in reducing moderate to severe vasomotor symptoms in a phase 3, double-blind placebo-controlled RCT including a diverse population of 527 otherwise healthy women in 97 international settings. In the treated population, symptoms abated in as little as one week and were significantly different from placebo at 4 and 12 weeks with efficacy persisting for the full 52 weeks of the trial. Side effects were rare, including headache and mildly elevated liver function tests, which reversed with discontinuation. Recent approval by the FDA has now made this treatment option available for the management of vasomotor symptoms (121–123).

Nonprescription 'Herbal' Remedies

Phytoestrogens are sterol molecules with weak estrogenic activity, which include isoflavones derived from plants including soy and red clover. They are available over the counter in concentrated nutraceuticals. They are not FDA regulated and may vary in their estrogen receptor agonist/antagonist properties. They are moderately effective in controlling vasomotor symptoms in some women. In vitro and animal studies have shown growth promotion in breast tissue and breast cancer tissue, but there has been no evidence of initiation or growth promotion in human breast cancer. Because of this potential, however, isoflavones are not recommended for women with or at high risk for breast cancer.

Isoflavones may impact thyroid function, reducing thyroid hormone synthesis, secretion, and binding to transport proteins, especially in the iodine-deficient state. In patients taking exogenous thyroid hormone, isoflavones and especially soy may interfere with its absorption. Neonates and people with subclinical hypothyroidism may be at greater risk of these effects (124).

Black cohosh is an unregulated herbal supplement available without a prescription, which has variable efficacy in treating vasomotor symptoms. Its mechanism of action may or may not be via estrogenic effects. A review and meta-analysis of human studies, which included 14 RCTs, 7 uncontrolled trials, and 5 observational studies, reported conflicting efficacy data. Overall, black cohosh showed a response when compared with baseline but not when compared with placebo (125). A Cochrane review found insufficient evidence to recommend its use (126). Its use is strongly contraindicated in women with breast cancer or at high risk for it. Liver toxicity has been reported, placing it in a 'do not use' category overall (127).

Other agents including Chinese herbs and primrose oil are available, but no high-quality studies support their efficacy.

Nonmedical interventions such as yoga, acupuncture exercise, and mindfulness are of uncertain benefit, while cognitive behavioral therapy may be of benefit.

Guidelines

With the accumulation of robust data from multiple trials, particularly the WHI but including other observational and epidemiologic studies, there is wide concordance among experts represented by multiple specialty societies. These conclusions inform recommendations for the use of HRT to alleviate vasomotor and genitourinary symptoms, with demonstrated safety in women under the age of 60 and/or less than 10 years from menopause with no inherent risk factors. Guidelines warn about contraindications to HRT as set forth by the FDA and inform about possible risks of HRT. HRT may carry a greater risk of CVD and stroke in older women. Risks of HRT including VTE and breast cancer (with combination therapy) are noted. Each guideline mentions the possible differences in outcomes with various formulations, doses, and routes of administration, as well as notes where strong evidence is lacking. HRT is not recommended for the prevention of chronic disease. Menopausal symptoms may be managed by alternative therapies rigorously studied and approved by the FDA, while unregulated and/or ineffective interventions are not recommended. All guidelines stress the importance of individualization of therapy and communication among women and their physicians.

Please see the specific guidelines from the following specialty societies:

American Association of Clinical Endocrinologists and American College of Endocrinology (89)
American College of Obstetrics and Gynecology (128)
North American Menopause Society (129)
The Endocrine Society (130)
French College of Gynecologists and Obstetricians (131).

MALE HYPOGONADISM

Masculinization is mediated by testosterone production in the testes and its action via androgen receptors in susceptible tissues. These effects include anabolic actions on bone, cartilage, and muscle; facilitation of pubertal growth spurt; maturation of external genitalia; and normal sperm production. Testosterone affects prostate growth and growth of beard and body hair, and permits scalp hair loss in genetically susceptible males.

Differentiation of the primordial gonad into a testis requires the presence of testis differentiating factors (SRY gene present on the Y chromosome), allowing differentiation of primordial cells into Sertoli cells, which, via multiple transcriptional regulators, cause differentiation of testosterone-producing Leydig cells. Regulation of testosterone is stimulated by pituitary LH, while sperm production in the seminiferous tubules is stimulated by FSH. Sertoli cells produce inhibin, which reduces hypothalamic GnRH and selectively reduces FSH. The KNDy neuron system in the hypothalamus regulates gonadotropin secretion, responding to input from other brain centers as well as feedback from testosterone, DHT, estradiol, and inhibin.

In peripheral tissues, testosterone is converted to estrogen by aromatization or to dihydrotestosterone, the active hormone in most target tissues, by 5-alpha reductase.

Primary hypogonadism, or testicular failure, may be the result of the lack of testicular tissue, enzymatic defects in testosterone synthesis, or its action. These may be congenital as a result of genetic abnormalities or acquired as a result of physical, radiation, or chemical damage, disease, or aging.

Secondary hypogonadism is the result of inadequate stimulation of the testis by pituitary gonadotropins and may be due to congenital or acquired disorders of the hypothalamic–pituitary system.

Androgen receptor defects may cause either a complete failure of masculinization of the male fetus (which then appears female) or partial failure resulting in ambiguous genitalia.

The clinical manifestations of hypogonadism depend upon the timing of its onset as well as its severity, individual susceptibility, and personal clinical concerns.

Problems occurring in the first trimester of intrauterine life result in ambiguous genitalia, while those beginning during the third trimester may cause cryptorchidism and microphallus. Male hypogonadism in the postnatal prepubertal period results in failure of development of the phallus and scrotal rogation, as well as failure of development of secondary sexual characteristics (male voice, muscle mass, beard, and body hair), eunuchoidal proportions (due to failure of epiphyseal closure), and reduced bone mass, as well as gynecomastia.

Postpubertal hypogonadism results in diminished libido, erectile dysfunction, and variable degrees of reduction in male hair distribution. Low testicular volume and abnormal texture may be noted. Gynecomastia may be present. Bone density and muscle mass may be reduced. Low 'energy' and measurements of physical stamina have been reported. Hypogonadism in the male has been linked to cardiovascular disease via poorly understood mechanisms.

Primary Hypogonadism: Congenital

In Klinefelter's syndrome, a chromosomal nondisjunction results in the XXY genotype, resulting in small firm testes with reduced seminiferous tubules, low sperm count, reduced testosterone production with failure of normal pubertal male secondary sexual characteristics, and infertility. Body habitus is eunuchoidal with long extremities due to failure of epiphyseal fusion during growth.

At birth, the syndrome may be suspected with a micropenis, hypospadias, or cryptorchidism. However, delayed diagnosis may occur:

(1) Teenage boys may present with delayed puberty, failure of secondary sexual characteristics, disproportionate growth of limbs, and gynecomastia.
(2) Learning disabilities and personality disorders may be present.
(3) Adult men often present with infertility and are noted to have small, fibrotic testes with azoospermia and androgen deficiency. The latter may result in osteoporosis.
(4) Comorbidities including dental abnormalities, facial abnormalities, increased CVD risk, MVP, varicose veins, COPD, Parkinson's disease, male breast cancer, and autoimmune disorders all have been linked to Klinefelter's syndrome. Although the relative risk is greater, absolute risks are still small.

Klinefelter's syndrome is diagnosed by physical examination, including small firm testes, eunuchoidal body habitus, and gynecomastia. Testosterone and free testosterone are low, LH and FSH are high, and the karyotype shows XXY. Some men have mosaicism, usually with milder clinical features. In this case, constitutional retardation of puberty, a benign self-limited condition with normal gonadotropins and karyotype should also be considered.

Other chromosomal abnormalities may cause inadequate testicular development, including a variety of nondisjunction abnormalities, mixed gonadal dysgenesis with the Y chromosome, or chimerism (2).

Incomplete Androgen Insensitivity Syndrome

This condition is caused by several different X-linked recessive mutations coding for the androgen receptor, resulting in abnormal androgen receptor structure and function. XY individuals present at birth with incomplete masculinization and ambiguous genitalia of variable severity, including hypospadias, micropenis, and bifid scrotum. Testes may be descended, inguinal, or intra-abdominal. Wolffian duct structures are variably developed. Müllerian duct–derived structures are absent or rudimentary, since testes produce

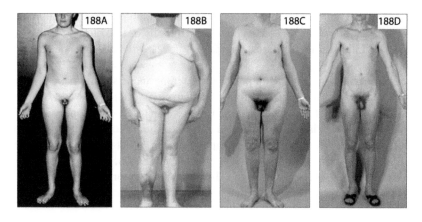

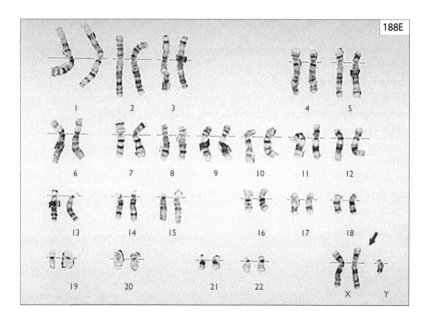

FIGURE 7.15 Klinefelter's syndrome patients: eunuchoid body habitus, decreased pubic hair, gynecomastia, karyotype (2). (Courtesy of Dr. Donald Gordon.)

AMH. Testosterone and LH levels are normal or high. Defective androgen-binding activity of genital skin fibroblasts may be demonstrated.

At puberty, gynecomastia and impaired spermatogenesis occur.

Most individuals with partial androgen insensitivity are raised as males. Treatment consists of genitoplasty, the success of which is dependent upon the amount of tissue available. Breast reduction surgery may be required.

If cryptorchid testes are present, gonadectomy is advised because of the 50% risk of gonadoblastoma development (132, 133).

(Complete androgen insensitivity results in female phenotype; see 'Amenorrhea' section.)

5-Alpha Reductase Deficiency

Deficiency of this enzyme, which converts testosterone to dihydrotestosterone, the active hormone that binds to androgen receptors, is inherited as an autosomal recessive trait with mutations in the SRD5A2 gene. During fetal life and childhood, this results in female or ambiguous external genitalia or a micropenis and hypospadias, despite the XY genotype and high levels of testosterone. Since AMH is present, there is regression of Müllerian ducts (uterus, vagina), while testosterone-dependent Wolffian duct structures are present.

During puberty, when the testicular output of testosterone increases dramatically, the enzyme deficiency is overcome, male external genitalia mature, and virilization occurs. However, male pattern baldness and prostate enlargement, both of which require DHT rather than testosterone, may fail to develop (134).

For individuals raised as girls, am orchidectomy may be advised to prevent virilization and testicular malignancy, while those raised as boys may anticipate virilization at puberty but may require surgical procedures to correct ambiguous genitalia. (See 'Amenorrhea' section, and References 26–31.)

Other causes of congenital primary hypogonadism include cryptorchidism, myotonic dystrophy, and gonadotropin receptor defect.

Acquired Primary Hypogonadism

Acquired primary hypogonadism may result from any damage to the testis, including:

Infections, especially mumps in adulthood
Radiation
Chemicals: suramin, ketoconazole, glucocorticoids, alkylating agents
Environmental toxins
Trauma
Testicular torsion
Autoimmune damage
Chronic systemic illnesses (which may cause secondary hypogonadism)
    Hepatic cirrhosis
    Chronic renal failure
    HIV
    Idiopathic

Secondary Hypogonadism

Congenital Secondary Hypogonadism

The most common form of congenital secondary hypogonadism is Kallmann syndrome, caused by various mutations of the KAL gene (Xp22.3) leading to failure of migration of GnRH neurons from the olfactory area to the hypothalamus resulting in hypothalamic hypogonadism and variable degrees of anosmia. Additional genetically diverse mutations have been described in multiple genes involved in the development and/or function of the hypothalamic gonadotropin regulatory pathway, including kisspeptin and its receptor, and GnRH and its receptor, some associated with nonreproductive developmental anomalies. There is variable inheritance, most commonly X-linked recessive.

Prader–Willi syndrome, caused by deletions of paternally derived critical genes on chromosome 15, is characterized by hypogonadotropic hypogonadism, neonatal hypotonia, and somatic features including narrow forehead, small hands and feet, short height, and light skin and hair. Uncontrollable hyperphagia and obesity ensue, often resulting in T2DM. Until now, management has been supportive only. Ongoing research into the specific genetic alterations and their consequences may offer more specifically targeted therapy, as much as a newly FDA-approved gene replacement treatment for other rare forms of genetic obesity has been reported (135–137).

Bardet–Biedermeier syndrome (BBS) is a rare multisystem genetic disease. In addition to hypogonadism, rod–cone dystrophy, obesity, polydactyly, hypogonadism, cognitive impairment, renal abnormalities,

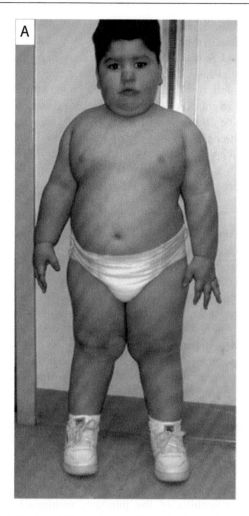

FIGURE 7.16   Young male with Prader–Willi syndrome. (From Butler MG, Angulo MA, Cataletto ME. Prader–Willi syndrome: A review of clinical, genetic, and endocrine findings. *J Endocrinol Invest* 1998;12(38):1249–1263. doi: 10.1007/s40618-015-0312-9.)

and defects in other organs have been described. Multiple genetic abnormalities and wide variability in phenotype have been reported (139).

Recently, the FDA has granted priority review of setmelanotide, a melanocortin-4 receptor agonist for patients with BBS as well as Alström syndrome, another extremely rare genetic disorder associated with hyperphagia and hypogonadotropic hypogonadism. It has already been approved for other rare genetic causes of obesity including POMC, PCSK1, or LEPRECHAUN deficiency (140).

Acquired Secondary Hypogonadism

Acquired secondary hypogonadism is caused by:

PATHOLOGIC: Hypothalamic/ pituitary disease,including tumors, infiltrative disease, and hyperprolactinemia (either by prolactin secreting adenomas, stalk compression or dopamine antagonists.

ACUTE ILLNESS: Since acute illness may cause transient secondary hypogonadism, men should not be investigated for hypogonadism until the inter-current illness has resolved. Low measurements of total testosterone concentrations are required on at least two separate occasions to confirm hypogonadism.

EXOGENOUS CHEMICALS: Opioid induced secondary hypogonadism and withdrawal from inappropriate use of exogenous androgens have become more common in clinical practice.

OBESITY IN YOUTH: Interestingly, given the rising incidence of obesity in children and adolescents, its impact on genital development may be noted early in life, just as gonadal function has been shown to be affected by obesity in older adults, perhaps as a result of insulin resistance.In a cross sectional study of 1130 (833 normal-weight and 297 obese) boys tested for testosterone level and a validated measure of penile length from birth to age 20, at general periodic examination,.. Age, height, weight, BMI, penile length and Tanner stage, gonadotropins and testosterone were recorded. Boys with genetic or endocrine pathology were excluded.

Puberty in obese young children started later and evolved more rapidly at more advanced Tanner stages. Testes volume was slightly smaller across pubertal stages in obese boys. Testosterone levels were approximately 50% lower in obese compared to normal-weight boys at all puberal stages. Penis length and testosterone are strongly related in children during puberty.

Penile growth is significantly decreased (by about 10%) in obese boys, another among the many rea- sons to emphasize healthy nutrition and exercise early in life (141).

HIV: Hypogonadism commonly affects HIV-positive men, especially those with advanced immunosuppression and sarcopenia. The introduction of antiretroviral therapy has lowered the incidence of hypogonadism among HIV-infected men. Free testosterone should be measured because it may be artifactually affected, as SSBG may be elevated in HIV men, beyond the effect of aging, while insulin resistance, obesity, and uncontrolled diabetes lower it.

Many common symptoms of hypogonadism in adult men are nonspecific, including fatigue, low mood, reduced libido, erectile dysfunction, reduced muscle mass, loss of body hair, weight loss, poor sleep, reduced concentration, memory difficulties, and increased risk of osteopenia, though conditions more common in HIV men or their treatment should be excluded.

Primary hypogonadism in HIV infection may be caused by upregulated tumor necrosis factor and interleukin-1, which impair testicular steroidogenesis and cause inflammation resulting in autoimmune testicular damage and the development of antisperm antibodies.

Secondary hypogonadism in HIV patients may be caused by cirrhosis, end-stage renal disease, lym- phoma or syphilis of the pituitary, meningeal or pituitary infection with Mycobacterium tuberculosis, or toxoplasmosis (with or without evidence of deficiency of other pituitary hormones).

Current Endocrine Society clinical practice guidelines suggest at least short-term testosterone therapy as adjunctive therapy in HIV-infected men with weight loss and low testosterone levels to promote gain in muscle strength and lean body mass. Bone density, fracture risk, strength, and quality of life may be improved (142).

Diagnostic Studies in Hypogonadism

Measurement of gonadotropins (LH and FSH) will distinguish between primary and secondary hypogonadism in the face of low testosterone. SSBG and/or free testosterone by equilibrium dialysis should be measured to exclude binding protein abnormalities yielding falsely high or low testosterone values. Prolactin should be measured to rule out hypogonadism caused by hyperprolactinemia. Karyotype analysis will assess genotype. When fertility issues are at stake, semen analysis is required.

An accurate testosterone assay by LC/MS/MS must be used. Reference ranges cross-calibrated by the Centers for Disease Control (CDC) are available.

Management of true hypogonadism should begin at the time of expected puberty in congenital cases and upon diagnosis in acquired cases. In prepubertal boys with proven hypogonadism of any etiology, once a diagnosis is established (and constitutional retardation of puberty excluded) testosterone therapy will result in normal virilization, appropriate growth, and establishment of healthy bone mass and musculature.

Treatment of low testosterone in adult men who have true 'organic' hypogonadism results in improved libido and potency, male body hair distribution, bone density, and lean body (muscle mass). It should be offered to all, excluding those with serious contraindications including prostate or breast cancer.

Testosterone levels should be kept at an age-appropriate normal range. Testosterone may be administered via intramuscular injection, by implantable pellets, and subcutaneously by patch or topical creams. Newly approved oral testosterone undecanoate is safe, unlike previous oral formulations.

Side effects of excess exogenous replacement include polycythemia, lower HDL cholesterol, and exacerbation of benign prostatic hyperplasia. Testosterone replacement does not appear to increase the risk of developing prostate cancer and may be safe in men with previously treated localized low-grade prostate cancer, but there is limited data concerning more aggressive disease. Thus individualization and caution are recommended for treatment in hypogonadal men in that situation. The prostate-specific antigen (PSA) will likely rise from low to normal levels in hypogonadal men treated with testosterone. This is of no concern if it remains in the normal range (143, 144).

Hypogonadism in the Aging Male

It has been reported that in the aging male, testosterone levels fall, while SSBG and gonadotropin levels rise, suggesting testicular failure or compensated testicular failure. Because of the rise of SSBG, the measurement of total testosterone may overestimate free bioactive testosterone (145).

A 2015 cross-sectional study of 1,093 Chinese men divided into 5-year age groups, from ages 20 to 87, however, showed slight increases in SSBG and LH, while total testosterone and calculated free testosterone fell slightly up to age 60, then rose so that levels were equivalent to the youngest men (146).

However, using data from four large epidemiologic studies of nonobese, nondiabetic men, and harmonized free testosterone levels performed by LC/MS/MS confirmed by CDC reference labs, the difference between the lowest and highest testosterone levels differed little by age. This fact suggests that many of the studies performed in aging males may be suspect simply based on assay use alone.

Because of previous conflicting or inconclusive studies, in 2003, an Institute of Medicine panel recommended a coordinated set of clinical trials to determine whether testosterone would benefit older men who had age-related low testosterone levels, including those with clinical conditions to which low testosterone might contribute or which conversely might cause low testosterone.

The T Trials were a series of placebo-controlled, RCTs of 790 men over age 65, with a serum total testosterone concentration of less than 275 ng/dL and symptoms suggesting hypoandrogenism, randomized to receive either testosterone gel or placebo gel for 1 year. To achieve relevance to real-world conditions, possibly contributing 'nongonadal' factors were not a basis for exclusion: 62.9% were obese, many were diabetic, 71.6% had hypertension, and 14.7% had a history of myocardial infarction. The two study groups had similar baseline characteristics, including those comorbidities. Of the testosterone-treated group, total testosterone rose to and was maintained at the normal range for men aged 19–40. Free testosterone, dihydrotestosterone, and estradiol also increased to midnormal for young men. (Critics of these studies have questioned whether young, normal-range testosterone levels are appropriate for older men or represent overtreatment, while others suggest that negative studies may have resulted from inadequate testosterone doses. See later.)

Testosterone compared with placebo resulted in significant effects on all measures of sexual function and some measures of physical function, mood, and depressive symptoms: all small to moderate degrees, consistent with the degree of testosterone deficiency; moderate benefit with respect to sexual function; some benefit with respect to mood and depressive symptoms; and no benefit with respect to vitality or

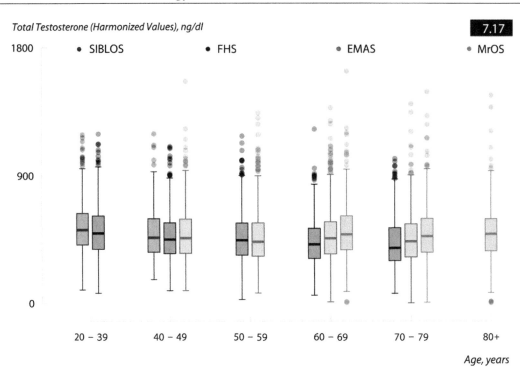

FIGURE 7.17 Box-and-whisker plots showing the distribution of total testosterone levels by decades of age in the four cohorts without harmonization (upper panel) and after harmonization (lower panel). The lower and upper boundaries of the box represent the 25th and 75th percentile values; the line inside the box represents the median. Independent adjustment of each study's measurements to the CDC (as shown in the lower panel) reduces the interstudy variation substantially over that observed in unstandardized measurements (shown in the upper panel). (From Travison, TG. et al. Harmonized reference ranges for circulating testosterone levels in men of four cohort studies in the United States and Europe. *J Clin Endocrinol Metab* 2017 April 1;102(4):1161–1173.)

walking distance. The number of participants was too few to draw conclusions about long-term risks including prostate cancer and cardiovascular outcomes (148).

In a subtrial trial, 211 participants (mean age 71, BMI 31, 86% Caucasian) were treated with the same aforementioned protocol. Spine and hip bone mineral density (BMD) were determined by quantitative computed tomography at baseline and 12 months. Bone strength was estimated by finite element analysis of quantitative computed tomography data. Areal BMD was assessed by dual-energy X-ray absorptiometry at baseline and 12 months. Testosterone treatment was associated with significantly greater increases than placebo in mean spine trabecular volumetric BMD (vBMD), spine peripheral vBMD, and hip trabecular and peripheral vBMD; and mean estimated strength of spine trabecular bone, spine peripheral bone, and hip trabecular and peripheral bone. The estimated strength increases were greater in trabecular than peripheral bone and greater in the spine than the hip. Testosterone treatment increased spine areal BMD but less than vBMD. No fracture data were reported. A larger, longer trial could determine whether this treatment also reduces fracture risk (149).

The T Trial investigators commented, "Unlike in previous studies where there T level was too low or there were not enough subjects, the T Trial trials yielded more statistically and clinically significant results. As expected, hemoglobin levels rose in treated patients. Sexual activity but not erectile function were improved by T in doses which were kept stable." (Although they did not comment on the use of a young normal range.) Testosterone compared with placebo did not improve cognitive function, physical function, or vitality, although using different assessment tools there was a modest improvement in vitality, mood, and depressive symptoms.

In this group of men with a high incidence of CVD and comorbidities, testosterone increased the noncalcified coronary plaque volume, compared with placebo, and was adjusted for the pretreatment scores in each group.

These findings, thought to be more methodologically sound in large RCTs than previous studies, have been used as the basis of many but not all new guidelines (150).

Metabolic Consequences of Hypogonadism and Its Treatment

Conflicting data have reported that low endogenous testosterone levels are associated with higher CVD, atrial fibrillation, and all-cause morbidity and mortality, perhaps in a bidirectional manner. Obesity and metabolic syndrome are strongly associated with low endogenous testosterone and may be responsible for changes in testosterone attributed to aging.

Androgen deprivation in men with prostate cancer has been associated with increased insulin resistance, worse glycemic control, and greater risk of diabetes. Low serum testosterone is associated with the development of metabolic syndrome and type 2 diabetes. SSBG has been inversely correlated with type 2 diabetes.

There is conflicting data on the risks and benefits of testosterone therapy with regard to morbidity (DM, MBS, MACE) and mortality.

Improvement in insulin sensitivity with testosterone treatment has been reported in healthy and diabetic adult men. In studies conducted in men with central adiposity, testosterone therapy has been shown to inhibit lipoprotein lipase activity in abdominal adipose tissue leading to decreased triglycerides (151).

Previously, lifestyle intervention alone had shown no benefit in improving body composition and function and created a concern for weight loss–induced exacerbation of age-related loss of muscle and bone. A 26-week RCT of testosterone versus placebo was conducted in men >65 years old with BMD >30, testosterone <300 ng/ml. A supervised diet providing an energy deficit of 500–750 kCal/day and 1 g/kg body weight, and nutritional counseling were instituted in both groups, plus supervised aerobic and resistance training resulting in 9% body weight loss. The treated group received transdermal testosterone to maintain healthy young (age 19–40) male levels. Testosterone increased aerobic capacity and minimized or prevented muscle and BMD loss that occurs with lifestyle therapy as well as improved sexual function, but did not further improve overall physical function or reduce frailty compared with lifestyle alone. There were no differences in adverse effects between the two groups (152).

In contrast, possibly because of the effect of weight loss, and with a longer follow-up period, a testosterone plus lifestyle program reduced the risk of T2DM in overweight and obese men (12.4% vs. 21% with placebo), with a small improvement in sexual function, but with a greatly increased risk of erythrocytosis and more adverse ischemic heart disease, cardiac arrhythmia syndrome, and benign prostatic hyperplasia, with similar mortality rates (153).

Meta-Analyses

A 2018 review of meta-analyses of placebo-controlled RCT risks and benefits of testosterone replacement found only four studies (of 2,807 reviewed) that met standards for inclusion. These studies included only men who met the ES guidelines for replacement (T <300, at least one definitive hypogonadal symptom). Treatment in all four studies consisted of transdermal testosterone to reach a normal level for age, for at least 12 weeks (12,16,52,12 weeks); one study included only men >65 years old. Only total, not free, testosterone was used and most studies used only one measurement. Within the appropriately treated group, meta-analyses revealed that testosterone treatment was associated with moderate improvement in sexual function. High-quality evidence shows that compared with placebo, testosterone therapy was associated with a small but substantial improvement in sexual desire (libido), erectile function, sexual activity, and sexual satisfaction in hypogonadal men. Treated men had more erythrocytosis but no effect on lower urinary tract symptoms and no statistically significant effect on energy.

None of the trials was long enough or large enough to have sufficient statistical power to determine the effects of testosterone replacement therapy on the incidence of prostate cancer, major adverse cardiovascular events, or bone fractures. The data on performance-based measures of physical function were available only in one trial, precluding a meta-analysis (154).

GUIDELINES

Based on a review of all studies in the aforementioned references, including the meta-analysis reviews, the Endocrine Society published its most current guidelines, still leaving room for physician–patient discussion of symptoms, levels, and individual risks and benefits.

By contrast, other societies' guidelines, while largely in agreement, differ in recommendations regarding indications for screening; testosterone measurement and cut points; classification and therapy in older men with obesity, T2DM, and MBS; and the use of a therapeutic trial of testosterone replacement in equivocal cases. A detailed granular review and comparison can be found in

Al-Sharefi and Quinton (155), which compares several guidelines from 2015 to 2018:

2015 International Society for Sexual Medicine (ISSM)
2017 British Society for Sexual Medicine (BSSM)
2015 Canadian Medical Association Journal (CMAJ)
2018 American Urological Association (AUA)
2018 European Association of Urology (EAU)
2018 Endocrine Society (ES)
2016 Endocrine Society of Australia (AUS)

Topics covered in this review of guidelines are:

Screening criteria – Criteria vary from those that advise testing only for men with specific clinical features of hypogonadism (AUS, ES), to those (CMAJ, AUA, ISSM and BSSM) that suggest screening in situations where the risk of male hypogonadism (MH) is high, even without symptoms. Some take account of the coexistence of aging, obesity, metabolic syndrome, and other comorbidities with MH, without the recognition that the latter may be a result of the former and thus possibly amenable to treatment of the underlying condition, while others recommend therapy with testosterone. Exposure to drugs, radiation, and HIV, along with other conditions, may be criteria for screening. While impaired spermatogenesis may be multifactorial, it is only part of the diagnostic criteria for MH in the ES and AUS, noting normal semen virtually rules out testosterone deficiency. Treatment of these men with normal testosterone but, abnormal semen with exogenous testosterone may exacerbate infertility by suppressing gonadotropins and intratesticular testosterone concentrations necessary for spermatogenesis.

Testosterone cut points – These vary by the guideline for MH. All agree that testosterone should be measured in the morning, but there is disagreement regarding whether the local laboratory normal range should be used rather than a universal cutoff lower limit of normal (see earlier) and what that should be, and whether it should be modified by age or other comorbidities. Even the requirements of fasting or confirming with a second sample are conflicting.

Measurement of bioavailable testosterone – Free testosterone calculation by mass action formula was recommended by the BSSM, ISSM, EAU, and ES. The EAU recommends calculating free testosterone in case of a discrepancy between serum (total) testosterone and symptoms, while the ES recommends the use of calculated free testosterone in the presence of conditions that alter SHBG levels or when serum testosterone levels are in the borderline range. The AUS is opposed to using calculated free testosterone because of its poor correlation to the measurement of free testosterone by equilibrium dialysis. The more recent ES guidelines recommend measuring total testosterone by LC/MS/MS with direct measurement of free testosterone by equilibrium dialysis, using calculated free testosterone only if the former is unavailable (156).

Approach to Low-Borderline Serum Testosterone Level – The ISSM and BSSM suggest that in symptomatic men with repeat serum testosterone in the 8 to 12 nmol/L (230–346 ng/dL) range, measurement of LH, SHBG, and prolactin should be undertaken, with either high levels of LH (indicating Leydig cell impairment) or SHBG affecting total, but not bioactive, testosterone. A therapeutic trial of testosterone (ISSM, 6 to 12 months; BSSM, 6 months) to determine whether this alleviates symptoms is recommended. The CMAJ likewise suggests considering a trial of testosterone replacement therapy for 3 months in the presence of a convincing clinical picture.

Apart from recommending prolactin measurement, neither the ISSM, BSSM, nor CMAJ address in any great depth the importance of identifying and treating potential causes of nongonadal illness (NGI) in men with sexual symptoms, low-normal testosterone and normal LH. Nor is a possible placebo effect from the testosterone trial considered.

The AUA suggests measuring prolactin levels in those with repeat low testosterone and low-normal LH levels (without measurement of free testosterone).

The AUA does not recommend measurement of free testosterone until later in their algorithm, e.g., after prolactin is measured and found to be normal in men with HH (hypothalamic hypogonadism). Since SSBG is affected in so many individuals with aging, obesity, liver disease, etc., it would seem more reasonable to first confirm that bioactive testosterone is indeed abnormal before proceeding with other investigations. They then suggest proceeding to treat with testosterone for MH if prolactin levels are normal, and only recommending further endocrine workup and pituitary magnetic resonance imaging if prolactin is elevated or testosterone <150 ng/dL, to rule out a structural pituitary lesion. (These arbitrary levels may miss cases of HH where prolactin is not elevated, is only minimally elevated, and not considering free testosterone, such as with nonsecretory pituitary adenomas, stalk compression, panhypopituitarism, and less severe impairment of testosterone.)

In addition to structural pituitary disease, investigating other potential causes of HH is recommended by some, but not all guidelines. For example, for hereditary hemochromatosis, a genetic disease causing pituitary iron overload, the ISSM, BSSM, AUA, EAU, and CMAJ provide no guidance on how best to approach men with hypogonadism secondary to opiate or exogenous androgens. The ES recommends only considering testosterone treatment of opiate-induced hypogonadism in men with distressing symptoms and in whom opiate withdrawal is not an option. The AUS stresses that opiates or androgens cause functional and reversible hypothalamic hypogonadism and that cessation of the offending drug should always be attempted first.

Aging, Obesity, and Other Comorbidities – All clinical practice guidelines acknowledge that the prevalence of subnormal serum testosterone levels increases with advancing age (despite the aforementioned recent data), either from age- or comorbidity-related decline in Leydig cell function, or from hypothalamic hypogonadism or nongonadal illness). The implications of this fact and the impact on recommendations for testosterone therapy vary widely and are a source of confusion to both physicians and patients. The ES considers advanced age to be a cause of primary but not secondary organic hypogonadism, whereas the AUS does not consider age to cause any form of hypogonadism and does not necessarily consider a raised LH level in an older man as indicating pathological MH requiring testosterone treatment. The ISSM and BSSM both defined low testosterone associated with comorbidity as a form of age-related MH, requiring treatment the same as those with classical organic hypogonadism.

The CMAJ, ISSM, and BSSM state that obesity, T2DM, and metabolic syndrome are all strongly associated with MH in a bidirectional manner, i.e., while they contribute to low testosterone, administration of testosterone may improve metabolic function, promoting muscle anabolism, lipolysis, and weight loss. Therefore, they recommend screening for hypogonadism in all men with these metabolic derangement syndromes and testosterone treatment for low testosterone associated with obesity, especially in people who are not likely to adhere to lifestyle modification. The AUA recommends screening for all men with diabetes and treatment of low testosterone if found, even if no hypogonadal signs or symptoms are present. (Note: This recommendation would result in a great deal more screening and likely more ambiguous conclusions regarding therapy. None of the guidelines give specific recommendations for the management of hypothalamic hypogonadism or nongonadal illness and MBS.)

The EUA, ES, and AUS all recommend lifestyle modification and addressing the underlying comorbid illness as a first-line intervention, with the EUA also recommending the use of PDE5 inhibitors as a first-line therapy ahead of testosterone for erectile dysfunction in symptomatic men with low serum testosterone. The ES and AUS concur that functional HH/NGI due to obesity can be reversed by addressing excess weight through diet and exercise. The AUS also noted only limited data from high-quality RCTs of testosterone, achieving clinically significant outcomes in older men – usually with chronic disease (such as obesity) – having low testosterone levels but no evidence of pathological MH. The AUS considers low testosterone in this context to be the marker of underlying poor health and does not support prescribing of testosterone in such settings. The T Trials, published after the AUS, were carefully performed placebo-controlled trials in hypogonadal older men with many comorbidities including diabetes, high blood pressure, obesity, and MBS. Their conclusions are reviewed earlier. More recent RCTs (152) have found no benefit in adding testosterone to lifestyle modification.

Testosterone and Cardiovascular Disease

Current guidelines state that there is no credible evidence that testosterone increases the risk of cardiovascular (CV) events, provided that it is prescribed appropriately to men with a well-founded diagnosis of male hypogonadism.

There have been no consistent results evaluating the relative risk of CVD in untreated older hypogonadal men because of differences in study populations, difference in assays, baseline testosterone levels, and study methodology, More importantly, results of morbidity and mortality in older men treated with testosterone have varied widely for similar reasons, as well as treatment dose, levels achieved, comorbidities, and trial length. Despite a multitude of studies, conclusions regarding CVD safety and efficacy in this group of men are therefore difficult to draw and likewise are difficult to form strong evidence for guidelines.

(An excellent detailed tabulation of epidemiological and observational studies, as well as basic science and preclinical animal studies, can be found in Gagliano-Juca and Basaria (157).)

Clinical trials raised CV safety concerns when testosterone was prescribed to older men having a primary diagnosis of age-related frailty or hypothalamic hypogonadism or nongonadal illness associated with obesity, T2DM, or metabolic syndrome. A 50% increased risk of CV thrombosis among men in the top 5% for hematocrit (0.48%), compared with the 25th to 50th centiles has been reported. Testosterone may shorten the cardiac QT interval as a potential contributing factor to CV risk, however, a possible role for testosterone to treat men predisposed to short QT–arrhythmias is currently being investigated.

Current recommendations from various guidelines therefore differ because of the lack of strong consistent evidence.

The ISSM recommends that hypogonadism in men with CVD be assessed and monitored in the same way as in other men, whereas BSSM recommends addressing CV risk factors and secondary prevention in men with established disease before starting testosterone therapy. The EAU suggests a greater need for caution in men with preexisting CVD and, potentially, considering echocardiography before initiation of testosterone.

The AUA recommends counseling patients before starting testosterone, explaining that the evidence is patchy and that it is unknown whether testosterone can increase or decrease the risk of any major adverse CV event. The CMAJ guideline makes a weak recommendation, based on low-quality evidence, that testosterone treatment in men with CVD be restricted to those with stable disease and only after a discussion of the potential risks and benefits. The AUA and ES caution against initiating testosterone since a recent CV or stroke event (3 to 6 months for the AUA and 6 months for the ES), while the AUS suggests the need for caution when using T in older men with known CVD.

The UK Society for Endocrinology has produced a brief position statement on testosterone in older men, discussing the uncertainty and potential risks of testosterone therapy in obese and/or older men with low testosterone. It notes, however, that the majority of older men retain Leydig cell function into old age and that, consequently, withholding testosterone treatment in symptomatic older men with a verified diagnosis of organic or syndromic MH is not warranted.

In the future, more reliable results should be available from the TRAVERSE study, the first randomized, controlled trial that was adequately able to evaluate the incidence of CV events with testosterone replacement therapy. A study sample of 6,000 men at high risk of CVD and with total testosterone of <300 was randomized to receive either testosterone gel or placebo for 5 years, beginning in 2018. The primary endpoint will be time to MACE (nonfatal myocardial infarction, nonfatal stroke, or death from cardiovascular causes). Secondary outcomes include time to occurrence of the composite cardiovascular end point (nonfatal myocardial infarction, nonfatal stroke, death from cardiovascular causes, or cardiac revascularization procedures including percutaneous coronary intervention and coronary artery bypass graft surgery). The findings of this trial will provide more definitive evidence about the cardiovascular safety of testosterone replacement therapy (157).

Indications for Testosterone Treatment

All guidelines affirm that testosterone replacement is indicated with a verified diagnosis of MH, i.e., the presence of characteristic symptoms combined with the unequivocal biochemical finding of low testosterone. According to the ES and AUS, hypogonadal men with a known organic pathologic hypogonadism, either primary or secondary, should be treated, absent contraindications. Some guidelines (particularly the ISSM, BSSM, and CMAJ) apply significantly lower thresholds for treatment and endorse trials of testosterone treatment with symptoms conceivably due to male hypogonadism, even when biochemistry is not entirely supportive, or potentially due to nongonadal illness.

None of the guidelines consider a high LH level, indicating a defect of Leydig cell function and physiological nongonadal illness or inappropriate sample collection time as a cause of lower serum testosterone.

The AUS emphasizes the importance of searching for organic pathologic causes of low testosterone.

Testosterone treatment is not generally recommended by the ES or AUS for men who have an intrinsically intact hypothalamic–pituitary–thyroid axis, but suppressed function due to other functional causes (e.g., obesity or other comorbidity). The ES defines these men as having functional MH, whereas the AUS does not consider them as having true hypogonadism at all.

In contrast, other guidelines do not differentiate between organic/classical/pathological MH and functional HH/NGI in terms of indications for treatment.

Aging, obesity, metabolic syndrome, and other comorbidities are acknowledged by all societies as a cause of low testosterone. But their approach to the significance of this, its pathophysiology, and the need for therapy is very divergent. The ES states that elevated LH denotes an age-related decline in Leydig cell function, while the AUS does not consider age to be a cause of any form of hypogonadism and does not indicate that elevated LH is not pathologic or requires testosterone replacement. The ISSM and BSSM regard low testosterone as age-related hypogonadism, even while recognizing that it may be due to comorbid conditions, and recommend treatment the same as organic/classical male hypogonadism.

The ES allows clinicians to individualize the decision to treat or not to treat with T based on careful consideration of the severity of symptoms, the degree of T deficiency, the confounding influence of the comorbid illness, patient preferences, and the uncertainty of the risks and benefits of testosterone therapy.

The authors of this cited guideline (157) stated that this recommendation "leaves open the possibility for prescribing T based solely upon patient expectations".

A careful reading of the ES recommendation, however, considers patient preference only in the setting of meeting other criteria, i.e., some older men with low testosterone counseled carefully may decide that the potential risks of therapy outweigh the benefits, especially in light of the unresolved issue of cardiovascular risk, while other men, particularly those with very low testosterone and distressing symptoms may decide that current benefit might outweigh the long-term risk.

The AUA offers the criticism that the ES does not recommend treatment for men over 65 years old. To this author, however, this criticism seems an oversimplification because the ES recommendation for older men is modified by clinical evaluation of hypogonadal symptoms and the degree of low testosterone as well as suggesting individualization and a possible therapeutic trial. This more nuanced recommendation takes into account the frequency of abnormal SSBG, the higher prevalence of obesity morbidities associated with low testosterone, and the unsettled question of CVD risk of treatment in older men, while allowing a discussion of therapy in men who have low free testosterone and low testosterone symptoms. https://doi.org/10.1038/s41443-021-0047

Testosterone Treatment and Androgen-Sensitive Cancers

All guidelines emphasize precautionary baseline PSA measurement and digital rectal examination (DRE), with periodic repeats during treatment. The ES advises against testosterone in men with prostate cancer, palpable prostate nodule, or induration; PSA level ≥4 ng/mL (or ≥3 ng/mL if combined with a high risk of prostate cancer such as African American origin and those with first-degree relatives with having prostate cancer); and without urological evaluation. In relatively younger men (age 55 to 69) with a life expectancy of ≥10 years or men aged 40 to 69 who have high risk, the ES suggests shared decision-making after discussing risks and benefits, and potential prostate monitoring. The ES advises that all men receiving testosterone treatment should have an urological evaluation upon the detection of a prostate nodule or induration, or a ≥40% rise in PSA level over the first year of treatment.

Most guidelines counsel against testosterone in patients with metastatic or locally advanced prostate cancer (PCa), any form of male breast cancer, and in patients at high risk for recurrent prostate cancer. The ISSM and AUA recommend a mutual decision to be made between the patient and the physician taking into account benefits versus the potential risks. The BSSM, EAU, and CMAJ recommend offering testosterone to symptomatic men with a history of treated localized low-risk PCa (Gleason score <8, stages 1–2, preoperative PSA levels <10 ng/mL, and not within 1 year of treatment with curative intent) and without evidence of active disease (based on measurable PSA level, DRE result, and imaging evidence of metastatic disease). The EAU advises that testosterone can be cautiously offered to patients who underwent brachytherapy or external beam radiation for low-risk prostate cancer.

Monitoring Testosterone Therapy

Testosterone levels, PSA, hematocrit, DRE, and symptoms should all be monitored while patients are being treated. The AUA in particular recommends a DRE, while others do not, suggesting that non-urologists may not be comfortable with the examination and/or that PSA will yield adequate information. To avoid testosterone-induced erythrocytosis, many guidelines counsel against initiating testosterone in patients with baseline elevated hematocrit, but advise it should be monitored during treatment even with a normal baseline (155).

For the sake of simplicity, recommendations from the Endocrine Society guidelines, most commonly used in the USA, are quoted (158), while recognizing that questions can be reasonably asked when comparing the other guidelines reviewed earlier.

Endocrine Society Guidelines

This guideline, which is the most commonly utilized in the United States, combines a practical approach to ensure that testosterone therapy is prescribed only in appropriate patients, by limiting its prescription to only those men who are hypogonadal by symptomatology and definitively low serum testosterone concentrations in accurate assays. Testosterone should be measured fasting in the morning and repeated for confirmation. Free testosterone by equilibrium dialysis and/or correction with a formula accounting for SSBG concentrations should be used. Most importantly, this guideline strongly recommends TESTING TO DETERMINE THE ETIOLOGY OF THE HYPOGONADISM, a feature not included in some of the other guidelines. The therapeutic goal is a testosterone in the mid-normal range. As in all guidelines, contraindications to testosterone therapy include breast or prostate cancer, or a high risk of the same, elevated PSA which has not been investigated, elevated hematocrit, untreated severe obstructive sleep apnea, severe lower urinary tract symptoms, uncontrolled heart failure, myocardial infarction or stroke within the last 6 months, or thrombophilia. The importance of patient counseling and regular follow-up to measure testosterone, hematocrit, PSA and symptoms is highlighted.

GYNECOMASTIA

Enlargement of the male breast is due to an elevated estradiol/testosterone ratio causing stimulation of normal breast tissue proliferation. This may be due to various alterations in production and/or clearance of both hormones, or changes in SSBG, as testosterone and DHT have a greater affinity for SSBG than does estradiol. Therefore, as SSBG rises with aging, free testosterone falls more significantly relative to free estradiol (159).

Though gynecomastia is usually bilateral, it can be asymmetric or unilateral, raising the differential diagnosis of male breast cancer (which is rare). True gynecomastia should be differentiated from breast enlargement caused by obesity. Usually, palpation can differentiate between the two. Gynecomastia occurs physiologically in pubertal boys in as many as 50% with careful examination. It is usually mild and self-limited. In older men, gynecomastia may be a manifestation of low testosterone levels caused by aging and or metabolic syndrome (see earlier). Pathologically elevated estrogen levels may be seen in liver disease, renal failure (because of decreased clearance), and excess estrogen production in tumors of the adrenal or testis.

Medication-induced gynecomastia is very common.

Management of gynecomastia depends upon the timing, severity, and associated signs and symptoms. In adolescents with mild gynecomastia and otherwise normal pubertal development, reassurance is all that is required. In aging men, evaluation of testosterone/estradiol and prolactin should be performed

TABLE 7.3   Mechanisms of Drug-Induced Gynecomastia

MECHANISM	DRUGS
Increases estrogenic activity or increases estrogen production	Anabolic steroids, conjugated and synthetic estrogens, hCG, digoxin, clomiphene, phenytoin, diazepam
Decreases androgen activity or decreases androgen production	Ketoconazole, metronidazole, cimetidine, ranitidine, omeprazole, spironolactone, flutamide, methotrexate, isoniazid, penicillamine
Increases androgen clearance	Alcohol
Causes hyperprolactinemia	Metoclopramide, phenothiazine, haloperidol
Increases SHBG	Phenytoin, diazepam

Source: Adapted from Ismail A, Barth J, Review: Endocrinology of gynaecomastia. *Ann Clin Biochem*, 2001;38(66):596–607.

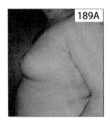

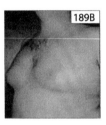

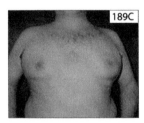

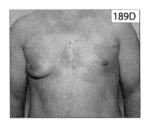

FIGURE 7.18   (A–C) Bilateral gynecomastia. (Courtesy of gynecomastia.org.) (D) Unilateral gynecomastia (2). (Courtesy of Dr. Donald Gordon.)

to exclude true pathology. If this is not found, counseling and reassurance are adequate. In men of all ages, the presence of significant hypogonadism, hyperprolactinemia, or other syndromic features should prompt further investigation and treatment as necessary. In those men whose gynecomastia is severe, uncomfortable, or psychologically stressful, surgical breast reduction may be performed.

HYPERPROLACTINEMIA

Prolactin, a peptide hormone secreted by lactotroph cells in the anterior pituitary gland, is predominantly regulated by tonic inhibition via hypothalamic dopamine release. Normal stimuli for secretion include TRH, GnRH, and vasoactive intestinal peptide, and nipple stimulation via reflex neurogenic input to the hypothalamus. Estrogen amplifies stimulation. Clinically, the most important function of prolactin is development of the mammary gland and milk secretion, although many other functions have been found that are outside the scope of this section.

Physiologically prolactin levels rise during pregnancy and lactation. Pharmacologic estrogenic stimulation, e.g., OCPs, causes appropriately elevated prolactin.

Etiology

Inappropriate excess production of prolactin may be caused by tumors of the lactotrophs or mixed pituitary tumors (cosecreting ACTH or GH) that cause autonomous secretion, or by disruption of the normal inhibitory action of dopamine, either by structural interruption of the pituitary stalk by non-prolactin-secreting pituitary adenomas, non-pituitary tumors, or infiltrative disease. Impaired clearance of prolactin in renal failure may cause elevated levels. Excess stimulation by TRH may be present in primary hypothyroidism. Prolactin elevation may be seen in PCOS and empty sella syndrome, while transient increases may be caused by nipple stimulation, stress, and exercise.

Medication-Induced Hyperprolactinemia

Hyperprolactinemia may be caused by the chemical suppression of dopamine or its action. Agents include dopamine receptor blockers, catecholamine or dopamine depleters, phenothiazine and other neuroleptics, antidepressants, antihypertensives (methyldopa, verapamil), metoclopramide, cimetidine, opiates, and exogenous estrogen.

Clinical Presentation

In females, hyperprolactinemia may present clinically with galactorrhea (inappropriate milk secretion) and/or oligomenorrhea or anovulation, with infertility. Low estrogen levels may lead to osteoporosis. Galactorrhea may be spontaneous and noticeable by the patient or may only be detected with breast expression. Since there are several types of breast secretion, if there is doubt whether the fluid is milk, an oil red stain may be done to demonstrate fat globules that only occur in milk.

In males, hyperprolactinemia may cause hypogonadism (both primary and secondary), impaired libido (possibly by a central mechanism), infertility, and low bone density as a result of low testosterone.

In either gender, large pituitary tumors may cause headaches or visual changes from compression of the optic chiasm.

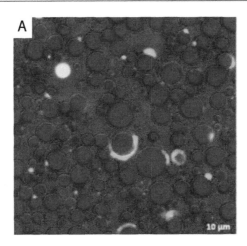

FIGURE 7.19 Human milk fat globules stained with Nile red. (From Post A, De Heijninga B, Actona D et al. A novel infant milk formula concept: Mimicking the human milk fat globule structure. *Colloids Surf B Biointerfaces* 2015;136(1):329–339.)

Measurement of prolactin is therefore mandatory in any of the aforementioned conditions. It is important to beware of pitfalls in measurement (see later) to properly assess clinical importance.

It has been stated that prolactin levels over 150–200 are nearly always a result of secretion from prolactinomas; however, 5% of those with drug-induced hyperprolactinemia had levels over 250, especially with haloperidol, phenothiazines, domperidone, and metoclopramide.

Laboratory Measurement

Immunometric assays are used to measure prolactin. Pitfalls in measurement may be caused by either overestimation because of the presence of big prolactin or underestimation due to the 'hook effect'.

Prolactin circulates in a monomeric chemically active form that binds to the prolactin receptor, causing its clinical effects. Inactive prolactin (including dimeric big prolactin), prolactin aggregates, and prolactin bound to antibodies may also be detected in immunoassays used to measure prolactin. This results in falsely elevated prolactin levels in patients with normal levels of monomeric prolactin, typically in patients with normal physiologic function. PEG (polyethylene glycol) precipitation will remove these large inactive forms. Assays report the percentage of macroprolactin (162).

The hook effect may return falsely low prolactin levels in double antibody 'sandwich' immunoassays. This occurs as a result of excess antigen concentration saturating available binding sites on the bivalent capture and detector monoclonal antibodies preventing the formation of a sandwich complex leading to a paradoxical loss of antigen signal intensity. If the sample is diluted, lowering the concentration of antigen, the hook effect may be resolved. This is particularly important in the case of known pituitary macroadenomas, as prolactinomas are treated differently from other tumors (163).

In well-differentiated pure prolactin-producing adenomas, the level of prolactin generally correlates well with the size of the tumor. Microprolactinomas are usually visible on dedicated high-resolution MRIs, and produce modest prolactin elevations; however, prolactin levels resulting from stalk compression from non-prolactin-secreting pituitary tumors, cystic prolactinomas, or nonpituitary masses (e.g., craniopharyngiomas, gliomas, meningiomas) of considerable size, and infiltration disease may also cause only modest elevations. Recognition of this fact is extremely important, as the decision to image the pituitary–hypothalamic area will depend at least in part upon this information. It should not be assumed that minimal elevations in prolactin indicate a microprolactinoma. Most authorities suggest imaging in nearly all cases of hyperprolactinemia in order not to miss a critical diagnosis.

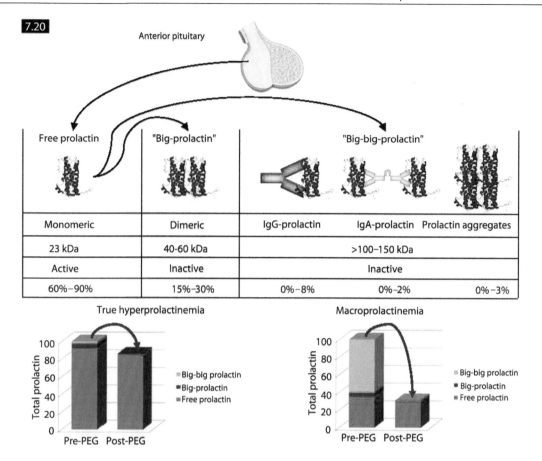

FIGURE 7.20   (From Saleem M, Martin H, Coates P. Prolactin biology and laboratory measurement: An update on physiology and current analytical issues. *Clin Biochem Rev* 2018;39(1):3–16.)

Imaging

Imaging is performed by MRI dedicated to the hypothalamic–pituitary area. It should be noted that occasionally very small microadenomas or lactotroph hyperplasia may not be apparent in even the most high-resolution studies.

Treatment

Not all patients with hyperprolactinemia require treatment. In patients with microadenomas or 'idiopathic hyperprolactinemia' without bothersome galactorrhea with adequate estrogen production and no desire for fertility, or in postmenopausal women, treatment may be withheld. Hypogonadal women or men may be treated with dopamine agonists to lower prolactin and prevent osteoporosis, or if this is not tolerated and/or fertility is not desired, estrogen in women or testosterone in men may be used instead to prevent osteoporosis. No RCTs have compared the efficacy of these treatments on bone. Microadenomas rarely grow and there is no evidence that growth is stimulated by exogenous estrogen or pregnancy. When pregnancy is confirmed in a patient with a microadenoma, dopamine agonists may be discontinued.

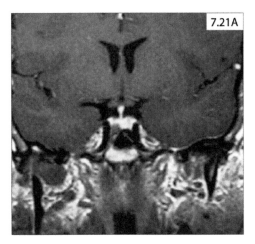
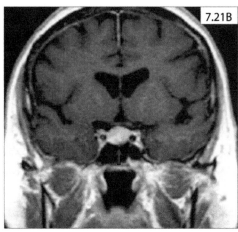

FIGURE 7.21   MRI of the sella showing a prolactinoma. (From Schlechte JA. Clinical practice: Prolactinoma. *N Engl J Med* 2003;349(21):2035–2041.)

Medical Therapy

Cabergoline, a second-generation dopamine agonist, is considered a first-line treatment, with better efficacy and tolerability and longer half-life than bromocriptine. It is taken once or twice a week and lowers prolactin levels to normal in 90% of those treated, usually within several weeks, while shrinkage of pituitary adenomas may take several weeks or months, particularly in large tumors. Visual field defects from macroadenomas may resolve promptly. The clinical consequences of hyperprolactinemia in both males and females resolve. In responsive patients with normal prolactin and no evidence of tumor on MRI, treatment may be continued for 2 years, before a trial of medication discontinuation may be instituted. About 20% will remain normoprolactinemic, while the rest will relapse and require reinstitution of therapy.

Side effects may include nausea and orthostatic hypotension, generally occurring just at the initiation of treatment. Although much higher doses used for the treatment of Parkinson's disease have been associated with valvular heart disease, there is only a questionable increase in mild asymptomatic tricuspid regurgitation in doses used in patients treated for hyperprolactinemia compared with the general population, leading to different guidelines for echocardiogram evaluation in the USA and Europe.

Treatment should be considered for all prolactin-secreting macroadenomas, because of mass effects, especially optic chiasm pressure, loss of other anterior pituitary hormones, and potential for further growth, including during pregnancy. Cabergoline is theoretically safe during pregnancy but has not been approved, so many authorities advise switching to bromocriptine for large tumors where medication is indicated throughout pregnancy. Prolactin levels will normally rise during pregnancy, thus there is no need to measure them. Tumor growth is assessed by clinical exam including visual fields. Routine MRIs are not recommended during pregnancy, but if headache or visual impairment occurs, may be required. Occasionally, pituitary surgery during pregnancy is required. There is controversy regarding the benefit of prepregnancy surgery for macroadenomas (165).

Previous concerns regarding the risk of cardiac valvular disease have been addressed by long-term studies with active echocardiogram surveillance, which has found no evidence of risk, unlike in Parkinson's disease treated with 3 mg/day cabergoline versus 0.5 mg one to two times a week for prolactinomas. In some dopamine agonist-resistant tumors, very large doses, e.g., up to 24 mg/week, have been tried with some success; here echocardiogram surveillance is advised.

After 2 years of successful treatment with normal prolactin and tumor shrinkage, a trial of medication withdrawal may be undertaken. Recurrence rates of 26% to 69% have been reported. If recurrence occurs, it is generally within 1 year, in larger tumors with higher pretreatment prolactin levels. Often there is no increase in tumor size but an elevation of prolactin and hypogonadism requiring resumption of therapy (166, 167).

Dopamine-Resistant Tumors

Dopamine-resistant tumors are defined as a failure to normalize prolactin with maximally tolerated doses, a failure to decrease macroprolactinoma tumor size by 50% (with other guidelines suggesting 30%), while others emphasize a reduction in the height of the tumor (i.e., the risk of chiasmatic pressure), and failure to achieve fertility, absent other causes. Failures occur in 10% of patients with microadenomas and 18% of macroprolactinomas that do not achieve normal prolactin with conventional doses of cabergoline. Resistant tumors are more common in men. The expression of estrogen receptor α is lower in men than in women, and is closely correlated to aggressiveness, in larger and or invasive tumors, and in prolactinomas associated with MEN 1 and AIRP syndromes. Bromocriptine has a failure rate of about 25%, while cabergoline fails in only about 10%. Some particularly aggressive tumors continue to grow and invade surrounding structures, with particular concern for the optic chiasm and cavernous sinuses. Even though these aggressive tumors may cause significant local effects, the definition of pituitary carcinoma is reserved for those with cerebrospinal fluid/systemic metastases and amounts to fewer than 100 cases in the world literature (168).

Histologic features that may be associated with more aggressive behavior include tumor invasiveness presence of more mitoses, Ki-67 index, p53 expression and apoptosis, and the density of somatostatin receptors (169).

The mechanism(s) of drug resistance are incompletely understood. Some tumors have a reduced number of D2 receptors, although apparently with normal binding affinity. No mutations in dopamine receptors have been found. It is postulated that defects downstream affect the regulation of tumor growth and secretion and thus may determine the response to dopamine agonists. Other factors, such as the expression of growth factors (vascular endothelial growth factor [VEGF] and epidermal growth factor [EGF]); the genes regulating invasion, differentiation, and proliferation; adhesion molecules (E-cadherin); matrix metalloproteinase 9; and chromosome abnormalities (chromosomes 11, 19, and 1) have also been correlated with aggressiveness (170).

Epigenetic studies have revealed high levels of methylation in invasive and large pituitary tumors. DNA methyltransferase overexpression has been detected in pituitary tumors, especially in macroadenomas. Methylation differences at CpG sites in promoter regions may distinguish several types of tumors from normal pituitary tissue. Histone modifications have been linked to increased p53 expression and longer progression-free survival in pituitary tumors. Upregulation in citrullinating enzymes may be an early pathogenic marker of prolactinomas. Numerous genes involved with cell growth and signaling show altered methylation status for pituitary tumors, including cell cycle regulators, components of signal transduction pathways, apoptotic regulators, and pituitary developmental signals (171).

After initial surgery and radiotherapy, watchful waiting on maximum-tolerated cabergoline may be reasonable as long as there is no threat to vision or other symptoms. Some authorities use up to 24 mg/week, while being mindful of cardiac valvular risk. If vital structures are jeopardized, repeat surgery is often attempted, with the surgical approach determined by the location and anatomy of the tumors.

Surgery

Surgical treatment is reserved for symptomatic patients; resistant to or intolerant of cabergoline; have macroadenomas but desire subsequent pregnancy; or, rarely, have a cerebrospinal fluid leak or apoplexy. Although microadenomas rarely grow during pregnancy, up to 35% of macroadenomas grow with anatomically, clinically significant effects. Tumor growth during pregnancy may be less likely with medical pretreatment for more than 1 year.

Various transsphenoidal approaches have been used for either initial or repeat surgery. A transcranial approach may be necessary in some cases with threatening superior extension. Success rates are measured by normalization of prolactin, tumor elimination (or debunking), and, in some guidelines, restoration of fertility. Adverse effects of surgery include diabetes insipidus, loss of other anterior pituitary hormones (especially with extensive surgery required for macroadenomas), and, less likely, damage to surrounding tissue, especially the cavernous sinus.

Successful surgery is best predicted by the experience of the neurosurgeon, moderately increased serum prolactin levels (<200 ng/mL), tumor size, and invasiveness. In a literature review involving more than 50 series, initial surgical remission, defined as the normalization of prolactin levels, occurred on average in 74.7% and 34% of patients with microprolactinomas and macroprolactinomas with a recurrence rate of 18% and 23%, respectively. Another report of surgical results from 13 published series, including at least 100 patients, has shown the control of prolactin levels to be achieved in approximately 73% of 1,211 microprolactinomas and 38% of 1,480 macroprolactinomas (165, 167)

Radiation

Radiation as the primary therapy is effective in reducing prolactin in only 30% of patients, with a very long lag period often decades. As an adjunct to medical and surgical therapy, radiation may be added to dopamine-resistant tumors and malignant prolactinomas. Radiation modalities may include conventional external beam radiation, stereotactic methods, and gamma knife, with the latter being preferred because of its more focused beam. Risks of radiotherapy include hypopituitarism: More than 50% of patients receiving pituitary radiotherapy will develop at least one anterior pituitary hormone deficiency within the following decade. Although very rare, cerebrovascular accidents, second brain tumors, and optic nerve injuries have been reported with conventional radiotherapy, the frequency of all increasing over time. Very rarely, encephalomalacia of surrounding tissues has been reported. Because of the narrower focus of gamma knife, the incidence of cerebrovascular accidents and encephalomalacia seems to be less, but the slow onset of action and eventual hypopituitarism are likely the same (172).

Alternative/Investigational Drugs

In patients who have failed conventional medical, surgical, and radiation therapy, alternative medical therapy may be added. Somatostatin analogues have been used. All somatostatin receptor (SSTR) types are present in prolactinomas; SSTR5 was particularly frequent. Trials using octreotide along with cabergoline have not normalized prolactin, but in a few cases have resulted in an 80% reduction and 90% reduction in tumor volume. Pasireotide, a second-generation somatostatin receptor antagonist, has a greater affinity for SSTR5 and shows promise in vitro. Very few patients have been reported, but with normalization of prolactin and either tumor shrinkage or stabilization (173, 174).

Temozolomide has been used with moderate success in 23 prolactinomas and 19 carcinomas resistant to all other therapy. Shrinkage was reported in 76% of patients. Reduced prolactin levels were observed in 75% of patients, while normalization of prolactin was reported in 8%. Temozolomide failure occurred in 20.6% of cases. Most patients exhibited no serious adverse effects (175).

Oral lapatinib, an ErbB1-epidermal growth factor receptor (EGFR)/ErbB2 or human EGFR2 (HER2) tyrosine kinase inhibitor, was tested for 6 months in four aggressive prolactinomas. None achieved the primary endpoint of a 40% reduction in any tumor dimension and normalization of prolactin. Three had stable disease. EGFR/HER2 expression did not correlate with treatment response. Lapatinib was well tolerated and might be an option for otherwise resistant tumors, but more study is necessary (176).

Guidelines

Endocrine guidelines for prolactinoma were published in 2006, 2011, and 2015. Their recommendations are incorporated in the preceding text. The most recently published guideline in 2020 of the European Society of Endocrinology emphasizes the need for histopathologic analysis, including evaluation of Ki-67 for proliferative activity and p53 and mitotic count if Ki-67 is greater than 3% (178). This guideline

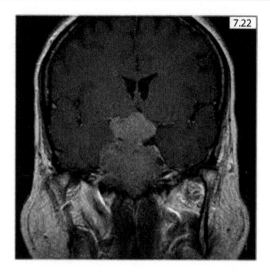

FIGURE 7.22 Invasive pituitary adenoma. (From Chuang CC, et al. Different volumetric measurement methods for pituitary adenomas and their crucial clinical significance. *Sci Rep* 2017;7:40792. doi: 10.1038/srep40792.)

focuses on aggressive tumors and recommends radiotherapy if tumors grow despite surgery and as adjuvant therapy in tumor postsurgical remnants with ominous markers. Temozolomide is recommended as chemotherapy for aggressive tumors and pituitary carcinomas with documented growth, often in combination with radiotherapy.

REFERENCES

1. Lynch KE, et al. Assessment of anovulation in eumenorrheic women: Comparison of ovulation detection algorithms. *Fertil Steril* 2014;102(2):511–518.
2. Cobin RH, Goodman NF, Jain S, Chapter 5, in *Reproductive disorders in evidence based endocrinology*, Camacho, P. et al. ed., 4th edition, pp. 166–265, Wolters Kluwer, Philadelphia, 2020, by permission of author.
3. Dunlop C, Anderson R. The regulation and assessment of follicular growth. *Scand J Clin Lab Investig* 2014;74(suppl 244):13–17.
4. Russell D, Robker R. Molecular mechanisms of ovulation: Co-ordination through the cumulus complex. *Hum Reprod Update* 2007;13(3):289–312.
5. Harrington J, Palmert M. Clinical review: Distinguishing constitutional delay of growth and puberty from isolated hypogonadotropic hypogonadism: Critical appraisal of available diagnostic tests. *J Clin Endocrinol Metab* 2012;97(9):3056–3067.
6. Lee KH, et al. Imperforate hymen: A comprehensive systematic review. *J Clin Med* 2019;8(1):56. Published 2019 Jan 7. doi:10.3390/jcm8010056.
7. Stone SM, Alexander JL. Images in clinical medicine. Imperforate hymen with hematocolpometra. *N Engl J Med* 2004;351(7):e6.
8. Robbins J, Broadwell C, Chow LC, Parry JP, Sadowski EA. Müllerian duct anomalies: Embryological development, classification, and MRI assessment. *J Magn Reson Imaging* 2014;41(1):1–12.
9. Biason-Lauber A, Konrad D, Navratil F, Schoenle EJ. A WNT4 mutation associated with Müllerian-duct regression and virilization in a 46,XX woman. *N Engl J Med* 2004;351(8):792–798.
10. Goldacre M, Seminog O. Turner syndrome and autoimmune diseases: Record-linkage study. *Arch Dis Child* 2013;99(1):71–73.
11. Turner's syndrome with neck webbing and shield chest. (Courtesy of Dr. Donald Gordon.) from ref 2.

12. Levitsky L, Luria AH, Hayes FJ, Lin AE. Turner syndrome: Update on biology and management across the life span. *Curr Opin Endocrinol Diabetes Obes* 2015;22(1):65–72.
13. Silberbach M, et al. Cardiovascular health in turner syndrome: A scientific statement from the American Heart Association. *Circ Genom Precis Med* 2018;11(10):e000048.
14. Dabrowski E, et al. Turner syndrome with Y chromosome: Spontaneous thelarche, menarche, and risk of malignancy. *J Pediatr Adolesc Gynecol* 2020 February;33(1):10–14. doi: 10.1016/j.jpag.2019.08.011. Epub 2019 Aug 26. PMID: 31465855; PMCID.
15. Reiter E, Blethen SL, Baptista J, Price L. Early initiation of growth hormone treatment allows age-appropria-teestrogen use in Turner's syndrome. *J Clin Endocrinol Metab* 2001;86(5):1936–1941.
16. Hogler, et al. Importance of estrogen on bone health in Turner syndrome: A cross-sectional and longitudinal stud using dual-energy Xray absorptiometry. *J Clin Endocrinol Metab* 2004;89(1):193–199.
17. Bakalov V, et al. Bone mineral density and fractures in Turner syndrome. *Am J Med* 2003;115(4):259–264.
18. Cabanes L, et al. Turner syndrome and pregnancy: Clinical practice. Recommendations for the management of patients with Turner syndrome before and during pregnancy. *Eur J Obstet Gynecol Reprod Biol* 2010;152(1):18–24.
19. Marrakchi A, Belhaj L, Boussouf H, Chraibi A, Kadiri A. Pure gonadal dysgenesis XX and XY: Observations in fifteen patients. *Ann Endocrinol (Paris)* 2005;66(6):553–556.
20. Weinberg-Shukron A, et al. A mutation in the nucleoporin-107 gene causes XX gonadal dysgenesis. *J Clin Invest* 2015;125(11):4295–4304.
21. Weinberg-Shukron A, et al. Essential role of BRCA2 in ovarian development and function. *N Engl J Med* 2018;379(11):1042–1049.
22. Gulía C, et al. Androgen insensitivity syndrome. *Eur Rev Med Pharmacol Sci* 2018;22(12):3873–3388.
23. Chauhan P, Rani A, Singh SK, Rai AK. Complete androgen insensitivity syndrome due to mutations in the DNA-binding domain of the human androgen receptor gene. *Sex Dev* 2018;12(6):269–274.
24. Hornig N, et al. Epigenetic repression of androgen receptor transcription in mutation-negative androgen insensitivity syndrome (AIS Type II). *J Clin Endocrinol Metab* 2018;103(12):4617–4627.
25. Nezzo M, De Visschere P, T'Sjoen G, Weyers S, Villeirs G. Role of imaging in the diagnosis and management of complete androgen insensitivity syndrome in adults. *Case Rep Radiol* 2013:Article ID 158484, 6 pages, 2013. doi: 10.1155/2013/158484.
26. Isfort A. 5 alpha reductase deficiency, 2021. *Medscape* https://emedicine.medscape.com/article/924291 -overview.
27. UPtoDate: https://www-uptodate-com.eresources.mssm.edu/contents/steroid-5-alpha-reductase-2-deficiency ?search=5%20alpha%20reductase%20deficiency&source=search_result&selectedTitle=1~12&usage_type =default&display_rank=1#H693108660.
28. Kumar G, Barboza-Meca JJ. 5 alpha reductase deficiency. [Updated 2022 October 17]. In: StatPearls [Internet], Treasure Island (FL): StatPearls Publishing; 2023 Jan. https://www.ncbi.nlm.nih.gov/books/NBK539904/.
29. Kang HJ et al. The first successful paternity through in vitro fertilization-intracytoplasmic sperm injection with a man homozygous for the 5a-reductase-2 gene mutation. *Fertil Steril* 2011 May;95(6):2125:e5–e8.
30. Imperato-McGinley J, Gautier T, Peterson RE, Shackleton C. The prevalence of 5 alpha reductase deficiency in children with ambiguous genitalia in the Dominican republic. *J Urol* 1986;136(4):867–873.
31. Cheng J, et al. Phenotype and molecular characteristics in 45 Chinese children with 5α-reductase type 2 deficiency from South China. *Clin Endocrinol (Oxf)* 2015;83(4):518–526.
32. https://www.ncbi.nlm.nih.gov/books/ NBK1334/table/kms.T.syndromes_associated_with_hypogona/.
33. Smikle C, Yarrarapu SNS, Khetarpal S, *Stat Pearls, Internet, 2023* https://www.ncbi.nlm.nih.gov/books/ NBK448088/.
34. Chon JC, Umair Z, Yoon MS. Premature ovarian insufficiency: Past, present, and future. *Front Cell Dev Biol* 10 May 2021, Sec. Molecular and Cellular Reproduction , Volume 9 - 2021.
35. Silva C, et al. Autoimmune primary ovarian insufficiency. *Autoimmun Rev* 2014;13(4–5):427–430.
36. Hoyos L, Thakur M. Fragile X premutation in women: Recognizing the health challenges beyond primary ovarian insufficiency. *J Assist Reprod Genet* 2016;34(3):315–323.
37. Fourman, LT, Fazeli PK. Neuroendocrine causes of amenorrhea—An update. *J Clin Endocrinol Metab* 2015;100(3):812–824.
38. Shufelt CL, Torbati T, Dutra E. Hypothalamic amenorrhea and the long-term health consequences. *Semin Reprod Med* 2017 May;35(3):256–262.
39. Misra M, et al. Physiologic estrogen replacement increases bone density in adolescent girls with anorexia nervosa. *J Bone Miner Res* 2011;26(10):2430–2438.
40. Fazeli P, Klibanski A. Effects of anorexia nervosa on bone metabolism. *Endocr Rev* 2018;39(6):895–910.

41. Goodman N, et al. Futterweit, W, American Association of Clinical Endocrinologists (AACE); American College of Endocrinology (ACE); androgen Excess and PCOS Society (AES): Disease state Clinical Review: Guide to the Best Practices in the Evaluation and Treatment of polycystic ovary syndrome, Part 1. *Endocr Pract* 2015 November;21(11):1291–1300.

42. Goodman N, et al. Futterweit, W, American Association of Clinical Endocrinologists (AACE); American College of Endocrinology (ACE); androgen Excess and PCOS Society (AES): Disease state Clinical Review: Guide to the Best Practices in the Evaluation and Treatment of polycystic ovary syndrome, Part 2. *Endocr Pract* 2015 December;21(12):1415–1426.

43. Tay C, et al. Updated adolescent diagnostic criteria forpolycystic ovary syndrome: Impact onprevalence and longitudinal body mass index trajectories from birth to adulthood. *BMC Med* 2020;18(1):389.

44. Murphy M, Hall E, Adams M. Polycystic ovarian morphology in normal women does not predict the development of polycystic ovary syndrome. *J Clin Endocirnol Metab* 2006;91(10):3878–3884.

45. Dapas M. et al. Family-based quantitative trait meta-analysis implicates rare noncoding variants in DENND1A in polycystic ovary syndrome. *J Clin Endocrinol Metab* 2019;104(9):3835.

46. Gorsic l, Dapas M, Legro R, Hayes MG, Urbanek M. Functional genetic variation in the anti-Müllerian hormone pathway in women with polycystic ovary syndrome. *J Clin Endocrinol Metab* 2019;104(7):2855.

47. Cimino I, et al. Novel role for anti-Müllerian hormone in the regulation of GnRH neuron excitability and hormone secretion. *Nat Commun* 2016;7:10055.

48. Barbotin AL, Peigné M, Malone SA, Giacobini P. Emerging roles of anti-Müllerian hormone in hypothalamic-pituitary function. *Neuroendocrinology* 2019;109(3):218–229.

49. Silva MSB, Giacobini P. New insights into anti-Müllerian hormone role in the hypothalamic-pituitary-gonadal axis and neuroendocrine development. *Cell Mol Life Sci* 2021 January;78(1):1–16.

50. Qu X, Donnelly R. Sex hormone-binding globulin (SHBG) as an early biomarker and therapeutic target in polycystic ovary syndrome. *Int J Mol Sci* 2020 November 1;21(21):8191.

51. Li Y, et al. Association between human SHBG gene polymorphisms and risk of PCOS: A meta-analysis. *Reprod Biomed Online* 2021 January;42(1):227–236.

52. Yilmaz B, Vellanki P, Ata B, Yildiz BO. Metabolic syndrome, hypertension, and hyperlipidemia in mothers, fathers, sisters, and brothers of women with polycystic ovary syndrome: A systematic review and meta-analysis. *Fertil Steril* 2018;109(2):356.e32–364.e32.

53. Yilmaz B, Vellanki P, Ata B, Yildiz BO. Diabetes mellitus and insulin resistance in mothers, fathers, sisters, and brothers of women with polycystic ovary syndrome: A systematic review and meta-analysis. *Fertil Steril* 2018;110(3):523.e14–533.e14.

54. Torchen L, et al. Increased antiMüllerian hormone levels and other reproductive endocrine changes in adult male relatives of women with polycystic ovary syndrome. *Fertil Steril* 2016;106(1):50–55.

55. Liu D, et al. Evidence for gonadotrophin secretory and steroidogenic abnormalities in brothers of women with polycystic ovary syndrome. *Hum Reprod* 2014;29(12):2764–2772.

56. Dapas M, et al. Distinct subtypes of polycystic ovary syndrome with novel genetic associations: An unsupervised, phenotypic clustering analysis. *PLOS Med* 2020;17(6):e1003132.

57. Kurman RJ, Ellenson LH, Ronnett BM, *Blaustein's Pathology of the Female Genital Tract*, Springer. doi: 10.1007/978-3-319-46334-6.

58. Giménez-Peralta I, Lilue M, Mendoza N, Tesarik J, Mazheika M. Application of a new ultrasound criterion for the diagnosis of polycystic ovary syndrome. *Front Endocrinol* 02 September 2022, Sec. Developmental Endocrinology.

59. Cobin RH, Fenichel R, Chapter 6, in *A Color Handbook, Clinical Endocrinology and Metabolism*, Canacho, P. ed., p. 151, Manson Publishing Ltd, London, 2011.

60. Gorsic L, et al. Pathogenic anti-Müllerian hormone variants in polycystic ovary syndrome. *J Clin Endocrinol Metab* 2017;102(8):2862–2872.

61. Graham R, Grahame H, Ewan R, Pearson E, The mechanisms of action of metformin. *Diabetologia* 2017;60(9):1577–1585.

62. Marinkovic-Radosevic J, Berkovic, Cigrovski,Kruez ME, Mrzljak A. Exploring new treatment options for polycystic ovary syndrome: Review of a novel antidiabetic agent SGLT2 inhibitor. *World J Diabetes* 2021 July 15;12(7):932–938.

63. Siamashvili M , Davis S. Update on the effects of GLP-1 receptor agonists for the treatment of polycystic ovary syndrome. *Expert Rev Clin Pharmacol* 2021;14(9):1081–1089.

64. Kakoly N, et al. Ethnicity, obesity and the prevalence of impaired glucose tolerance and type 2 diabetes in PCOS: A systematic review and meta-regression. *Hum Reprod Update* 2018;24(4):455–467.

65. Pelanis R, et al. The prevalence of Type 2 diabetes is not increased in normal-weight women with PCOS. *Hum Reprod* 2017;32(11):2279–2286.

66. Kiconco S, Teede, Earnest A et al. Menstrual cycle regularity as a predictor for heart disease and diabetes: Findings from a large population-based longitudinal cohort. *Clin Endocrinol (Oxf)* 2021, November 24. doi: 10.1111/cen.14640. Online ahead of print.
67. Solomon CG. et al. Menstrual cycle irregularity and risk for future cardiovascular disease. *J Clin Endocrinol Metab* 2002 May;87(5):2013–2017.
68. de Groot P, Dekkers OM, Romijn JA, Dieben SW, Helmerhorst FM. PCOS, coronary heart disease, stroke and the influence of obesity: A systematic review and meta-analysis. *Hum Reprod Update* 2011;17(4):495–500.
69. Anderson S, Barry JA, Hardiman PJ. Risk of coronary heart disease and risk of stroke in women with polycystic ovary syndrome: A systematic review and meta-analysis. *Int J Cardiol* 2014;176(2):486–487.
70. Zhao L. et al. Polycystic ovary syndrome (PCOS) and the risk of coronary heart disease (CHD): A meta-analysis. *Oncotarget* 2016;7(23):33715–22721.
71. Zhou Y. et al. Association between polycystic ovary syndrome and the risk of stroke and all-cause mortality: Insights from a meta-analysis. *Gynecol Endocrinol* 2017;33(12):904–910.
72. Kiconco S, et al. Natural history of polycystic ovary syndrome: A systematic review of cardiometabolic outcomes from longitudinal cohort studies. *Clin Endocrinol (Oxf)* 2021 December 11. doi: 10.1111/cen.14647. Online ahead of print.
73. Azziz R, et al. The androgen Excess and PCOS Society criteria for the polycystic ovary syndrome: The complete task force report. *Fertil Steril* 2009;91(2):456–488.
74. Dewailly D, et al. Definition and significance of polycystic ovarian morphology: A task force report from the Androgen Excess and Polycystic Ovary Syndrome Society. *Hum Reprod Update* 2014;20(3):334–352.
75. Dumesic D, et al. Scientific statement on the diagnostic criteria, epidemiology, pathophysiology, and Molecular Genetics of polycystic ovary Syndrome. *Endocr Rev* 2015;36(5):487–525.
76. ACOG Committee on Practice Bulletins, with Richard S, Legro MD, ACOG Practice Bulletin. *Obstet Gynecol* 2018, 131(6):e157–e171.

PEDIATRIC ENDOCRINE SOCIETY

77. Ibáñez L, et al. An International Consortium Update: Pathophysiology, Diagnosis, and Treatment of Polycystic Ovarian Syndrome in Adolescence, IInternational Consortium of Paediatric Endocrinology (ICPE). *Horm Res Paediatr* 2017;88(6):1–25.
78. Williams T, Mortada M, Porter S. Diagnosis and treatment of polycystic ovary syndrome. *Am Fam Physician* 2016;94(2):106–113.
79. Teede H, Misso M, Costello M et al., on behalf of the International PCOS Network. International evidence-based guideline for the assessment and management of polycystic ovary syndrome, Monash University, Melbourne Australia, 2018. monash.edu/medicine/sphpm/mchri/pcos.
80. International evidence based guidelines for assessment and management of polyystic ovarian syndrome. *Clin Endocrinol (Oxf)* 2018 September;89(3):251–268. doi: 10.1111/cen.13795. Epub 2018 Jul 19.
81. Kiconco S, Teede, HJH, Azziz R, Joham AE. The need to reassess the diagnosis of polycystic ovary syndrome (PCOS): A review of diagnostic recommendations from the international evidence-based guideline for the assessment and management of PCOS. *Semin Reprod Med* 2021 July;39(3–04):71–77.
82. Al Wattar B et al. Clinical practice guidelines on the diagnosis and management of polycystic ovary syndrome: A systematic review and quality assessment study. *J Clin Endocrinol Metab* 2021;106(8):2436–2446.
83. Li H, Zhang Y, Lu L, Yi W. Reporting quality of polycystic ovary syndrome practice guidelines based on the RIGHT checklist. *Medicine* 2020;99(42):(e22624).
84. Kiconco S, et al. PCOS phenotype in unselected populations study (P-PUP): Protocol for a systematic review and defining PCOS diagnostic features with pooled individual participant data. *Diagnostics (Basel)* 2021 October 21;11(11):1953.
85. Muka T, et al. Age at natural menopause and risk of type 2 diabetes: A prospective cohort study. *Diabetologia* 2017;60(10):1951–1960.
86. Ley S, et al. Duration of reproductive life span, age at menarche, and age at menopause are associated with risk of cardiovascular disease in women. *J Am Heart Assoc* 2017;6(11).
87. Kuh D, Cooper R, Moore A, Richards M, Hardy R. Age at menopause and lifetime cognition: Findings from a British birth cohort study. *Neurology* 2018;90(19):e1673–e1681.

88. Svejme O, Ahlborg HG, Nilsson JÅ, Karlsson MK. Early menopause and risk of osteoporosis, fracture and mortality: A 34-year prospective observational study in 390 women. *BJOG* 2012;119(7):810–818.

89. Cobin R, Goodman N. American Association of Clinical Endocrinologists and American College of Endocrinology position statement on menopause–2017 update. *Endocr Pract* 2017;23(7):869–880.

90. https://www.fda.gov/consumers/free-publications-women/menopause-medicines-help-you.

91. Galson S. PharmacyCompounding/CompoundingofBio-identicalHormoneReplacement therapies. Testimony before the senate special committee on aging, 2017. https://wayback.archive-it.org/7993/20170723044115/https://www. fda.gov/NewsEvents/ Testimony/ucm154031.htm.

92. https://www.accessdata.fda.gov/drugsatfda_docs/label/2021/210132s006lbl.pdf.

93. Preventive Services Task Force recommendation statement: Hormone therapy for the primary prevention of chronic conditions in postmenopausal persons. *JAMA* 2022;328(17):1740–1746.

94. Henderson VW, Lobo RA. Hormone therapy and the risk of stroke: Perspectives 10 years after the Women's Health Initiative trials. *Climacteric* 2012 June;15(3):229–234.

95. Canonico M, et al. Postmenopausal hormone therapy and risk of stroke: Impact of the Route of Estrogen Administration and Type of Progestogen. *Stroke* 2016;47(7):1734–1741.

96. Carrasquilla G, et al. Postmenopausal hormone therapy and risk of stroke: A pooled analysis of data from population-based cohort studies. *PLOS Med* 2017;14(11):e1002445.

97. Løkkegaard E, Nielsen LH, Keiding N. Risk of stroke with various types of menopausal hormone therapies: A national cohort study. *Stroke* 2017;48(8):2266–2269.

98. Manson J, et al. Menopausal hormone therapy and long-term all-cause and cause- specific mortality. *JAMA* 2017;318(10):927–938.

99. Asi N, et al. Progesterone vs. synthetic progestins and the risk of breast cancer: A systematic review and meta-analysis. *Syst Rev* 2016;5(1):121.

100. Stute P, Wildt L, Neulen J. The impact of micronized progesterone on breast cancer risk: A system- atic review. *Climacteric* 2018;21(2):111–122.

101. Bakken K et al. Menopausal hormone therapy and breast cancer risk: Impact of dif- ferent treatments. The European prospective investigation into cancer and nutrition. *Int J Cancer* 2010;128(1):144–156.

102. Brusselaers N, et al. Different menopausal hormone regimens and risk of breast can– cer. *Ann Oncol* 2018;29(8):1771–1776.

103. Savolainen-Peltonen H, et al. Use of postmenopausal hormone therapy and risk of Alzheimer's disease in Finland: Nationwide case-control study. *BMJ* 2019;364:l665.

104. Coughlan GT, et al. Association of age at menopause and hormone therapy use with tau and β-amyloid positron emission tomography. *JAMA Neurol.* Published online April 3, 2023. doi: 10.1001/jamaneurol.2023.0455.

105. Saleh R, Hornberger M, Ritchie CW, Minihane AM. Hormone replacement therapy is associated with improved cognition and larger brain volumes in at-risk APOE4 women: Results from the European Prevention of Alzheimer's Disease (EPAD) cohort. *Alzheimers Res Ther* 2023;15(1):10. doi: 10.1186/s13195-022-01121-.

106. Stuenkel C. Menopause, hormone therapy and diabetes. *Climacteric* 2017;20(1):11–21.

107. Grossman D, et al. Hormone therapy for the primary prevention of chronic conditions in postmenopausal women: US Preventive Services Task Force Recommendation Statement. *JAMA* 2017;318(22):2224.

108. Grodstein F, et al. Hormone therapy and coronary heart disease: The role of time since menopause and age at hormone initiation. *Obstet Gynecol Surv* 2006;61(6):392–394.

109. Manson J, et al. Menopausal hormone therapy and health outcomes during the intervention and extended post-stopping phases of the women's health initiative randomized trials. *JAMA* 2013;310(13):1353–1368.

110. Manson JE, et al. Anderson GL; WHI investigators. Menopausal hormone therapy and long-term all-cause and cause-specific mortality: The Women's Health Initiative randomized trials. *JAMA* 2017 September 12;318(10):927–938.

111. Wild R, et al. Coronary heart disease events in the Women's Health Initiative hormone trials. *Menopause* 2012;20(3):254–260.

112. Shufelt C, et al. Hormone therapy dose, formulation, route of delivery, and risk of cardiovascular events in women. *Menopause* 2014;21(3):260–266.

113. Poornima I, et al. Coronary artery calcification (CAC) and post-trial cardiovascular events and mortality within the Women's Health Initiative (WHI) estrogen-alone trial. *J Am Heart Assoc* 2017;6(11).

114. Miller V, Hodis HN, Lahr BD, Bailey KR, Jayachandran M. Changes in carotid artery intima-media thickness 3 years after cessation of menopausal hormone therapy. *Menopause* 2019;26(1):24–31.

115. Shams T, et al. SSRIs for hot flashes: A systematic review and meta-analysis of ran- domized trials. *J Gen Intern Med* 2013;29(1):204–213.

116. Binkhorst L, et al. Unjustified prescribing of CYP2D6 inhibiting SSRIs in women treated with tamoxifen. *Breast Cancer Res Treat* 2013;139(3):923–929.
117. Pinkerton J, et al. Phase 3 randomized controlled study of gastroretentive gabapentin for the treatment of moderate-to-severe hot flashes in menopause. *Menopause* 2014;21(6):567–573.
118. LiL, et al. Comparative efficacy of nonhormonal drugs on menopausal hot flashes. *Eur J Clin Pharmacol* 2016;72(9):1051–1058.
119. Hervik J, Stub T. Adverse effects of non-hormonal pharmacological interventions in breast cancer survivors, suffering from hot flashes: A systematic review and meta- analysis. *Breast Cancer Res Treat* 2016;160(2):223–236.
120. Sharifi M, Lewiecki E. Conjugated estrogens combined with Bazedoxifene: The first approved tissue selective estrogen complex therapy. *Exp Rev Clin Pharmacol* 2014;7(3):281–291.
121. Lederman S, Ottery F, et al. Fezolinetant for treatment of moderate-to-severe vasomotor symptoms associated with menopause (SKYLIGHT 1): A phase 3 randomized controlled study. *Lancet* 2023;401(10382):1091–1102.
122. Johnson KA, Martin N, Nappi RE, Neal-Perry G, Shapiro M, Stute P, Thurston RC, Wolfman W, English M, Franklin C, Lee M, Santoro N. Efficacy and safety of fezolinetant in moderate to severe vasomotor symptoms associated with menopause: A Phase 3 RCT. *J Clin Endocrinol Metab* 2023;108(8):1981–1997.
123. Johnson KA, Martin N, Nappi RE, Neal-Perry G, Shapiro M, Stute P, Thurston RC, Wolfman W, English M, Franklin C, Lee M, Santoro N. Efficacy and safety of fezolinetant in moderate to severe vasomotor symptoms associated with menopause: A phase 3 RCT. *J Clin Endocrinol Metab* 2023;108(8):1981–1997. doi: 10.1210/clinem/dgad058. PMID: 36734148; PMCID: PMC10348473. https://www.astellas.com/en/system/files/news/2023-02/20230220_en_1.pdf.
124. Hüser S, et al. Effects of isoflavones on breast tissue and the thyroid hormone system in humans: A comprehensive safety evaluation. *Arch Toxicol* 2018;92(9):2703–2748.
125. Fritz H, et al. Black cohosh and breast cancer: A systematic review. *Integr Cancer Ther* 2013;13(1):12–29.
126. Leach M, Moore V. Black cohosh (Cimicifuga spp.) for menopausal symptoms. *Cochrane Database Syst Rev* 2012;9(9):CD007244.0004386954.INDD 259 8/27/2019 1:55:16 PM.
127. Brown A. Liver toxicity related to herbs and dietary supplements: Online table of case reports. Part 2 of 5 series. *Food Chem Toxicol* 2017;107(A):472–501.
128. American College of Obstetrics and Gynecology (ACOG), Practice Bulletin No. 141. *Obstet Gynecol* 2014;123(1):202–216.
129. North American Menopause Society (NAMS), The 2022 hormone therapy position statement of the North American menopause society Advisory Panel. The 2022 hormone therapy position statement of The North American Menopause Society. *Menopause* 2022 July 1;29(7):767–794.
130. The Endocrine Society (TES), et al. Treatment of symptoms of the menopause: An Endocrine Society clinical practice guideline. *J Clin Endocrinol Metab* 2015 November;100(11):3975–4011.
131. French College of Gynecologists and Obstetricians. Trémollieres FA, et al. Management of postmenopausal women: Collège National des Gynécologues et Obstétriciens Français (CNGOF) and Groupe d'Etude sur la Ménopause et le Vieillissement (GEMVi) Clinical Practice Guidelines 2022 September;163:62–81.
132. Mohan S, Garima Kapoor G, Raman DK. Partial androgen insensitivity syndrome: A diagnostic and therapeutic dilemma. *Armed Forces India Med J* 2011;67(4):382–384.
133. Hannema SE, Hughes I. A: Regulation of Wolffian duct development. *Horm Res* 2007;67(3):142–151.
134. https://rarediseases.info.nih.gov/diseases/5680/5-alpha-reductase-deficiency.
135. Mendiola AJP, LaSalle JM. Epigenetics in Prader-Willi syndrome. *Front Genet* 2021 February 15;12:624581.
136. Bochukova EG. Transcriptomics of the Prader-Willi syndrome hypothalamus. *Handb Clin Neurol* 2021;181:369–379.
137. https://www.ncbi.nlm.nih.gov/books/NBK367946/#dup15q.Genetically_Related_Disordersis.
138. Butler MG, Angulo MA, Cataletto ME. Prader-Willi syndrome: A review of clinical, genetic, and endocrine findings. *J Endocrinol Invest* 1998;12(38):1249–1263. doi: 10.1007/s40618-015-0312-9.
139. Castro-Sánchez S, Álvarez-Satta M. Laurence-Moon-Biedel syndrome, generalized congenital hypothalamic deficiency which presents with microphallus and neonatal hypoglycemia, and midline craniofacial developmental defects. *J Pediatr Genet* 2013.
140. https://ir.rhythmtx.com/news-releases/news-release-details/rhythm-pharmaceuticals-announces-fda-acceptance-filing-and.
141. Mancini M, et al. Obesity is strongly associated with low testosterone and reduced penis growth during development. *J Clin Endocrinol Metab* 2021;106(11):3151–3159.
142. Wong M, Levy M, Stephenson M. Hypogonadism in the HIV-infected man. *Curr Treat Options Infect Dis* 2017;9(1):104–116.
143. Kaplan A, Hu C, Morgentaler A. Testosterone therapy in men with prostate cancer. *Eur Urol* 2016 May;69(5):894–903.

144. Lenfant L et al. Testosterone replacement therapy (TRT) and prostate cancer: An updated systematic review with a focus on previous or active localized prostate cancer. *Urol Oncol* 2020 August;38(8):661–670.

145. Araujo A, Wittert G. Endocrinology of the aging male. *Best Pract Res Clin Endocrinol. Metab.* 2011;25(2):303–319.

146. Liu Z et al. Dynamic alteration of serum testosterone with aging: A cross-sectional study from Shanghai, China. *Reprod Biol Endocrinol* 2015;13:111. doi: 10.1186/s12958-015-0107-z.

147. Travison, TG. et al. Harmonized reference ranges for circulating testosterone levels in men of four cohort studies in the United States and Europe. *J Clin Endocrinol Metab* 2017 April 1;102(4):1161–1173.

148. Snyder P, et al. Effects of testosterone treatment in older men. *N Engl J Med* 2016;374(7):611–624.

149. Snyder PJ, et al. Effect of testosterone treatment on volumetric bone density and strength in older men with low testosterone: A controlled clinical trial. *JAMA Intern Med* 2017;177(4):471–479.

150. Snyder PJ, et al. Lessons from the tes- tosterone trials. *Endocr Rev* 2018;39(3):369–386.

151. Araujo AB, Wittert GA. Endocrinology of the aging male. *Best Pract Res Clin Endocrinol Metab* 2011;25(2):303–319.

152. Barnouin Y. Testosterone replacement added to intensive lifestyle intervention in older men with obesity and Hypogonadis. *Jclinendometab* 2021 March;106(3):e1096–e1110.

153. Practice Update. ADA, 2020: Testosterone plus lifestyle program reduced risk of type 2 diabetes in overweight and obese men (Internet). Amsterdam: Elsevier; c2020 [cited 2020 August 4]. https://www.practiceupdate. Com/Content/ada-2020-testosterone-plus-lifestyle-program- Reduced -Risk-of-type-2-diabetes-in-overwei ght-and-obese- Men/102636)}}.

154. Ponce O et al. The efficacy and adverse events of testosterone replacement therapy in hypogonadal men: A systematic review and meta-analysis of randomized, placebo-controlled TrialsJ. *J Clin Endocrinol Metab* 2018 May;103(5):1745–1754.

155. Al-Sharefi, A, Quinton, R. Current national and international guidelines for the management of male hypogonadism: Helping clinicians to navigate variation in diagnostic criteria and treatment recommendations. *Endocrinol Metab (Seoul)* 2020 September;35(3):526–540.

156. Zucker IJ, Masterson TA. Comparison of American Urological Association and Endocrine Society guidelines on testosterone replacement. *Int J Impot Res* 2021. doi: 10.1038/s41443-021-0047.

157. Gagliana-Jura, B. Testosterone Replacement therapy and cardiovascular Risk. *Nat Rev Cardiol* 2019 September;16:555.

158. Bhasin S et al. Testosterone therapy in men with hypogonadism: An Endocrine Society* clinical practice guideline. *J Clin Endocrinol Metab* 2018;103(5):1715–1744.

159. Laurent MR et al. Sex hormone-binding globulin regulation of androgen bioactivity in vivo: Validation of the free hormone hypothesis. *Sci Rep* 2016;6:35539. doi: 10.1038/srep35539.

160. Ismail A, Barth J, Review: Endocrinology of gynaecomastia. *Ann Clin Biochem*, 2001;38(6):596–607.

161. Post A, De Heijninga B , Actona D et al. A novel infant milk formula concept: Mimicking the human milk fat globule structure. *Colloids Surf B Biointerfaces* 2015;136(1):329–339.

162. Saleem M, Martin H, Coates P. Prolactin biology and laboratory measurement: An update on physiology and current analytical issues. *Clin Biochem Rev* 2018;39(1):3–16.

163. Ross, GMS, Filippini, D, Nielen, MWF, Gert IJ. Salentijn, unraveling the hook effect: A comprehensive study of high antigen concentration effects in sandwich lateral flow immunoassays, *Anal Chem* 2020;92(23):15587–15595.

164. Schlechte JA. Clinical practice: Prolactinoma. *N Engl J Med* 2003;349(21):2035–2041.

165. Vilar L. et al. Controversial issues in the management of hyperprolactinemia and prolactinomas – An overview by the Neuroendocrinology Department of the Brazilian Society of Endocrinology and Metabolism. *Arch Endocrinol Metab* 2018;62(2):236–263.

166. Casanueva F. *et al.* Guidelines of the Pituitary Society for the diagnosis and management of prolactinomas. *Clin Endocrinol (Oxf)* 2006;65(2):265–273.

167. Melmed S. et al. Diagnosis & treatment of hyperprolactinemia: An endocrine society clinical practice guideline. *J Clin Endocrinol Metab* 2011;96(2):273–288.

168. Maiter D. Management of dopamine agonist resistant prolactinomas. *Neuroendocrinology* 2019;109(1):42–50.

169. Kontogeorgos G. Predictive markers of pituitary adenoma behavior. *Neuroendocrinology* 2006;83(3–4):179–188.

170. Trouillas J, et al. Clinical, pathological, and molecular factors of aggressiveness in lactotroph tumours. *Neuroendocrinology* 2019;109(1):70–76.

171. Hauser B, Lau A, Sacksham S, Bi WL, Dunn IF. The epigenomics of pituitary adenoma. *Front Endocrinol (Lausanne)* 2019 May 14;10:290.

172. Frederic Castinetti F, et al. Long-term results of stereotactic radiosurgery in secretory pituitary adenomas. *J Clin Endocrinol Metab* 2009;94(9):3400–3407.

173. Souteiro P, Karavitaki N. Dopamine agonist resistant prolactinomas: Any alternative medical treatment? *Pituitary* 2020;23(1):27–37.
174. Raverot G, Vasiljevic A, Jouanneau E, Lasolle H. Confirmation of a new therapeutic option for aggressive or dopamine agonist-resistant prolactin pituitary neuroendocrine tumors. *Eur J Endocrinol* 2019 August;181(2):C1–C3.
175. Almalki M et al. Temozolomide therapy for resistant prolactin-secreting pituitary adenomas and carcinomas: A systematic review. *Hormones (Athens)* 2017;16(2):139–149.
176. Cooper O, et al. EGFR/ErbB2-targeting lapatinib therapy for aggressive prolactinoma. *J Clin Endocrinol Metab* 2021;106(2):e917–e925.
177. Chuang CC. et al. Different volumetric measurement methods for pituitary adenomas and their crucial clinical significance. *Sci Rep* 2017;7:40792. doi: 10.1038/srep40792.
178. Raverot G et al. The European Society of Endocrinology, European Society of Endocrinology Clinical Practice Guidelines for the management of aggressive pituitary tumours and carcinomas. *Eur J Endocrinol* 2018;178(1):G1–G24.

Lipid Disorders

8

Fatima Kazi and Francis Q. Almeda

LIPID DISORDERS

Definition/Overview

Atherosclerotic cardiovascular disease (ASCVD) is the leading cause of mortality in industrialized nations, and cardiac event rates remain significant despite major advances in cardiovascular care. Abnormalities in lipid metabolism increase the risk for the development and progression of coronary heart disease (CHD) and the diagnosis and treatment of patients with lipid disorders has been shown to significantly reduce the risk of future adverse cardiac events. In general, the intensity of risk reduction therapy should approximate the individual's absolute risk, and thus the accurate assessment of the patient's overall cardiovascular risk status is the central component for the optimal treatment of individuals with dyslipidemia.

Dyslipidemia comprises a range of conditions, primarily defined by elevations in lipoprotein cholesterol, including high-density lipoprotein cholesterol (LDL-C) and non-high-density lipoprotein cholesterol (HDL-C), as well as elevated triglycerides. All of these conditions independently increase the risk of ASCVD. The American Association of Endocrinology and American College of Endocrinology (AACE/ACE) released a consensus statement in 2020 outlining risk categories and treatment goals (Table 8.1).

The Executive Summary of the Third Report of the National Cholesterol Education Program (NCEP) Expert Panel on detection, evaluation, and treatment of high blood cholesterol in adults (Adult Treatment Panel III [ATP III]) provides evidence-based recommendations for the diagnosis and management of high cholesterol and related disorders in high-risk populations and primary prevention in patients with multiple risk factors. Table 8.2 summarizes the definitions for elevated total cholesterol (TC), LDL, HDL, and triglycerides (TAGs).

Etiology

Lipid disorders can be classified into primary (genetic or inherited) (see Tables 8.3 and 8.4) or secondary (due to disease or environmental factors). Severe hypercholesterolemia has been associated with genetic abnormalities such as familial hypercholesterolemia with mutations in the LDL receptors,

DOI: 10.1201/9781003100669-8

TABLE 8.1   ASCVD Risk Categories and Treatment Goals

RISK CATEGORY	RISK FACTORS AND 10-YEAR RISK	TREATMENT GOALS (Mg/dL)			
		LDL-C	NON-HDL-C	APOB	TG
Extreme risk	– Progressive ASCVD including unstable angina – Established clinical ASCVD plus diabetes or CKD ≥3 or heterozygous familial hypercholesterolemia – History of premature ASCVD (<55 years, male; <65 years, female)	<55	<80	<70	<150
Very high risk	– Established clinical ASCVD or recent hospitalization for ACS, carotid or peripheral vascular disease, or 10-year risk >20% – Diabetes with ≥1 risk factor(s) – CKD ≥3 with albuminuria – Heterozygous familial hypercholesterolemia	<70	<100	<80	<150
High risk	– ≥2 risk factor and 10-year risk 10%–20% – Diabetes or CKD ≥3 with no other risk factors	<100	<130	<90	<150
Moderate risk	– <2 risk factors and 10-year risk<10 %	<100	<130	<90	<150
Low risk	No risk factors	<130	<160	Not recommended	<150

TABLE 8.2   ATP III Lipid and Lipoprotein Classification

I. Total Cholesterol Mg/dL (Mmol/L)			**III. HDL Cholesterol mg/dL (mmol/L)**		
<200	(5.2)	Desirable	<40 (1.0) <50 (1.3)	(males) (females)	Low
200–239	(5.2–6.2)	Borderline high	≥60 (1.5)		High
≥240	(6.2)	High			
II. LDL Cholesterol Mg/dL (Mmol/L)			**IV. Triglycerides (mg/dL)**		
<100	(2.6)	Optimal	<150	(1.6)	Normal
100–129	(2.6–3.3)	Near optimal/above optimal	150–199	(1.6–2.1)	Borderline high
130–159	(3.4–4.1)	Borderline high	200–499	(2.2–5.4)	High
160–189	(4.2–4.9)	High	≥500	(5.5)	Very high
≥190	(5.0)	Very high			

TABLE 8.3 Clinical History, Physical Examination, and Laboratory Evaluation of Hyperlipoproteinemias

HYPERLIPOPROTEIN EMIA	MOLECULAR DEFECT	LIPOPROTEINS	MAJOR DENSITY CLASS	CLINICAL HISTORY	PHYSICAL EXAMINATION	EVALUATION
Familial chylomicronemia syndrome	LPL (lipoprotein lipase) deficiency	ApoC-II deficiency	Chylomicrons elevated TGLs, VLDL/IDL elevated	Occurs in approximately 1 in a 1,000,000 Pancreatitis Dry eyes and mouth Numbness or tingling of the extremities Neuropsychiatric symptoms (depression and memory loss)	Eruptive xanthoma Lipemic plasma Lipemia retinalis Hepatosplenomegaly	Very high TAG >1500 mg/dL (15 mmol/L)
Familial hypercholesterolemia (FH)	Structural defect or absence of LDL receptor	Elevated plasma apoB	LDL elevated	Occurs in 1 in 500 Premature CAD	Tendon xanthomas (in the dorsum of the hands and Achilles tendons) Xanthomas Xanthelasmas and xanthomas of the eyes Arcus juvenilis	Heterozygous FH; LDL range (325–450 mg/dL [8.5–12 mmol/L]) Homozygous FH with very high LDL (500–1000 mg/dL [13–26 mmol/L]); normal TAG
Dysbetalipoproteinemia (type III hyperlipoproteinemia)	Delayed clearance of remnants of TAG-rich lipoproteins	ApoE deficiency	TGLs/cholesterol elevated VLDL/IDL elevated	Premature CAD Peripheral vascular disease Relatively common (up to 2% of population)	Palmar xanthomas (pathognomonic) Tuberous xanthomas Xanthelasma Premature CAD	Elevated TC and TAG
Familial combined hyperlipidemia (FCH)	To be established	Increased apoB-100	LDL/VLDL elevated Often HDL reduced	Premature CAD Common comorbidity includes diabetes, hypertension, and obesity	No tendon xanthomas Xanthelasma Arcus juvenilis Eruptive xanthomas	Varying patterns of high LDL with moderate elevations of TAG and low HDL
Familial defective apoB-100 (FDB)	ApoB-100 mutation	Defective apoB-100 (the mutation affects the receptor-binding domain of the protein decreasing the affinity of the mutant apoB-100 for its receptor to 3%–5% of normal; the result is decreased receptor-mediated clearance of LDL from the circulation)	LDL elevated	Premature CAD	Arcus juvenilis Tendon xanthomas Xanthelasma	Elevated TC Elevated LDL

resulting in impaired clearance of LDL and elevated LDL-C levels. Important secondary factors that result in altered lipid metabolism include hypothyroidism, diabetes mellitus, renal disease, obstructive liver disease, and alcohol intake. In addition, several medications, including estrogens/progestins, glucocorticoids, thiazides, isotretinoin, and cyclosporine, have been associated with mild to moderate hypercholesterolemia.

Pathophysiology

The central concept of lipid transport is that plasma lipids circulate in lipoprotein particles. Lipoproteins are large complexes that transport lipids (mainly cholesterol esters, TAGs, and fat-soluble vitamins) between the vasculature and various body tissues. The plasma lipoproteins are divided into major classes based on their relative densities: chylomicrons, very low-density lipoproteins (VLDLs), intermediate-density lipoproteins (IDLs), LDLs, HDLs, and lipoprotein (a) (Lp(a)). There are ten major human plasma apolipoproteins (Table 8.5).

Lipoprotein metabolism occurs through two basic mechanisms: the transport of dietary lipids to the liver and peripheral tissues (exogenous pathway), and the production and delivery of hepatic lipids into the circulation and peripheral tissues (endogenous pathway). In the exogenous pathway, dietary cholesterol is acted upon by the intestinal cells to form cholesterol esters through the addition of fatty acids (Figure 8.1). TAGs from the diet are hydrolyzed by pancreatic lipases within the intestine and emulsified with bile acids to form micelles. Longer-chain fatty acids are incorporated into TAGs and complexed with other particles such as cholesterol esters and phospholipids to form chylomicrons (which have a high concentration of TAG). These particles are acted upon by lipoprotein lipase along the capillary endothelium, and the TAGs are hydrolyzed releasing free fatty acids, most of which are taken up by adjacent adipocytes or myocytes, and the remaining particles (chylomicron remnants) are transported to the liver.

In the endogenous pathway, VLDL is transformed into IDL and then into LDL through hepatic metabolism (Figure 8.2). VLDL particles are similar to chylomicrons but have a higher ratio of cholesterol to TAG and contain apolipoprotein B-100. The TAG of VLDL is hydrolyzed by lipoprotein lipase and the particles continue to become smaller and denser and transform into IDL, which is composed of similar amounts of cholesterol and TAG. The hepatic cells remove approximately half of VLDL remnants and IDL. The remainder of IDL is modified by hepatic lipase to form LDL. LDL is composed of a core of primarily cholesterol esters, surrounded by a surface of phospholipids, free cholesterol, and apolipoprotein B. The majority of circulating LDL is cleared through LDL-mediated endocytosis in the liver. Modified (oxidized) plasma LDL accumulates in the intima and is acted upon by activated macrophages (foam cells) and through complex mechanisms involving cytokines, growth factors, smooth cell proliferation, and inflammation, and results in atheroma formation (Figure 8.3). The process of transferring cholesterol from peripheral cells to the liver for removal from the body by biliary secretion is called reverse cholesterol transport. The role of HDL in enhancing reverse cholesterol transport is one of the mechanisms by which HDL protects against the process of atherosclerosis (Figure 8.4). The major protein of HDL is apo A-1.

TABLE 8.4 Clinical History, Physical Examination, and Laboratory Evaluation of Hypolipoproteinemias

HYPOLIPOPROTEINEMIA	MOLECULAR DEFECT	LIPOPROTEINS	MAJOR DENSITY CLASS	CLINICAL HISTORY	PHYSICAL EXAMINATION	LABORATORY EVALUATION
Tangier disease	ABCA1 transporter mutation	Decreased apoA-I	HDL <5 mg/dL 0.1 mmol/L)	Modest increased risk of premature CAD	Orange-yellow tonsils (pathognomonic) Corneal opacities Peripheral neuropathy	TC1 <120 mg/dL (3.1 mmol/L) Normal or elevated TAG Low HDL
Abetalipoproteinemia (autosomal recessive)	Defect in assembly and secretion of apoB-containing lipoproteins	ApoB-100 deficiency ApoB-48 deficiency	Absence of ALDL/IDL, LDL	cardiac arrhythmias	Neurologic dysfunction Nystagmus Retinitis pigmentosa Progressive blindness	TC <50 mg/dL (13 mmol/L) Low TAG Vitamin A and E deficiency Hemolytic anemia (acanthocytes)
Familial hypobetalipoproteinemia	ApoB gene mutation	ApoB-48 and apoB-100 deficiency	Deficiency of chylomicrons and VLDL	Mild malabsorption	Absence of neurologic dysfunction Progressive degeneration	Mild deficiency of fat-soluble vitamins
Sitosterolemia	ABCG5 or ABCG8 mutation	Defective transporter (ABCG5 or ABCG8); this transporter preferentially transports plant and shellfish sterols from the intestine or liver into the gastrointestinal tract thus preventing absorption of the plant and shellfish sterols	Elevated plant and fish sterols	Premature CAD Arthralgia Arthritis at a young age	Tendon xanthomas Tuberous xanthomas Hypersplenism	Elevated TC Elevated plant and fish sterols (500–600 mg/dL [13–15.6 mmol/L]) Hemolytic anemia

TABLE 8.5 Major Human Plasma Apolipoproteins

APOLIPOPROTEIN	MAJOR DENSITY CLASS
A-I	HDL
A-II	HDL
A-IV	Chylomicrons, HDL
B-100	VLDL, IDL, LDL
B-48	Chylomicrons, VLDL, IDL
C-I	Chylomicrons, VLDL, IDL, HDL
C-II	Chylomicrons, VLDL, IDL, HDL
C-III	Chylomicrons, VLDL, IDL, HDL
E	Chylomicrons, VLDL,
Apo(a)	Lp(a)-density LDL to HDL

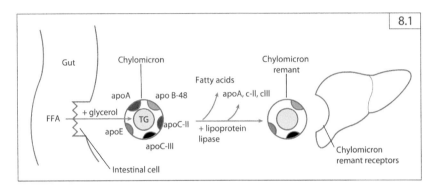

FIGURE 8.1 Exogenous pathway of lipid metabolism. Free fatty acids are absorbed in the gastrointestinal tract and combine with glycerol in the intestinal cell to form triglycerides. These triglycerides combine with a variety of apolipoproteins including apoA, apoB-48, apoC-II, apoC-III, and apoE, the main one being apoB-48. This combination forms a very large particle called a chylomicron to carry the dietary lipid. The enzyme lipoprotein lipase hydrolyzes the core and releases fatty acids. The remnant is then taken up and cleared by the liver.

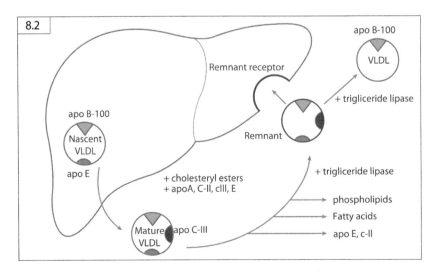

FIGURE 8.2 Endogenous pathway of lipid metabolism. Nascent VLDL is synthesized by the liver. It becomes mature VLDL after the addition of cholesterol esters and several apolipoproteins (the main ones as shown in the diagram). At this point, lipoprotein lipase breaks down the VLDL into smaller remnants. The smaller VLDL remnants can then proceed down one of two paths: they can be taken up and cleared by the liver, or hydrolyzed and released as LDL.

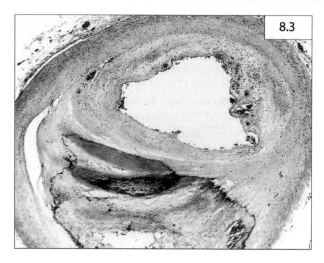

FIGURE 8.3 Magnified view (10×) of atheroma seen in atherosclerosis. At this level, intima, media, and adventitia are evident. Blue areas in the media represent calcification. (Courtesy of Drs. J.H. Lim and C. Oyer.)

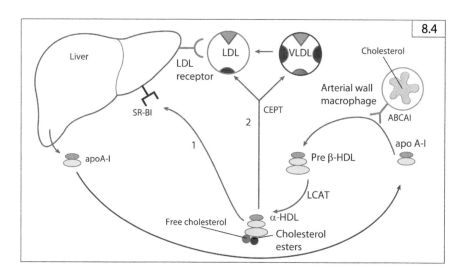

FIGURE 8.4 HDL metabolism. The liver produces lipid-poor apolipoprotein A-I, which removes excess cellular cholesterol by interacting with ABCAI. LCAT then esterifies this more lipid-rich particle into cholesterol esters, which can either return to the liver directly to be taken up by SRB-I (1) or they can transfer the cholesterol to VLDL and LDL (2). LDL can then be taken up by the liver via its receptor. ABCI, ATP-binding cassette transporter; CEPT, cholesterol ester transfer protein; HDL, high-density lipoprotein; LCAT, lecithin cholesterol acyltransferase; LDL, low-density lipoprotein; SRB-I, scavenger receptor class B, type I; VLDL, very low-density lipoprotein.

Clinical Presentation

There are two kinds of genetic dyslipoproteinemia, which result in abnormal plasma levels of several classes of plasma lipoproteins: hyperlipoproteinemias and hypolipoproteinemias. The clinical presentation, physical exam, differential diagnosis, and laboratory evaluation of lipoproteinemias are summarized in Tables 8.3 and 8.4. Important clinical findings in patients with significant hypercholesterolemia include xanthomas (Figures 8.5 and 8.6), xanthelasma (Figure 8.7), arcus juvenilis (Figure 8.8), and lipid keratopathy (Figure 8.9). The chylomicronemia syndrome results in very high triglyceride levels of >1500 mg/dL (15 mmol/L) and is associated with eruptive xanthoma (Figures 8.10 and 8.11), a creamy layer on top of plasma left overnight in a refrigerator (Figure 8.12), and lipemia retinalis (Figure 8.13). Palmar xanthomas (Figure 8.14) are often demonstrated in patients with dysbetalipoproteinemia.

Elevated LDL, low HDL, and elevated TAG are associated with progressive atherosclerosis in the coronary, carotid, cerebral, and peripheral vasculature (Figure 8.15). Acute myocardial infarction (MI) often occurs in coronary plaques with 'mild' stenosis (<50%), and factors associated with plaque rupture include a large lipid core, a thin fibrous cap, and activated macrophages and inflammatory cytokines. Rupture often occurs at the lateral edge or 'shoulder' at the interface of plaque and normal intima. Acute MI usually occurs when a 'vulnerable' atherosclerotic plaque ruptures with subsequent thrombosis and

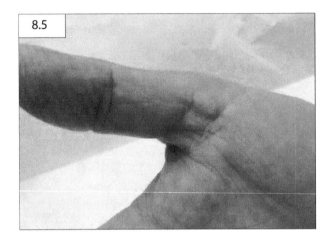

FIGURE 8.5   A 7 × 4 mm firm nodule representing a xanthomatous nodule of the flexor pollicis brevis in a patient with hypercholesterolemia. (Courtesy of foto@finlay-online.org.)

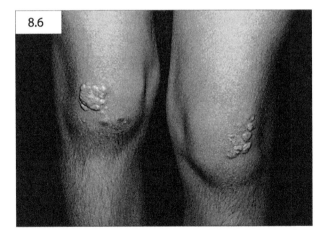

FIGURE 8.6   Cutaneous xanthomas in homozygous familial hypercholesterolemia. (From Teruel JL, Lasunción MA. Images in clinical medicine. Cutaneous xanthoma in homozygous familial hypercholesterolemia. *N Engl J Med* 1995:**332**(17):1137. Copyright 1995 Massachusetts Medical Society. All rights reserved.)

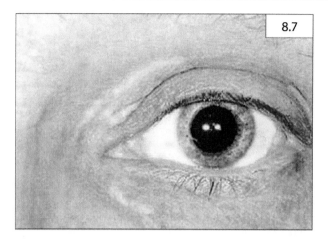

FIGURE 8.7 Xanthelasma in the periorbital region of a patient with hypercholesterolemia. (Reprinted from *Dorland's Dictionary*, 30th ed. Copyright 2004, with permission from Elsevier.)

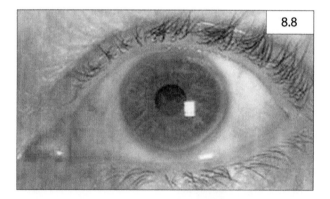

FIGURE 8.8 Arcus juvenilis is an opaque circle around the cornea, identical to arcus senilis but occurring in young people. Deposits of lipids cause a white ring around the periphery of the cornea and when seen in a young person it can be associated with hypercholesterolemia. (Courtesy of www.argy-bargey.blogspot.com.)

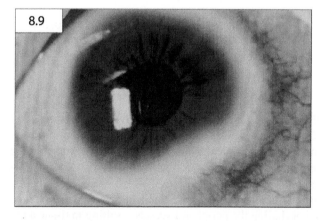

FIGURE 8.9 Lipid degeneration of the cornea, also known as lipid keratopathy, appears as a dense yellow-cream-colored opacification or cholesterol crystals on the corneal stroma surrounding blood vessels as a result of cholesterol or free fatty acid infiltration. The primary form is often bilateral and can occur in conditions such as Tangier disease. (Courtesy of www.eyeatlas.com.)

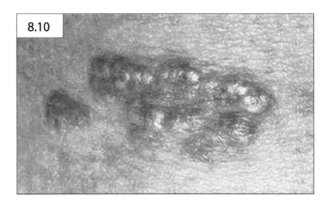

FIGURE 8.10   Close-up of an eruptive xanthoma in a patient with hypercholesterolemia. (Reprinted from *Dorland's Dictionary*, 30th ed. Copyright 2004, with permission from Elsevier.)

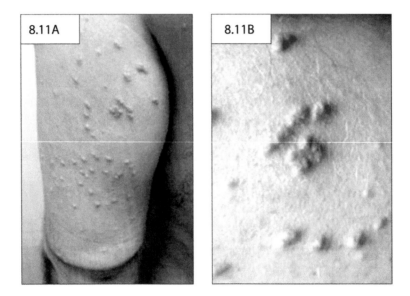

FIGURE 8.11   Eruptive xanthomas on the (A) arm and (B) upper torso in a patient with severe hypertriglyceridemia. (From Nayak KR, Daly RG. Images in clinical medicine. Eruptive xanthomas associated with hypertriglyceridemia and new-onset diabetes mellitus. *N Engl J Med* 2004:**350**(12):1235. Copyright 2004 Massachusetts Medical Society.)

occlusion of coronary flow (Figure 8.16), and is treated with either thrombolytic therapy or percutaneous coronary intervention. Cholesterol emboli syndrome may occur after any invasive arterial procedure and may also occur spontaneously. The clinical syndrome may involve worsening renal function, hypertension, and distal ischemia, and may be associated with characteristic dermatologic and ophthalmologic findings (Figures 8.17 and 8.19). The pathophysiology of this syndrome may involve cholesterol crystals showering the distal vascular beds with the associated local vasospastic mediators, or larger cholesterol plaques breaking off and occluding the peripheral vessels resulting in tissue and organ ischemia.

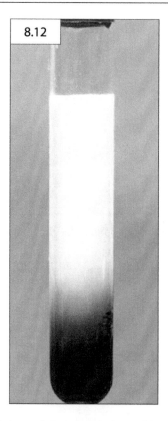

FIGURE 8.12 Creamy layer on top of plasma left overnight in a refrigerator, usually occurs when triglycerides are over 1500 mg/dL. (From Fred HL, Accad M. Images in clinical medicine. Lipemia retinalis. *N Engl J Med* 1999:**340**(25):1969. Copyright I999 Massachusetts Medical Society.)

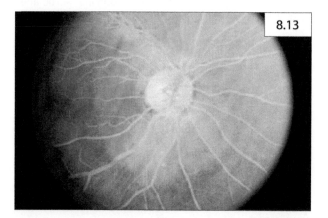

FIGURE 8.13 Lipemia retinalis, characterized by the creamy white appearance of retinal vessels, is a fundoscopic finding occurring with very high triglyceride levels that can be seen in chylomicronemia syndrome. (From Fred HL, Accad M. Images in clinical medicine. Lipemia retinalis. *N Engl J Med* 1999:**340**(25):1969. Copyright 1999 Massachusetts Medical Society.)

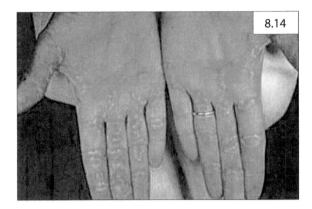

FIGURE 8.14 Palmar xanthomas are pathognomonic for dysbetalipoproteinemia type III. (Courtesy of Dr. Pham Thi Thu Thuy.)

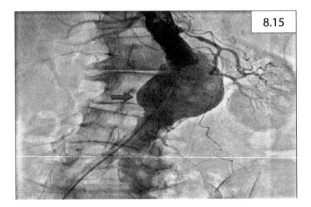

FIGURE 8.15 Aortogram demonstrating a large infrarenal abdominal aortic aneurysm measuring approximately 6.0 cm (arrow) with an associated severe stenosis of the proximal left renal artery.

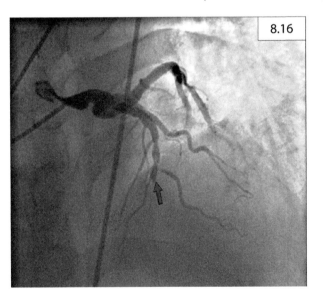

FIGURE 8.16 Coronary angiogram in a patient who presented with chest pain and an acute ST segment elevation myocardial infarction, demonstrating a large thrombus totally occluding the mid-left anterior descending artery (arrow).

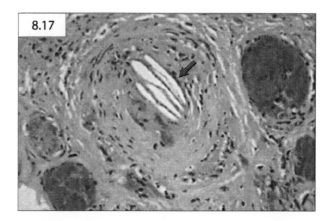

FIGURE 8.17 Characteristic needle-shaped clefts (arrow) resulting from atheroembolism. (From Bradley M. Images in clinical medicine. Spontaneous atheroembolism. *N Engl J Med* 1995:**332**(15):998. Copyright 1995 Massachusetts Medical Society.)

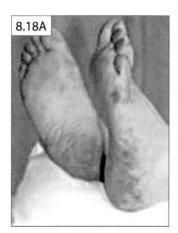 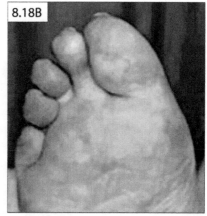

FIGURE 8.18 Cholesterol emboli demonstrated by livedo reticularis on the legs and a bluish discoloration of the toes in a patient 12 hours after cardiac catheterization. (From Rana O, McCrea W. Cholesterol emboli after coronary angioplasty. *N Engl J Med* 2006;**354**(12):1294. Copyright 2006 Massachusetts Medical Society. All rights reserved.)

Differential Diagnosis

The diagnosis of elevated lipoproteins can be established with the appropriate laboratory tests. If an underlying genetic abnormality is present, the diagnosis is suggested by the severity and pattern of the lipoprotein abnormalities, the family history, and the presence of premature atherosclerotic vascular disease. The history, physical examination, and laboratory evaluation remain crucial for the proper diagnosis as well as the appropriate treatment (Tables 8.3 and 8.4). Certain clinical features, such as tendon xanthomas, help distinguish familial hypercholesterolemia (present) from familial combined hypercholesterolemia (absent) (Figures 8.20 and 8.21). Some of the rare entities have pathognomonic or characteristic clinical findings, such as orange-yellow tonsils. Tangier disease (Figures 8.22 and 8.23). It is essential to rule out secondary factors that result in altered lipid metabolism, including hypothyroidism, diabetes mellitus, renal disease, obstructive liver disease, and alcohol intake, and medications such as estrogens/progestins, glucocorticoids, thiazides, and cyclosporine.

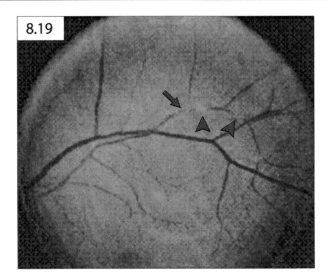

FIGURE 8.19 Fundoscopic examination showing a cholesterol emboli (arrow) at the bifurcation of a retinal and vascular sheathing distal to the occlusion (arrowheads). (From Bradley M. Images in clinical medicine. Spontaneous atheroembolism. *N Engl J Med* 1995;**332**(15):998. Copyright 1995 Massachusetts Medical Society.)

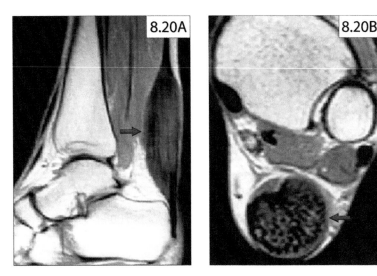

FIGURE 8.20 Sagittal proton-weighted magnetic resonance imaging showing a homogeneously enlarged Achilles tendon with increased signal intensity (arrow, A) and axial T-2 weighted magnetic resonance imaging revealing diffuse stippled pattern (arrow, B). Both are characteristic of xanthomas in this patient with hypercholesterolemia. (From van den Bosch HC, Vos LD. Images in clinical medicine. Achilles' tendon xanthoma in familial hypercholesterolemia. *N Engl J Med* 1998;**338**:1591. Copyright 1998 Massachusetts Medical Society.)

Diagnosis

The diagnosis of dyslipidemia is established by laboratory data and supported by comprehensive history and physical exam.

Significant dyslipidemia often results in progressive cardiovascular disease, and various imaging modalities for measuring clinical and subclinical atherosclerotic vascular disease include exercise and

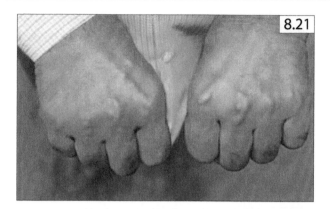

FIGURE 8.21 Tendon xanthomas in a patient with hypercholesterolemia. (From *JIACM* 2003;**4**(1):69. With permission.)

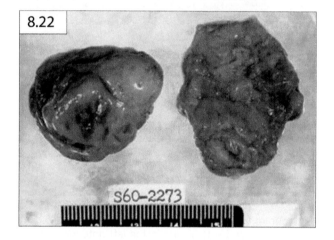

FIGURE 8.22 Enlarged tonsils seen in Tangier disease. (Courtesy of the National Institutes of Health.)

chemical stress testing, arterial Doppler evaluation, MRI, and conventional coronary and peripheral angiography. The availability of cardiac CT/coronary calcium scan provides an excellent noninvasive tool for the evaluation of the degree and extent of coronary plaque and imparts incremental value for risk stratification (Figure 8.24).

Management/Treatment

The largest body of evidence exists for improved outcomes with LDL lowering, and thus LDL remains the major therapeutic target for intervention. Large epidemiologic studies have confirmed the continuous and graded association between total serum cholesterol and coronary heart disease. Large, placebo-controlled, randomized trials have confirmed the benefit of LDL lowering in reducing long-term cardiac event rates in both primary and secondary prevention. Although LDL remains the primary lipid lowering priority, a low HDL and high TAG have been associated with increased cardiac risk and are potential targets for therapeutic intervention. Pooled data from several studies estimate a 2%–3% reduction in cardiovascular risk for every 1 mg/dL increase in HDL. If the TAG level is ≥500 mg/dL (5.6 mmol/L), then treatment of TAG takes priority over LDL reduction due to the desire to lower the risk of acute pancreatitis.

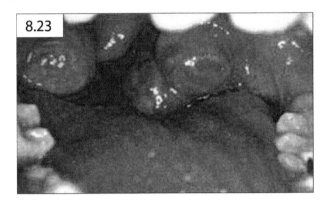

FIGURE 8.23   Enlarged orange-yellow tonsils in a patient with Tangier disease.

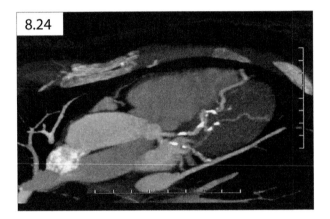

FIGURE 8.24   Coronary angiogram using a 64-slice computed tomography, demonstrating severe atherosclerosis with multiple mixed calcified and soft plaque in the left anterior descending artery and circumflex artery.

The central principle of management of the patient with dyslipidemia is that the intensity of risk reduction should be commensurate with the individual's absolute cardiovascular risk (Table 8.6). The major risk factors (exclusive of LDL cholesterol) include age ≥45 years in men and >55 years in women, cigarette smoking, hypertension (defined as >140/90 mmHg or on antihypertensive medication), low HDL cholesterol (<40 mg/dL [1 mmol/L] in males, <50 mg/dL in females [1.3 mmol/L]), family history of premature coronary heart disease in a first-degree relative (≥55 years in male relative, and <65 years in female relative). The 10-year risk of a cardiac event is assessed by using Framingham scoring, which takes into account these factors and may be calculated using tables or handheld and internet-based online calculators (www.cvriskcalculator.com or www.nhlbi.nih.gov/guidelines/cholesterol). The highest risk group includes those patients with established cardiovascular disease or a 'CHD risk equivalent'. This group is comprised of patients with known coronary artery disease; other clinical forms of atherosclerotic vascular disease including peripheral vascular disease, carotid artery disease, abdominal aortic aneurysm, and diabetes mellitus; and patients with multiple risk factors that confer a risk for a major cardiac event of >20% over 10 years. The identification of subclinical atherosclerotic disease such as high coronary calcification, significant carotid intimal medial thickness, or significant atherosclerotic burden on CT angiography likewise warrants aggressive and intensive lipid lowering.

Recent trials have demonstrated incremental reductions in risk for adverse cardiac events with LDL levels lowered to below 100 mg/dL (2.6 mmol/L). Overall, these data suggest that there is no clear-cut

TABLE 8.6 Major Atherosclerotic Cardiovascular Disease Risk Factors

MAJOR RISK FACTORS	ADDITIONAL RISK FACTORS	NONTRADITIONAL RISK FACTORS
• Advancing age • Elevated total serum cholesterol • Elevated non-HDL-C • Elevated LDL-C • Low HDL-C • Diabetes mellitus • Hypertension • Chronic kidney disease stages 3, 4 • Cigarette smoking • Family history of ASCVD	• Obesity, abdominal obesity • Family history of hyperlipidemia • Elevated small dense LDL-C • Elevated apoB • Elevated LDL particle concentration • Hypertriglyceridemia • PCOS • Dyslipidemia triad	• Elevated Lp(a) • Elevated clotting factors • High inflammatory markers • Elevated homocysteine levels • Apo E4 isoform • Elevated uric acid • Elevated TG-rich remnants

identifiable threshold for LDL level for risk reduction and that 'lower is better'. Based on these new trials demonstrating reduced cardiovascular event rates with lower LDL levels, the current recommendation for optimal LDL is <70 mg/dL (1.8 mmol/L) and ideally <55 mg/dL (1.4 mmol/L) in patients with the highest risk, including those with established ASCVD and CHD equivalents, and multiple major risk factors. No major safety issues have been identified thus far with lowering LDL in the range of 50–70 mg/dL (1.3–1.8 mmol/L) and even extremely low levels of about 20 mg/dL (0.5 mmol/L) are well tolerated and appear to be free of adverse effects.

Therapeutic Modalities for Dyslipidemia

A summary of the available agents for hypercholesterolemia is provided in Table 8.7.

Dietary Modification
Lifestyle and dietary modification remain the cornerstone of therapy, and reduced intake of saturated fat and cholesterol, increased physical activity, and weight control for all patients are strongly recommended. All patients should be advised to adopt therapeutic lifestyle changes including reduced intake of saturated fats (<7% of total calories) and cholesterol (<200 mg/d), increased intake of soluble fiber (10–25 g/day), weight reduction, and increased physical activity. However, although dietary modification should be a mainstay of any LDL-lowering strategy, the average LDL reduction from diet alone is in the range of 5% to 10%. HDL levels have been shown to increase with weight reduction, regular aerobic exercise, modest alcohol consumption, and smoking cessation. Typically, one may expect a 1 mg/dL increase in HDL for every 3 kg weight loss. Regular aerobic exercise may increase HDL by 10%–20% in sedentary adults.

Statins (3-Hydroxy-3-Methylglutaryl Coenzyme A Reductase Inhibitors)
Statins lower serum LDL levels through intracellular inhibition of the rate-limiting step in cholesterol production, which reduces cholesterol biosynthesis in the liver and upregulates LDL receptors to increase clearance of LDL from the blood. The statins lower the LDL by 18%–55%, increase HDL by 5%–15%, and lower TAG by 7%–30% (Table 8.2). At the currently available doses, rosuvastatin and atorvastatin are the most potent statins followed in order of LDL-lowering potency by simvastatin, lovastatin, pravastatin, and fluvastatin. Each doubling of a statin dose achieves an approximately 6% additional reduction in serum LDL (the 'rule of 6s'). A large meta-analysis involving 14 randomized, placebo-controlled trials with 90,056 patients showed that lowering LDL cholesterol levels by 39 mg/dL (1 mmol/L) with statin therapy significantly reduces the 5-year risk of major coronary events, coronary revascularization, and stroke by 21%. Although treatment with statins has resulted in major reductions in cardiac event rates, the amount of plaque regression demonstrated has been modest at most, raising the possibility that the

TABLE 8.7 Effects of LDL-C Lowering Agents

AGENT	LDL-C REDUCTION	SIDE EFFECTS/DRUG INTERACTIONS
Moderate Intensity Statins		
Atorvastatin 10–20 mg	–29% to –52%	Increased risk of myopathy with itraconazole, ketoconazole, erythromycin, clarithromycin, HIV protease inhibitors, nefazodone, amiodarone, verapamil, or large quantities of grapefruit juice (>1 quart [<1L] daily); may raise hepatic levels
Pravastatin 40–80 mg	–34% to –37%	
Simvastatin 20–40 mg	–29% to –41%	
Rosuvastatin 5–10 mg	–45% to 52 %	
High Intensity Statins		
Atorvastatin 40–80 mg	50% to 60%	
Rosuvastatin 20–40 mg	–55% to 63%	
Cholesterol Absorption Inhibitor (Ezetimibe 10 mg daily)	–12% to –17%	Side effects include headache and diarrhea; myopathy and hepatitis rare
Fibric Acids		
Gemfibrozil 600 mg twice per day	–5% to –20%	Side effects include rash and dyspepsia; potentiates the action of warfarin; contraindicated in patients with gallstones, or severe renal insufficiency/hemodialysis; variable effects on serum LDL and may increase LDL
Fenofibrate (48–145 mg or 43–130 mg daily)		
PCSK9 Inhibitors		
Evolocumab 140 mg q2w or 420 q4w	–63% to –71%	Nasopharyngitis, headache, hypertension, skin rash, diabetes mellitus
Alirocumab 75–150 mg q2w	–48% to –58%	
Bile Acid Sequestrants		
Colesevelam (3750–4375 mg daily)	–8% to 16%	Common side effects include nausea, constipation and bloating; associated with increased TAG levels
Bempedoic Acid	–17 to –18%	Rise in serum uric acid, tendon rupture (rare)
Small Interfering RNA Therapy		
Inclisiran 248 mg Subq 6 months	–52%	Local injection site reaction, antibody development, arthralgia, bronchitis

beneficial effects extend over and beyond LDL lowering, including anti-inflammatory, antithrombotic, immunomodulatory, and vascular effects.

Statins are generally well tolerated; however, common minor side effects include muscle and joint aches (up to 5%), fatigue, dyspepsia, and headaches. More serious side effects, such as severe myositis with generalized muscle pain and weakness and elevated creatine kinase (rarely leading to rhabdomyolysis and acute renal failure) or severe hepatitis, may occur infrequently. Adverse drug interactions should be carefully monitored, particularly at higher doses and in elderly patients with low body weight, and in patients with impaired renal function or on combination therapy with fibrates and/or nicotinic acid.

Ezetimibe (Cholesterol Absorption Inhibitor)
Ezetimibe acts through inhibition of intestinal cholesterol absorption in the small intestine leading to a reduction in hepatic cholesterol stores, increasing clearance of cholesterol from the blood. As monotherapy, ezetimibe effectively decreases LDL by 12%–17%. The combination of ezetimibe and a statin provides a dual effect by inhibiting cholesterol intestinal absorption and cholesterol production in the liver, respectively. This combination lowers the LDL by as much as an additional 25%, with potentially fewer side effects. Large randomized clinical trials evaluating the effect of the combination of ezetimibe

and simvastatin compared with simvastatin alone on 'hard' clinical end points such as mortality and MI are currently underway.

Bile Acid Sequestrants (Resins)
Bile acid sequestrants act through binding bile acids in the intestine resulting in increased excretion in the stool, stimulating greater intrahepatic cholesterol utilization for bile acid synthesis. This results in upregulation of the LDL receptor, which enhances the clearance of LDL in the bloodstream. In general, resins lower LDL by 15%–30%. The available bile acid sequestrants include cholestyramine, colesevelam, and colestipol. Treatment with cholestyramine has been associated with a reduction in the progression of atherosclerosis compared to control. Since resins are not systemically absorbed, they are extremely safe; however, they are associated with side effects including nausea, constipation, and bloating. Other medications should be taken either 1 hour before or 4 hours after the resins due to binding and decreased absorption (i.e., warfarin, digoxin). Resins may significantly raise the TAG level and should be avoided in patients with hypertriglyceridemia.

PCSK9 Inhibitors
The development of monoclonal antibody inhibitors of PCSK9, a protein that regulates the recycling of LDL receptors, has revolutionized the treatment of hyperlipidemia with profound LDL lowering in the range of 60%. Inhibiting PCSK9 results in more LDL receptors being recycled to the surface of the hepatocyte leading to increased clearance of LDL cholesterol from the circulation. Alirocumab and evolicumab are the two subcutaneous injections available, and have been shown to reduce cardiovascular outcomes and all-cause deaths by 15% in high-risk patients (ODYSSEY OUTCOMES trial NEJM 2018 and FOURNIER trial NEJM 2017). PCSK9 inhibitors should be considered for use in conjunction with statin therapy for LDL-C lowering in individuals with clinical cardiovascular disease who are unable to reach goal LDL-C/non-HDL-C levels with maximally tolerated statin, for individuals with familial hypercholesterolemia, or as monotherapy in statin-intolerant individuals. These drugs have a favorable safety profile and tolerability. Nasopharyngitis is the most reported side effect of both formulations.

Bempedoic Acid
Bempedoic acid is an oral inhibitor of adenosine triphosphate citrate lyase, an enzyme in the cholesterol biosynthesis pathway. Bempedoic acid alone or in combination with statin or ezetimibe lowers LDL-C by approximately 20% by upregulating LDL receptors. Side effects noted from the use of bempedoic acid include a rise in serum uric acid. Therefore, patients with active gout should be stabilized before starting bempedoic acid. Tendon rupture has also been rarely reported, and this risk may be increased in patients over 60 years of age, patients taking corticosteroids or fluoroquinolones, or with prior tendon disorders (CLEAR Harmony trial NEJM 2019).

Small Interfering RNA (siRNA) Therapy/Inclisiran
Inclisiran is a first-in-class small interfering RNA (siRNA) therapy that is administered subcutaneously and is selectively taken up by hepatocytes. The drug is slowly released into the cytoplasm and loads onto the RNA-induced silencing complex (RISC) and works with RISC to sequentially cleave multiple copies of PCSK9 protein mRNA, thus preventing PCSK9 protein production. As a result, there is upregulation of the LDL receptor on the surface of the hepatocyte, which leads to increased clearance of circulating LDL in the bloodstream. In patients with atherosclerotic cardiovascular disease with elevated LDL despite statin therapy, subcutaneous administration of inclisiran every 6 months has been shown to result in sustained and effective reduction of LDL cholesterol in the range of 52% (ORION-10 and ORION-11 trials NEJM 2020). Inclisiran was well tolerated for over 18 months and the most common side effect was injection site reaction (8.2%).

Nicotinic Acid
Nicotinic acid, or niacin, is a B-complex vitamin that raises HDL by 15%–35%, decreases TAG by 20%–50%, and modestly lowers LDL (approximately 5%–20%). Niacin raises HDL through metabolic pathways that increase the pre-β, apoA-I–rich HDL particles, which are the cardioprotective subfraction of HDL. Treatment with niacin reduced the risk of nonfatal MI even after 15 years of follow-up. The most common side effect is cutaneous flushing, and the major adverse side effect is hepatotoxicity.

Fibric Acids
Fibrates are agonists of PPARa, which is a nuclear receptor involved in the modulation of lipid and carbohydrate metabolism. Fibrates increase the hydrolysis of TAG by enhancing lipoprotein lipase activity, increasing clearance of TAG-rich lipoproteins from the plasma, and decreasing the rate of release of free fatty acids from adipocytes. Fibrates are the most effective agents for reducing TAG (20%–55%) and effectively raising HDL (10%–20%). These agents have variable effects on the serum LDL, and treated patients with hypertriglyceridemia may have an increase in their LDL. Fibrates are the drug of choice in patients with severe hypertriglyceridemia (>1000 mg/dL [11 mmol/L]). These drugs are beneficial in both primary prevention and in patients with established coronary artery disease.

Omega-3 Fatty Acids
Fish oils contain a high concentration of polyunsaturated fatty acids and have been shown to significantly reduce plasma triglycerides, by up to 45%. Omega-3-acid ethyl esters are available as an adjunct to the diet for the reduction of very high TG levels (≥500 mg/dL [5.5 mmol/L]) in adults. The mechanism of action is poorly defined but may involve the inhibition of acyl Coa:1,2- diacylglycerol acyltransferase and increased peroxisomal β-oxidation in the liver. Icosapent ethyl (Vascepa) has gained much attention in the last few years since this pure form of eicosapentaenoic acid at 2 grams twice a day was superior to placebo in lowering triglycerides, cardiovascular events, and cardiovascular death (31% relative risk reduction) among patients with high triglycerides and either known cardiovascular disease or those at high risk of developing it, and who were already on statin therapy with relatively well-controlled LDL levels (REDUCE-IT trial NEJM 2019). Conversely, adding a carboxylic acid formulation of omega 3-3 fatty acids (eicosapentaenoic acid and docosahexaenoic acid) in statin-treated patients with high cardiovascular risk resulted in no significant difference in the composite outcome of major cardiovascular events compared with placebo (STRENGTH trial JAMA 2020).

Nonpharmacologic Strategies for Lowering LDL Cholesterol
LDL apheresis involves the direct removal of LDL from the plasma and may be the preferred option in severe drug-resistant or refractory hyperlipidemia. Partial ileal bypass surgically depletes the enterohepatic supply of bile acids resulting in upregulation of the LDL receptor in the liver increasing LDL clearance, and may be an option for patients with severely elevated LDL and normal TAG refractory to maximal medical management who are not candidates for LDL apheresis.

New Treatment Options for Raising HDL
Cholesterol ester transfer protein (CETP) is a plasma glycoprotein produced in the liver that circulates in the bloodstream bound to HDL that facilitates the transfer of cholesterol esters between lipoproteins. CETP inhibition is a potential new therapy. CETP activity is potentially atherogenic and results in the net transfer of cholesterol esters from HDL to VLDL and LDL, thereby decreasing the concentration of HDL and increasing the concentration of LDL. Pharmacologically inhibiting CETP has been shown to increase the reverse cholesterol transport to the liver by increasing HDL and enhancing the hepatic uptake of cholesterol via scavenger receptor B-1 (SRB-1). However, CETP inhibition with torcetrapib was associated with increased mortality in a phase III clinical trial diminishing the enthusiasm for this class of drugs.

Other novel therapies under investigation for raising HDL include direct infusions of plasma-derived or synthetic apolipoprotein A-1 and agents that augment the expression of scavenger receptors.

LIPOPROTEIN (A)

Lipoprotein (a) (Lp(a)) is a lipoprotein similar to LDL in lipid and protein concentration but is composed of two protein particles – apolipoprotein (Apo) B-100 and apolipoprotein (a). The precise role of Lp(a) in the pathogenesis and progression of atherosclerosis remains controversial, but potential mechanisms of Lp(a) include binding to proinflammatory oxidized phospholipids, decreased nitric oxide synthesis, increased leukocyte adhesion and smooth muscle proliferation, and inhibition of the fibrinolytic system. However, there remains substantial uncertainty regarding the role of Lp(a) in clinical practice, although an elevated level might warrant more aggressive treatment in patients who have high-risk family histories but few other risk factors. Treatment options for patients with elevated Lp (a) include aspirin, statins, and PCSK9-I. Niacin is no longer recommended by National Lipid Association guidelines.

Studies evaluating the use of antisense oligonucleotide (ASO) administered subcutaneously (where a single DNA strand binds to messenger RNA), as well as siRNA therapy, which results in marked reductions in lipoprotein (a) levels are currently underway (APOLLO trial NEJM 2020).

Monoclonal Antibodies against ANGPTL3

Angiopoietin-like proteins (ANGPTLs) are regulators of lipoprotein metabolism. ANGPTL3 is a hormone produced by the liver that inhibits lipoprotein lipase. Evinacumab is a fully human monoclonal antibody against ANGPTL3 approved by the US Food and Drug Administration in 2021 for the treatment of familial hypercholesterolemia. It causes about a 50% reduction in LDL-C. The approved dose is 15 mg/kg IV infusion every 4 weeks. Nasal congestion, upper respiratory infection, and fatigue were the most common side effects of evinacumab reported.

FUTURE DIRECTIONS

The optimal diagnostic and therapeutic approach to lipid disorders remains a crucial component of contemporary clinical practice. The increasing prevalence of obesity, metabolic syndrome, and diabetes mellitus continues to fuel the need for comprehensive treatment strategies for dealing with multiple lipid and metabolic disorders. LDL cholesterol will remain the primary target for intervention, and new therapies targeting specific genetic pathways will continue to evolve. The proper identification and assessment of the patients at increased risk for the development and progression of atherosclerotic cardiovascular disease and the selection of the appropriate goals for therapy will continue to be the focus of basic science research and clinical trials in the future.

Neuroendocrine Tumors and Genetic Endocrine Disorders

9

Multiple Endocrine Neoplasia Type 1

Norma Lopez, Ikram Haque, and Shanika Samarasinghe

DEFINITION/OVERVIEW

Multiple endocrine neoplasia type 1 (MEN1), or Wermer's syndrome, is a complex autosomal dominant tumor syndrome with >95% penetrance by the fifth decade. It predisposes patients to more than 20 endocrine and non-endocrine tumors (Table 9.1); however, the primary manifestations are the occurrence of parathyroid, enteropancreatic, and anterior pituitary tumors. Duodenopancreatic neuroendocrine tumors, particularly nonfunctional neuroendocrine tumors, with their malignant potential represent the leading cause of death in patients with MEN1 followed by thymic neuroendocrine tumors.

PATHOPHYSIOLOGY

A germline inactivating mutation in the MEN1 gene located on chromosome 11q13.1 encodes a 610 amino acid protein called menin. More than 700 different germline and somatic mutations in the MEN1 gene

DOI: 10.1201/9781003100669-9

TABLE 9.1   Tumors Associated with MEN1

TUMOR	ESTIMATED PENETRANCE
Endocrine	
Parathyroid	90%
Enteropancreatic Tumors	
• Gastrinoma	40%
• Insulinoma	10%
• Nonfunctional, PPoma	20%–50%
• Glucagonoma	<1%
• VIPoma	<1%
Pituitary Adenomas	
• Prolactinoma	20%
• Somatotropinoma	10%
• Corticotropinoma	<5%
• Nonfunctioning	<5%
Adrenal	
• Adrenal cortical tumor	25%
• Pheochromocytoma	<1%
Foregut Carcinoid	
• Gastric enterochromaffin NET	10%
• Thymic NET	4%
• Bronchopulmonary NET	2%
Non-Endocrine	
Angiofibromas	85%
Collagenomas	70%
Lipomas	30%
Meningiomas	8%
Leiomyomas of uterus or esophagus	30%
Ependymoma	1%
Predisposition to breast cancer*	

Source: Adapted from Thakker RV et al., *JCEM* (2012), The Endocrine Society, with permission. * From Dreijerink, KMA, *NEJM*, 371, 2014.

have been reported since its cloning in 1997. Menin is primarily a nuclear protein involved in essential cell functions such as transcription, regulation, proliferation, DNA repair, cell division, and cell cycle control. Germline MEN1 mutations are not sufficient per se to develop clinical MEN1, and loss of the unaffected MEN1 allele is necessary for tumorigenesis. There is no clear genotype–phenotype correlation to date and approximately 10% of patients have a de novo mutation.

DIAGNOSIS

The clinical diagnosis of MEN1 is based upon the occurrence of two or more primary MEN1 tumor types (parathyroid gland, anterior pituitary, or enteropancreatic) or at least one MEN1-related tumor and a first-degree relative with a confirmed MEN1 gene mutation. It can also be diagnosed by identifying a germline MEN1 mutation in an individual or asymptomatic family member in whom the clinical diagnosis is not yet clearly established.

The optimal role of mutational analysis in MEN1 is not well defined. Guidelines suggest testing in any index patient with clinical MEN1, all first-degree relatives of known MEN1 carriers to identify those who require tumor screening, and individuals with suspicious MEN1 such as manifestations in young patients (<30 years) or those with multiple lesions in the same gland (multigland parathyroid disease or multiple pancreatic neuroendocrine tumors [pNETs]). All patients with gastrinoma should have MEN1 mutational analysis given that 25%–35% of patients will have MEN1 and its malignant potential.

PROGNOSIS AND SCREENING

Despite advances in diagnosis and management, this syndrome has a decreased life expectancy with a mean age of death of 55–60 years. The most common cause of death has shifted from complications of hormone excess states mainly due to gastrinomas to malignant neuroendocrine tumors (NETs). A monitoring program has been developed for patients and asymptomatic carriers with testing suggested as early as age 5, to detect and prevent significant morbidity and mortality (Table 9.2).

TABLE 9.2 Suggested Surveillance for MEN1-Associated Tumors

TUMOR	AGE TO BEGIN (YEARS)	BIOCHEMICAL TESTING ANNUALLY	IMAGING
Parathyroid	8	Calcium, PTH	None
Gastrinoma	20	Gastrin (±pH)	None
Insulinoma	5	Fasting glucose, insulin	None
Other enteropancreatic	<10	CgA, PPP, glucagon, VIP	MRI, CT or EUS (annual)
Anterior pituitary	5	Prolactin, IGF-1	MRI (every 3 years)
Adrenal	<10	None unless symptoms or tumor >1 cm seen on imaging	MRI or CT (annual with pancreatic imaging)
Thymic and bronchial carcinoid	15	None	CT or MRI (every 1–2 years)

Source: Adapted from Thakker RV et al., *JCEM* (2012), The Endocrine Society, with permission.

CLINICAL PRESENTATION AND MANAGEMENT

Parathyroid

Primary hyperparathyroidism (PHPT) is the most common manifestation, occurring in almost all patients by age 50. Differences in PHPT associated with MEN1 include an earlier age of onset (by 25 years vs. 55 years), greater reduction in bone mineral density, an equal male/female ratio (1:1 vs. 1:3), and multiple gland involvement. Preoperative localization with Tc99 sestamibi scintigraphy or neck ultrasound offers limited value since all parathyroid glands may be impacted and bilateral neck exploration is often required.

The recommended surgical approach is subtotal parathyroidectomy with the removal of 3.5 glands. Parathyroid tumors can be asynchronous and differ in size, each tumor likely representing a different clonal adenoma (Figure 9.1). MEN1-associated PHPT has a high recurrence rate that reaches up to 50% at 12 years compared to a 4%–16% recurrence rate in sporadic cases. As such, a less favored option would be total parathyroidectomy with autotransplantation of a parathyroid graft in the forearm or neck in those with extensive disease or at repeat surgery, but this is associated with higher rates of hypoparathyroidism (up to 46%). A thymectomy is also recommended in patients with MEN1, as additional glands are detected in 6%–20% of MEN1 patients with intrathymic parathyroid tissue as a cause as well as due to the risk of thymic carcinoid.

Enteropancreatic

MEN1 is the most common hereditary syndrome associated with pancreatic NET with a prevalence of 30%–80% depending on the series. These tumors are either nonfunctional or can be associated with a hormonal syndrome producing gastrin, insulin, vasoactive intestinal polypeptide (VIP), glucagon, or somatostatin. PNETs have an earlier age of onset in MEN1 (10–50 years vs. 50–80 years in sporadic cases), tend to be small (<2 cm) and multiple, and can lead to diffuse microadenomatosis (tumors <0.5 cm) (Figure 9.2). Nonfunctional tumors are increasingly recognized as the most frequent pNETs associated with MEN1 and tend to carry a worse prognosis.

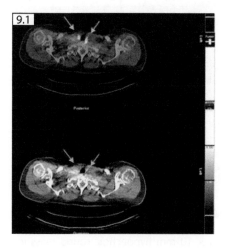
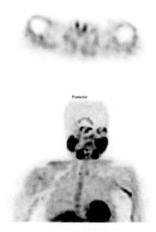

FIGURE 9.1 Parathyroid-SPECT shows synchronous multigland parathyroid adenomas in the two inferior glands. Faint uptake is also seen in the right superior gland. (Courtesy of the Nuclear Medicine Team, Loyola University.)

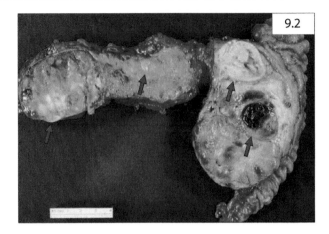

FIGURE 9.2   Multiple pancreatic islet cell tumors (arrows).

Diagnosis of NET depends on systematic imaging studies and hormonal measurements (Table 9.2). Endoscopic ultrasound (EUS) is the most sensitive method but is invasive and operator dependent (Figure 9.3). MRI is more sensitive than CT with less radiation. The role of functional imaging is uncertain, but 68Ga-DOTATATE PET/CT seems to have increased sensitivity in detecting NETs in MEN1, and FDG PET/CT may provide risk stratification in determining the malignant potential of pNETs (Figure 9.4).

Insulinomas, glucagonomas, and VIPomas are usually treated surgically once the tumor is localized. Figures 9.5 and 9.6 show CT images and resection of a pancreatic glucagonoma. Pancreatic cystic islet cell tumors in a MEN1 patient are shown in Figure 9.7. Figures 9.8 and 9.9 show imaging and histopathology in a patient with metastatic insulinoma. Gastrinomas are typically treated medically with proton-pump inhibitors, histamine 2-receptor blockers, and/or somatostatin analogues. Correction of concomitant hyperparathyroidism is associated with a decrease in gastrin levels and improvement in symptoms. Nonfunctional NETs larger than 2 cm or with rapid growth should be considered for resection given the concern for metastatic spread, whereas watchful waiting is reasonable for smaller tumors.

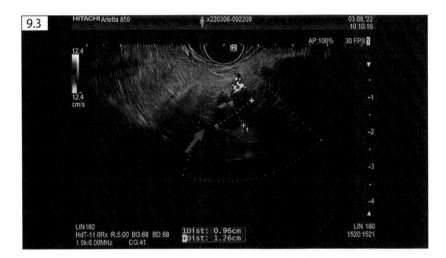

FIGURE 9.3   Endoscopic ultrasound depicts a 12 mm × 10 mm hypoechoic round mass in the pancreatic tail of a patient with MEN1. The endosonographic borders were well-defined. An intact interface was seen between the mass and the adjacent structures suggesting a lack of invasion. Fine needle aspiration demonstrated a well-differentiated NET. (Courtesy of Nuclear Medicine Team, Loyola University.)

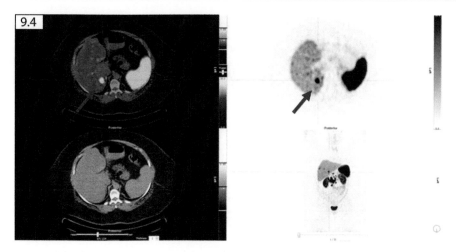

FIGURE 9.4 68Ga-DOTATATE PET/CT demonstrating a pancreatic neuroendocrine tumor with metastatic disease to the liver. (Courtesy of Nuclear Medicine Team, Loyola University.)

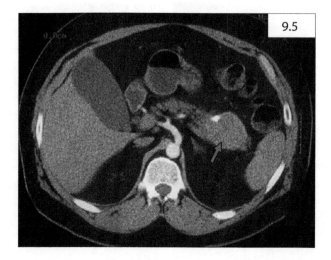

FIGURE 9.5 Pancreatic glucagonoma. A 6 cm solid mass with peripheral calcification at the tail of the pancreas is seen.

Pituitary

Hormonal studies including prolactin, IGF-1, and imaging with MRI of the sella (Figure 9.10) should be done at regular screening intervals. The management of pituitary adenomas in MEN1 patients is the same as those with sporadic tumors, although some reports suggest these tumors may be less responsive to medical management.

Cutaneous Lesions

Angiofibromas and collagenomas may be a strong sign in diagnosing MEN1 and tend to be multiple and more common in these patients (64% vs. 8% in the general population and 62% vs. 5%, respectively) (Figure 9.11).

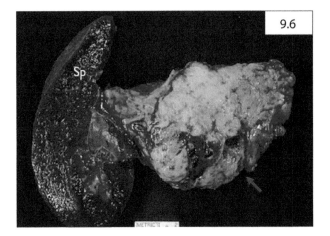

FIGURE 9.6   Tail of resected pancreas glucagonoma (arrow) from a patient with MEN1. Spleen (Sp) is seen on the left.

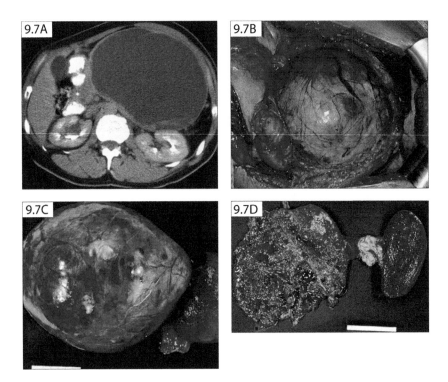

FIGURE 9.7   Cystic islet cell tumor in a MEN1 patient. (A) Exceptionally large homogeneous low-attenuation mass on the scan with thickened irregular wall, arising from the body of the pancreas. (B) Intraoperative photograph. (C) Gross resected pancreas, with tumor on the left, spleen on the right. (D) Dissected tumor on the left, spleen on the right.

Other

Adrenal tumors are common in MEN1. These lesions are usually bilateral, nonfunctional hyperplasia, although hyperaldosteronism, Cushing's syndrome, pheochromocytoma, and adrenocortical carcinoma have all been reported in up to 15% of MEN1-associated tumors. Recent studies from the Dutch MEN1

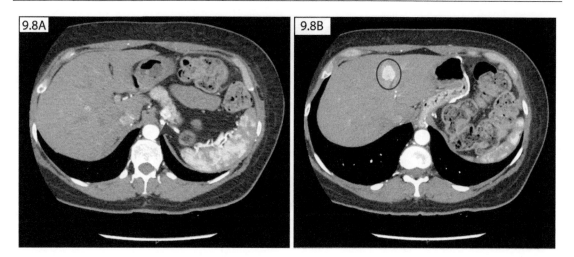

FIGURE 9.8   CT imaging in a patient with metastatic insulinoma with MEN1. (A) CT pancreas with contrast, showing a pancreatic body lesion measuring 1.4 × 1.2 × 1.5 cm (red arrowhead) with central hypodense cystic area. (B) A hyperenhancing liver lesion measuring 1.8 × 1.8 cm (red circle). ([A] From Poku C, Amjed H, Kazi F, Samarasinghe S. Metastatic insulinoma presenting after bariatric surgery in a patient diagnosed with MEN1. *Clinical Case Reports.* 2022 Feb;10(2). [B] From Poku C, Amjed H, Kazi F, Samarasinghe S. Metastatic insulinoma presenting after bariatric surgery in a patient diagnosed with MEN1. *Clinical Case Reports.* 2022 Feb;10(2).)

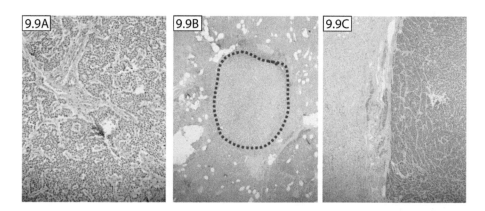

FIGURE 9.9   Histopathology in metastatic insulinoma. (A) Well-differentiated pancreatic neuroendocrine tumor. (B) Separate neuroendocrine microadenoma surrounded by normal pancreas. (C) Metastatic, well-differentiated neuroendocrine tumor within the liver (left, normal liver; right, metastatic tumor). (From Poku C, Amjed H, Kazi F, Samarasinghe S. Metastatic insulinoma presenting after bariatric surgery in a patient diagnosed with MEN1. *Clinical Case Reports.* 2022 Feb;10(2).)

database have shown an increased risk of breast cancer in female patients with a risk ratio of 1.96 (95% CI 1.33–2.88) compared to the general population. MEN1-associated carcinoid tumors include thymic, bronchial, and gastric enterochromaffin NETs (Table 9.1) and are discussed elsewhere in the chapter.

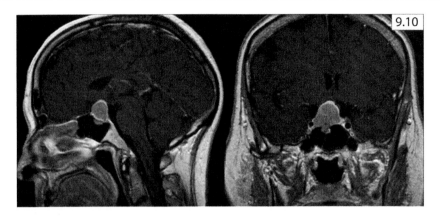

FIGURE 9.10   A pituitary macroadenoma measuring 1.5 × 1.9 × 1.8 cm, with slight elevation of the optic chiasm and invasion into the right cavernous sinus seen on MR of sella.

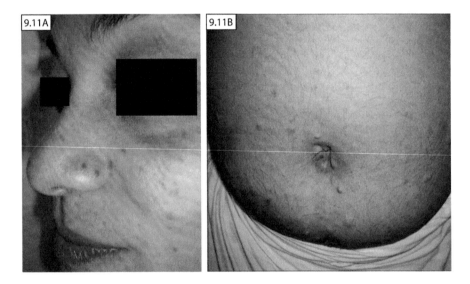

FIGURE 9.11   Cutaneous lesions are common in MEN1. (A) Angiofibromas are benign tumors that consist of acneiform papules that do not regress. (B) Collagenomas are round and firm and range from a few mm to several centimeters. (From A. Vashi, N. et al. *Dermatology Online Journal*, 18(12); B. Simi SM et al. *Indian J Dermatol*, 2012: 57:304-7.)

MULTIPLE ENDOCRINE NEOPLASIA TYPE 2

Definition/Overview

Multiple endocrine neoplasia type 2 is an autosomal dominant syndrome that can be classified into MEN2A, MEN2B, and familial medullary thyroid cancer (FMTC). These are rare genetic cancer syndromes involving multiple endocrine organ systems, more commonly the thyroid, adrenal, and parathyroid glands. First-degree relatives of patients with MEN2 have a 50% risk of inheriting the gene mutation leading to the syndrome. The prevalence of all MEN2 worldwide is 1 in 35,000.

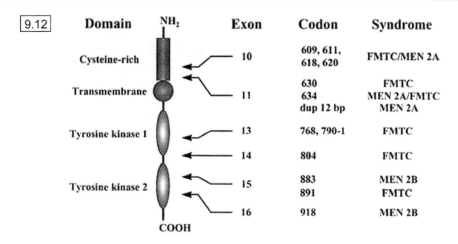

9.12	Domain	NH₂	Exon	Codon	Syndrome
	Cysteine-rich		10	609, 611, 618, 620	FMTC/MEN 2A
	Transmembrane		11	630	FMTC
				634	MEN 2A/FMTC
				dup 12 bp	MEN 2A
	Tyrosine kinase 1		13	768, 790-1	FMTC
			14	804	FMTC
	Tyrosine kinase 2		15	883	MEN 2B
				891	FMTC
		COOH	16	918	MEN 2B

FIGURE 9.12   Representation of RET gene showing codons identified in MEN2 families. (From Jhiang, S.M. The RET proto-oncogene in human cancers. *Oncogene*, 2000: 19(49):5590–5597.)

MEN2A is characterized by medullary thyroid carcinoma (MTC), pheochromocytoma (Pheo), and hyperparathyroidism (HPT). Those affected by MEN2B display a more aggressive MTC and present with Pheo and ganglioneuromas but not with HPT. FMTC only manifests with MTC (characteristic features can be found in Brandi ML, et al., CONSENSUS: Guidelines for diagnosis and therapy of MEN type 1 and type 2, *Journal of Clinical Endocrinology & Metabolism*, 2001 Dec;86(12):5658–71.)

Pathophysiology

The pathophysiology for MEN2 involves the RET (rearranged during transfection) protooncogene. The RET gene is located on chromosome 10. It is expressed in neuroendocrine and neural cells where it encodes receptor-type tyrosine kinase in extracellular, transmembrane, and intracellular tyrosine kinase domains. Missense mutations in this gene are the cause of MEN2. A specific RET mutation has been identified in over 95% of families with MEN2A (Figure 9.12).

Clinical Presentation

Patients with classic MEN2A will almost all develop MTC (90%–100%). A lower number of patients develop Pheo (up to 50%) and HPT (up to 30%) with risk and penetrance depending on the RET gene mutation. Most MEN2A RET mutations involve codon 609, 611, or 620 of exon 10 or codon 634 of exon 11 with the latter being the most common mutation. MEN2B is associated with MTC (100%) presenting at an earlier age, Pheo (up to 50%) depending on gene mutation, and no demonstration of HPT. The most common mutation in MEN2B is M918T, which is present in over 95% of MEN2B patients. Patients with MEN2B also manifest extra-adrenal features of intestinal ganglioneuromas, ophthalmologic signs, mucosal neuromas, and marfanoid body habitus. Patients with FMTC present with medullary thyroid cancer and RET germline mutation but without Pheo, HPT, or other somatic abnormalities (Figures 9.13–9.15).

MEN2A includes rare variants with cutaneous lichen amyloidosis (CLA) and MEN2A with Hirschsprung's disease. CLA is an intense itchy rash consisting of raised spots that are scaly and brown on the shins, thighs, feet, and forearms. Hirschsprung's disease presents at birth due to missing nerve endings in an infant's colon resulting in gastrointestinal symptoms such as constipation, vomiting, diarrhea, or the more serious condition of toxic megacolon.

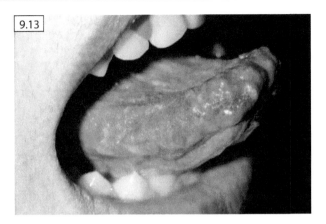

FIGURE 9.13   Mucosal neuromas of the tongue. (From NCI Visuals Online, Edward Cowen, National Cancer Institute. Available from https://visualsonline.cancer.gov/details.cfm?imageid=12516.)

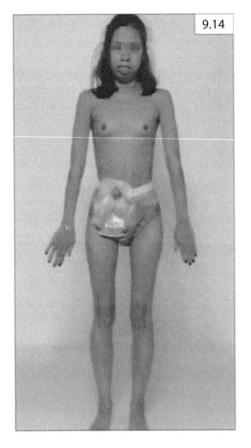

FIGURE 9.14   Marfanoid body habitus, typical facial features, and colostomy due to megacolon complications.

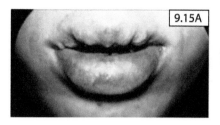
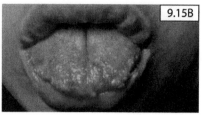

FIGURE 9.15   Neuromas in MEN2B. (A) Thick, lumpy lips. (B) Mucosa neuromas of the tongue and lips.

MEDULLARY THYROID CANCER

Medullary thyroid carcinoma (MTC) originates from parafollicular C-cells of the thyroid. These cells secrete calcitonin (Ct). Medullary thyroid cancer represents 3%–5% of all thyroid cancers with most cases being sporadic (75%) and 25% associated with MEN2. Advances in genetic analysis of tumor cells have shown that there is a difference in levels of regulators of genetic expression called microRNAs (miRNAs) in hereditary MTC compared to sporadic disease. Investigators have found higher levels of miRNAs associated with worse clinical outcomes, and persistent and metastatic disease.

MTC presents in the first few years of life in MEN2B and presents about 10 years earlier on average than in MEN2A. MTC in MEN2 is usually multifocal and bilateral, and exhibits c-cell hyperplasia, known to be a precursor to tumors. This differs from sporadic MTC, which is usually unifocal and unilateral (Figure 9.16).

Diagnosis

Medullary thyroid cancer is suspected on fine needle aspiration specimen and confirmed on thyroidectomy specimen. Guidelines recommend immunohistochemical analysis for the presence of markers such as calcitonin, chromogranin, and CEA, and the absence of thyroglobulin in surgical specimens suspected of MTC due to its variance of histologic appearance. More than 14 different histological variants of MTC have been described; usually, epithelioid cells predominate, however, spindle cells may be seen (Figure 9.17). Medullary thyroid cancer can often be confused with other types of thyroid tumors

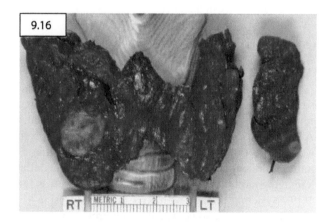

FIGURE 9.16   Gross specimen of MTC in MEN2A. Pathologic specimen from a thyroidectomy. Right MTC (1.5 cm) and multiple small foci of MTC in a patient with MEN2A.

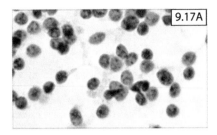
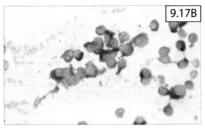

FIGURE 9.17   (A) Spindle-shaped cells can be seen in MTC (H&E ×300). (B) Positive calcitonin immunostaining, consistent with MTC (H&E ×150).

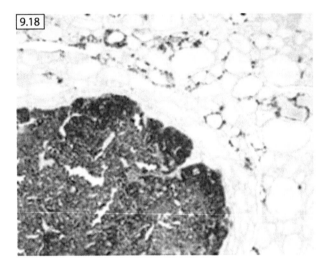

FIGURE 9.18   Strong immunoreactivity with calcitonin in MTC tumor with diffuse reactivity in surrounding thyroid parenchyma with C-cell hyperplasia. (From Thompson L. Pathology Clinic. Available from https://lester-thompsonmd.com/pdf/ENTJ-2010-07_Medullary%20thyroid%20carcinoma.pdf.)

including papillary and follicular thyroid cells. Concurrent serum Ct and CEA should be measured in all patients with MTC. Levels of Ct and CEA are used for prognosis and surveillance. High CEA in relation to Ct as well as low levels of Ct and CEA in advanced disease are associated with poorly differentiated tumors (Figure 9.18).

Management and Treatment

The treatment of MTC is resection of the thyroid tumor and resection of locoregional metastasis in both sporadic as well as hereditary forms of MTC. Postoperative management and staging depend on the postoperative Ct and CEA levels. Most guidelines recommend checking tumor markers 2–3 months postoperatively when levels would expect to nadir. Systematic additional imaging to search for metastasis is recommended if postoperative Ct remains above 500 pg/ml. Metastatic medullary thyroid cancer can be found using cross-section imaging modalities such as CT and MRI as well as functional imaging such as DOPA/PET-CT (Figure 9.19). Systemic therapy with RET-targeted tyrosine kinase inhibitors (TKIs) is not curative but offers promising results for some patients with progressing or symptomatic disease.

Genetic testing is recommended for early screening of patients at risk for MEN2. The decision to perform prophylactic thyroidectomy based on RET mutation testing alters the clinical course of MTC and

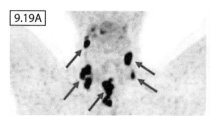
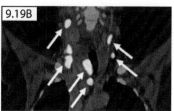

FIGURE 9.19   PET/CT DOPA MTC with DOPA-positive disease in the right thyroid lobe and central and bilateral lymph node metastasis. (From Rasul S, Hartenbach S, Rebhan K, Göllner A, Karanikas G, Mayerhoefer M, et al. [18F]DOPA PET/ceCT in diagnosis and staging of primary medullary thyroid carcinoma prior to surgery. *European Journal of Nuclear Medicine and Molecular Imaging.* 2018 [cited 2023 Feb 28];45(12):2159–69. Available from https://www.ncbi.nlm.nih.gov/pmc/articles/PMC6182401/.)

early thyroidectomy can be curative in MEN2. Prophylactic thyroid surgery is recommended based on the youngest age at the first diagnosis of MEN2 according to a specific codon. Medullary thyroid cancer, however, remains the main cause of mortality in patients with both MEN2A and MEN2B due to improved diagnosis and treatment of other associated conditions involving the syndrome including Pheo.

Prognosis

The RET-specific mutations determine the phenotypic expression of MEN2 and the aggressiveness of the medullary thyroid cancer component. Specific mutations have been shown to correlate with the age of onset of MTC as well as the risk of developing Pheo or HPT. Investigators determined that there is a moderate, high, or highest risk of development and growth of MTC based on the distinct point mutation of RET in MEN2. This discovery led to an improved ability to predict clinical course and optimize treatment and management based on RET mutation risk. Moderate- and high-risk mutations have similar rates of overall survival and distant metastatic disease, therefore, experts suggest early-onset versus late-onset MTC in MEN2 should be considered in predicting clinical course.

PHEOCHROMOCYTOMA IN MEN2

Diagnosis

Pheochromocytoma (Pheo) is the second most common disease in MEN2 and is seen in approximately 50% of patients. The penetrance of Pheo in this syndrome depends on the specific RET mutation and varies in penetrance from 10% to 80%. It is important to note that in families with known MEN2, early thyroidectomy greatly decreases the risk of MTC; therefore, Pheo remains the main disease requiring close surveillance.

Penetrance of Pheo is higher in RET mutations in codons 634, 883, and 918. Due to the progressive nature of Pheo in MEN2, bilateral disease diagnosis may be synchronous or metachronous, thereby requiring prolonged surveillance.

One-third of patients with MEN2 and Pheo were asymptomatic at the time of diagnosis, therefore, most are identified during Pheo screening due to known MEN2. Pheochromocytoma in MEN2 secrete both metanephrines and normetanephrines, therefore, both should be checked every year even in asymptomatic patients. Adrenal CT can be used to detect Pheo and usually reveals an unenhanced density of >10 HU (with washout >50%).

Functional imaging may be reserved for consideration of multifocal or rarely metastatic Pheo.

Management and Treatment

Surgery is the only treatment option for patients with Pheo in MEN2. Experienced centers have reported data suggesting adrenal-sparing surgery has advantages over bilateral adrenalectomies, sparing patients from lifelong steroid dependence. Moreover, current application of laparoscopic adrenalectomy has reduced surgical morbidity (Figures 9.20–9.23).

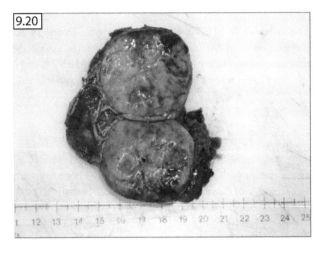

FIGURE 9.20   Gross specimen of pheochromocytoma. Note the vascular and dusky appearance of the tumor, a characteristic of Pheo. (Courtesy of Dr. Steven De Jong.)

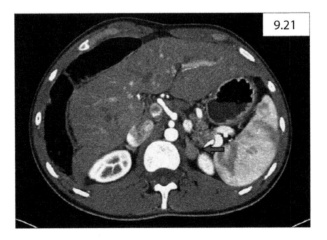

FIGURE 9.21   CT scan of abdomen in a patient with MEN2B demonstrating a pheochromocytoma. The 2 cm left adrenal pheochromocytoma (arrow) was subsequently removed by laparoscopic adrenalectomy.

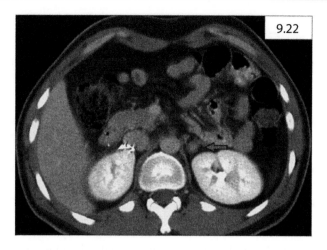

FIGURE 9.22 Left adrenal nodule (arrow) in an asymptomatic patient with MEN2A. Biochemistry was negative for Pheo. Note surgical clips from previous right adrenalectomy due to Pheo.

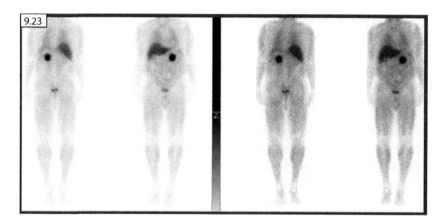

FIGURE 9.23 MIBG demonstrating a left Pheo. Increased MIBG uptake in the left upper abdomen corresponding to previously seen mass on MRI and consistent with a left 7 cm pheochromocytoma postoperatively. (Courtesy of Nuclear Medicine Team, Loyola University.)

PRIMARY HYPERPARATHYROIDISM IN MEN2

Diagnosis and Management

Primary hyperparathyroidism has been reported in as high as 20%–30% of MEN2A syndromes with some series detailing lower prevalence. All patients with MEN2 syndrome should be screened for HPT. The peak age of presentation is the third decade, a younger presentation compared to non-syndrome-related HPT. Parathyroid tumors do not usually occur in MEN2B. The workup and clinical indication for surgery are similar to sporadic cases of HPT. Most cases are asymptomatic and are diagnosed with a finding of asymptomatic hypercalcemia. The surgical approach considers the possibility of multigland disease, both hyperplasia and adenoma presenting in the same patient, and the possibility of only a single adenoma.

CARCINOID SYNDROME

Definition and Etiology

Carcinoid syndrome is the most frequent of the ectopic hormone syndromes. It describes a constellation of symptoms including cutaneous flushing, diarrhea, bronchospasms, and skin changes arising from tumoral secretion of a variety of biogenic amines and peptides such as serotonin, 5-hydroxytryptophan, kallikrein, histamine prostaglandins, and VIP. Over 40 types of secretary products have been implicated in carcinoid syndrome.

Not all carcinoid tumors produce carcinoid syndrome; frequency varies from 1.7% to 18.7% in some series, whereas prior series describe it in 8% of patients. The frequency of carcinoid varies with the location of the carcinoid tumor. The most common locations causing the syndrome are found in parts of the small intestine, pulmonary tract, certain types of gastric carcinoid tumors, and Meckel's diverticulum. Midgut carcinoids account for a mean of 72% of carcinoid syndrome cases.

Pathophysiology

The dominant culprit substance produced by a tumor explains the symptoms of carcinoid syndrome. Serotonin and its precursors affect gut motility and secretion and cause bowel hypermotility and diarrhea. Tumor vasoactive products stimulate myofibroblast proliferation and deposits of extracellular matrix, which is thought to be the mechanism of carcinoid heart disease. Histamine, kallikrein, and prostaglandin secretion cause peripheral vasodilation leading to spells of flushing and even hypotension. Niacin deficiency is not uncommon and can cause symptoms in carcinoid syndrome, although severe niacin deficiency causing pellagra is uncommon. Niacin and serotonin share the precursor tryptophan, therefore, niacin deficiency can ensue when there is a large amount of serotonin synthesis.

Clinical Presentation

The most common symptoms of carcinoid syndrome are flushing and secretory diarrhea. The frequency of flushing is up to 90%; and can be long lasting and purple or violaceous in hue with foregut tumors, or short lasting and pink to red in hue for midgut tumors. Diarrhea is reported in anywhere from 60% to 80% of cases of carcinoid syndrome and is spontaneous or a result of alcohol or tyramine-containing foods, and occurs with or without abdominal pain. Bronchospasms occur with 15% frequency and manifest with wheezing. Pellagra is rare but can manifest as dermatitis, diarrhea, or dementia in carcinoid syndrome (Figure 9.24). Carcinoid heart disease has been reported in 19%–60% of carcinoid cases and may manifest as dyspnea or a murmur indicating valvular disease (Figure 9.25).

Diagnosis

Initial testing to confirm the diagnosis of suspected carcinoid syndrome most frequently consists of a 24-hour urine assessment for 5-HIAA after avoiding serotonin-rich foods and potentially interfering drugs. This measurement has a sensitivity of 73%–93% and a specificity of 100%. Plasma and serum 5-HIAA have similar sensitivity and specificity compared to urine and can be used for the diagnosis and surveillance of carcinoid syndrome as long there is consideration of renal function given that there was an inverse relationship between serum 5-HIAA levels and eGFR. Echocardiography is required to diagnose

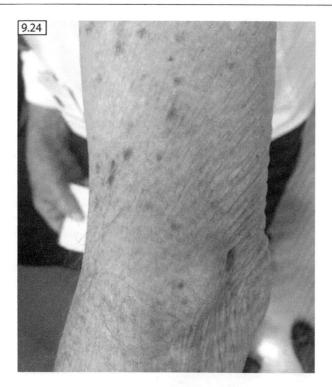

FIGURE 9.24 Pellagra skin findings. Dry skin and scratches in a patient with pellagra. (From Anezka C. Rubin de Celis Ferrari, João Glasberg, Rachel P Riechelmann, Carcinoid syndrome: Update on the pathophysiology and treatment, *Clinics*, 73, Suppl 1, 2018, https://doi.org/10.6061/clinics/2018/e490s.)

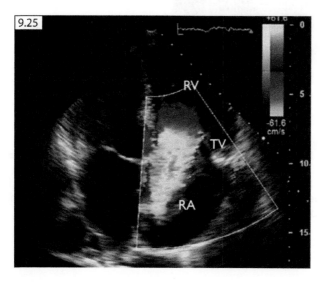

FIGURE 9.25 Carcinoid valvular disease. Severe tricuspid regurgitation as seen in Doppler resulting from thickened tricuspid valve (TV).

carcinoid heart disease and experts recommend using echocardiography for screening in patients with known carcinoid syndrome.

Management and Treatment

Somatostatin analogues are considered standard treatment in carcinoid syndrome both for controlling symptoms and for their antigrowth effect on the carcinoid tumor. Octreotide and lanreotide are somatostatin analogues that bind to somatostatin receptors to inhibit the hormones and vasoactive substances that cause the symptoms in carcinoid syndrome. They have been shown to reduce the frequency of diarrhea and flushing in 70%–90% of patients with carcinoid symptoms. Octreotide-LAR and Lanreotide Autogel are longer-acting agents requiring monthly administration. Pasireotide LAR has a different pharmacodynamic profile than octreotide and lanreotide and has shown similar symptom control.

Promising studies have been undertaken in patients with somatostatin analogue-resistant disease. Alternative therapies and methods include the mTOR inhibitor everolimus, PRRT (peptide-directed radiotherapy) using ^{177}Lu-DOTATATE with octreotide-LAR, cytoreductive therapy, liver-directed therapies such as radiofrequency ablation of the tumor, as well as the tryptophan hydroxylase (TPH) inhibitor telotristat ethyl. These alternative therapies can be considered for refractory disease or to palliate severe symptoms (Figures 9.26 and 9.27).

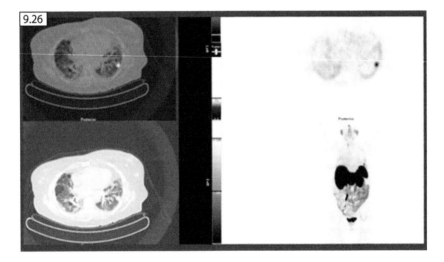

FIGURE 9.26 PET/CT DOTATATE of lung carcinoid. Abnormal PET/CT DOTATATE study demonstrating DOTATATE avid left lower lobe lung nodule, compatible with a lung carcinoid tumor. (Courtesy of Nuclear Medicine Team, Loyola University.)

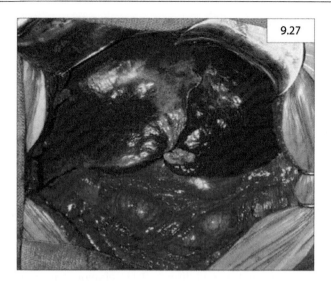

FIGURE 9.27 Carcinoid metastasis to the liver.

AUTOIMMUNE POLYENDOCRINE SYNDROMES

Definition/Etiology

Autoimmune polyglandular syndrome (APS) is a hereditary, diverse group of clinical syndromes of endocrine deficiencies caused by autoantibody-mediated destruction of endocrine and non-endocrine organs.

APS type I, also called autoimmune polyendocrinopathy–candidiasis–ectodermal dystrophy (APECED) syndrome, can be inherited in both the autosomal recessive and autosomal dominant fashion. It is associated with a mutation in the autoimmune regulator gene (AIRE) on chromosome 21q22.3. This usually presents in early childhood and is noted to have a higher prevalence in certain populations such as those living in Finland, Sardinia, and Persian Jews in Israel.

APS type II, also called Schmidt's syndrome, is likely polygenic and is more prevalent than APS type I. There is a female predominance, and the disease has a later onset than APS type I, usually manifesting in adulthood.

IPEX (immunodysregulation, polyendocrinopathy, enteropathy, X-linked) is an extremely rare inherited syndrome. IPEX has an earlier onset than APS type I and usually manifests in infancy. It has a high mortality rate if treatment is not started promptly in the first few years of life.

Pathophysiology

The main abnormalities are loss of immune tolerance due to defects in the AIRE gene leading to lymphocytic infiltration of affected organs, along with the generation of autoantibodies to various components of the affected organs. These include antibodies to adrenocortical enzymes such as 21-hydroxylase or 17-alpha-hydroxylase, glutamic acid decarboxylase (GAD), islet cell antibodies (ICA), thyroid peroxidase (TPO), and type 1 interferon autoantibodies. The result of the aforementioned dysregulated processes leads to autoimmune destruction of the glands and endocrine insufficiency.

Also, the use of an immune checkpoint inhibitor for cancer therapy has been identified as a new trigger for autoimmune polyendocrine syndromes. For example, colitis is common, and autoimmune thyroiditis has frequently been seen in patients treated with both CTLA-4 and PD-1 immune checkpoint blockade, with an incidence of more than 10%.

Clinical Presentation

Characterizing APS can be challenging due to the large heterogeneity and overlap of clinical manifestations and the broad spectrum. Table 9.1 summarizes the broad characteristics and classification of APS.

APS Type I

APS-I is characterized by the development of at least two of three cardinal components during childhood: chronic mucocutaneous candidiasis, hypoparathyroidism, and primary adrenal insufficiency (Addison's disease). Other manifestations include primary hypogonadism, type 1 diabetes mellitus, autoimmune gastritis and other gastrointestinal problems, skin conditions such as alopecia and vitiligo, keratoconjunctivitis, autoimmune hepatitis, and thyroid disease (less common than in APS type II). Ectodermal dystrophies may manifest as tooth enamel hypoplasia and nail dystrophy (Figure 9.28).

APS Type II

APS-II is far more prevalent than APS-I and IPEX. Patients with APS-II have courses characterized by at least two of the following three endocrinopathies: type 1 diabetes, autoimmune thyroid disease, and Addison's disease. Other autoimmune diseases may also be present such as celiac disease, alopecia, vitiligo, primary ovarian insufficiency, and pernicious anemia. Additional manifestations are more frequent among patients with APS-II who have Addison's disease. Unlike APS-I, APS-II usually manifests in adulthood, most commonly in the third and fourth decades of life, and is more common in females.

IPEX

IPEX is an extremely rare inherited syndrome manifesting during infancy characterized by early-onset type 1 diabetes; autoimmune enteropathy with intractable diarrhea and malabsorption; and dermatitis that

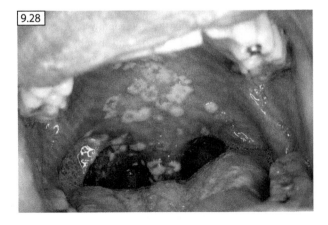

FIGURE 9.28 Secondary oral pseudomembranous candidiasis infection. (From Centers for Disease Control and Prevention, Sol Silverman Jr., DDS, ID 6053.)

may be eczematiform, ichthyosiform, or psoriasiform. Eosinophilia and elevated IgE levels are seen often in patients with IPEX. Renal involvement, most often with membranous glomerulonephritis or interstitial nephritis, is also common.

Diagnosis

There is no universally accepted diagnostic protocol for APS. However, once APS is suspected, testing for autoantibodies is indicated. Organ-specific autoantibodies predict for preexisting, or a potential for, insufficiency of that endocrine gland. These include ICA and GAD for type 1 diabetes, TPO for thyroid disease, 21-hydroxylase for Addison's disease, and antismooth muscle antibody for autoimmune hepatitis. Patients with IPEX have autoantibodies against harmonin and villin, proteins that are found in the microvilli of the intestinal brush border. Endocrine organ-specific function can be evaluated by measuring fasting glucose (pancreas), calcium and phosphorus (parathyroid hormone [PTH] if indicated), TSH, early morning cortisol, gonadotropins with sex steroids, and hemoglobin (pernicious anemia).

Management/Treatment

The general theme in the management of APS syndromes is hormone replacement as needed and treatment of complications. All patients with the disease and asymptomatic carriers should have endocrine organ function evaluation at least twice annually. Siblings of all patients with APS-I should be screened for the disease. Patients with IPEX can be cured with allogenic bone marrow transplantation.

Chronic mucocutaneous candidiasis is treated with oral mycostatin and oral amphotericin B to avoid drug resistance associated with continuous azole use. In addition, azoles inhibit steroid synthesis, which increases the risk of precipitating adrenal insufficiency in patients with undiagnosed Addison's disease.

Immunosuppressants, such as prednisone, azathioprine, and cyclosporine, are used for the treatment of autoimmune hepatitis, keratitis, pneumonitis, and enteritis.

McCUNE–ALBRIGHT SYNDROME

Definition/Overview

Fibrous dysplasia/McCune–Albright syndrome (FD/MAS) is a rare disease typified by skeletal lesions, skin hyperpigmentation, and variable hyperfunctioning endocrinopathies. The classic triad includes fibrous dysplasia of the bone, café-au-lait skin macules, and precocious puberty. It results from an embryonic post-zygotic activating mutation in the GNAS gene, which encodes the α-subunit of the G_s signaling protein. This leads to constitutive $G\alpha_s$ activation, ligand-independent signaling of the G_s-coupled protein receptor, and inappropriate cAMP production. The clinical presentation is determined by the extent and site of the mutation-bearing tissue, and there is a high degree of variability between individuals. FD/MAS is not inherited and there are no known genetic or environmental triggers.

Pathophysiology

Constitutive signaling through LH, FSH, TSH, GnRH, and ACTH receptors results in endocrinopathies. These include precocious puberty due to activation of ovarian or testicular tissue, thyroid enlargement, nodules with or without hyperthyroidism, growth hormone (GH) excess, and neonatal hypercortisolism. In bone, $G\alpha_s$ activation impairs differentiation of skeletal stem cells, leading to replacement of normal bone with fibrotic stroma and immature woven bone. These FD lesions can also secrete increased fibroblastic growth factor 23 (FGF-23), which can lead to renal phosphate wasting. Increased cAMP signaling in the skin stimulates melanin production, resulting in café-au-lait macules.

Clinical Presentation

Characteristic café-au-lait macules show jagged and irregular borders ('coast of Maine') and are often the first clinical sign. Location respects the midline of the body with distribution reflecting patterns of embryonic cell migration (Figure 9.29). FD ranges from monostotic disease affecting one bone to polyostotic and can involve any combination of the craniofacial, axial, or appendicular skeleton (Figure 9.30). Radiographs show a characteristic lesion of thinning cortex and intramedullary ground glass. The proximal femur is a frequently involved site and may develop a classic 'shepherd's crook' deformity (Figure 9.30A). Lesions of the craniofacial region can present with painless facial asymmetry or, in rare cases, malocclusion, hearing, or visual impairment.

GNAS activation in ovarian tissue results in recurrent estrogen-producing cysts leading to early breast development, vaginal bleeding, and growth acceleration. Precious puberty is less common in boys and presents with macroorchidism and ultrasonographic abnormalities such as focal testicular heterogeneity, masses, and microlithiasis. Approximately 10%–15% of such boys show signs of early pubic and axillary hair, acne, aggressive behavior, and early growth. Thyroid abnormalities occur in approximately 50% of patients with sonographic findings of diffuse thyroid enlargement and mixed cystic and solid

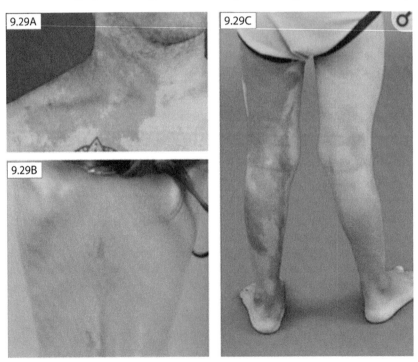

FIGURE 9.29 Characteristic café-au-lait macules show jagged and irregular borders ('coast of Maine'). Location respects the midline of the body with distribution reflecting patterns of embryonic cell migration. (From Javaid MK, Boyce A, Appelman-Dijkstra N, Ong J, Defabianis P, Offiah A, et al. Best practice management guidelines for fibrous dysplasia/McCune-Albright syndrome: A consensus statement from the FD/MAS international consortium. *Orphanet Journal of Rare Diseases*. 2019 Jun 13;14(1).)

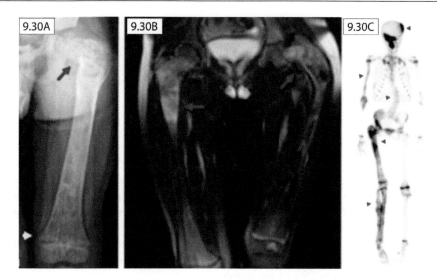

FIGURE 9.30 Fibrous dysplasia. (A) Radiographs show a characteristic lesion of thinning cortex and intramedullary ground glass. (B) The proximal femur is a frequently involved site and may develop a classic 'shepherd's crook' deformity. (C) FD ranges from monostotic disease affecting one bone to polyostotic, and can involve any combination of the craniofacial, axial, or appendicular skeleton. (From Javaid MK, Boyce A, Appelman-Dijkstra N, Ong J, Defabianis P, Offiah A, et al. Best practice management guidelines for fibrous dysplasia/McCune-Albright syndrome: A consensus statement from the FD/MAS international consortium. *Orphanet Journal of Rare Diseases*. 2019 Jun 13;14(1).)

lesions interspersed with areas of normal-appearing tissue. In the pituitary, GNAS activation results in somatolactotroph cell hyperplasia, leading to excessive growth hormone and prolactin production in 15% of patients (Figure 9.31). A clinical sign in these patients is the expansion of craniofacial FD, which is

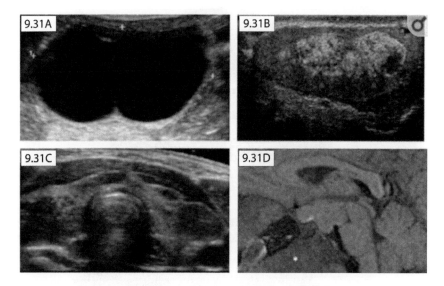

FIGURE 9.31 (A) Pelvic ultrasound in 5-year-old girl with large ovarian cyst and clinical signs of precocious puberty. (B) Testicular ultrasound in a patient with macroorchidism. (C) Thyroid ultrasound showing multiple hyper and hypoechoic nodules. (D) A pituitary MRI in a patient with growth hormone excess revealing a pituitary macroadenoma. (From Javaid MK, Boyce A, Appelman-Dijkstra N, Ong J, Defabianis P, Offiah A, et al. Best practice management guidelines for fibrous dysplasia/McCune-Albright syndrome: a consensus statement from the FD/MAS international consortium. *Orphanet Journal of Rare Diseases*. 2019 Jun 13;14(1).)

sensitive to the effects of GH. Hypercortisolism is the rarest complication arising from GNAS activation in the fetal adrenal gland and presents during the first year of life. There are no medical therapies that can alter the disease course of FD, however, treatment of underlying endocrinopathies can help lessen skeletal complications.

CARNEY COMPLEX

Carney complex (CNC) is a rare multiple endocrine neoplasia syndrome that is a constellation of distinctive pigmented lesions of the skin and mucosal surfaces, cardiac and noncardiac myxomatous tumors, and multiple endocrine tumors. It was previously known as NAME (nevi, atrial myxoma, ephelides) and LAMB (lentigines, atrial myxoma, blue nevi) syndrome.

CNC is inherited in an autosomal dominant pattern with high penetrance but heterogeneous expression. It is mostly associated with mutations in the PRKAR1A gene. It can also occur sporadically due to de novo mutations (approximately 25% of the cases).

Lentiginous skin pigmentation is the hallmark lesion of CNC, found in about 70%–80% of the patients, with perioral and periocular distribution. About 40% of patients have multiple blue nevi. Café-au-lait macules, nevus spilus, and, rarely, Spitz nevus can also be seen in patients with CNC (Figure 9.32).

Cutaneous myxomas of the head, neck, and trunk are seen in less than half of patients, but when present strongly suggest a diagnosis of CNC (Figure 9.33).

Endocrine tumors such as large-cell calcifying Sertoli cell tumors (LCCSCTs), primary pigmented nodular adrenocortical disease (PPNAD), and GH-secreting pituitary adenomas, are frequent manifestations of CNC. Almost 75% of male patients with CNC have LCCSCTs, which often leads to prepubertal gynecomastia. Cushing's syndrome secondary to PPNAD can be seen in 25%–45% of patients.

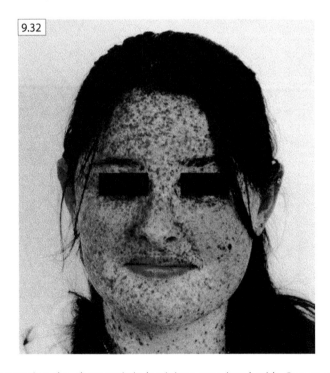

FIGURE 9.32 Demonstrating the characteristic lentigines associated with Carney syndrome in the facial region. (From *British Journal of Plastic Surgery*. With permission.)

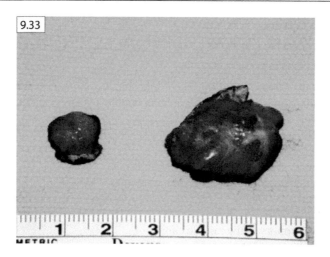

FIGURE 9.33   Cutaneous myxomas associated with Carney syndrome. (From *British Journal of Plastic Surgery*. With permission.)

GH-secreting pituitary adenomas are the least common, occurring only in 10%–15% of patients. Approximately 75% of patients with CNC have thyroid nodules, however, the incidence of thyroid cancer is less than 10%.

Hallmark non-endocrine tumors associated with CNC include cardiac myxomas (most frequent), psammomatous melanotic schwannomas, breast myxomas and ductal adenomas, and osteochondromyxomas.

Diagnosis is made on clinical suspicion. Treatment consists of surgical resection of various tumors. For surveillance, an annual echocardiogram for myxomas and annual ultrasounds of the thyroid and testes for nodules is recommended. Annual measurement of urinary free cortisol, IGF-1, and prolactin beginning in adolescence is also recommended to screen for cortisol excess and pituitary overactivity (Figure 9.34).

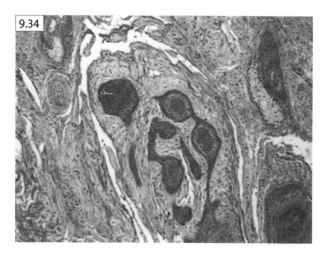

FIGURE 9.34   Histologic examination of the myxoma pictured in Figure 9.33. (From *British Journal of Plastic Surgery*. With permission.)

VON HIPPEL–LINDAU DISEASE

Von Hippel–Lindau (VHL) disease is an inherited, autosomal dominant syndrome characterized by a variety of benign and malignant tumors. The disease can manifest at any point in a patient's life; the mean age at initial presentation is about 26.

The spectrum of VHL-associated tumors includes:

- Hemangioblastomas of the brain (cerebellum) and spine
- Retinal capillary hemangioblastomas (retinal angiomas)
- Clear cell renal cell carcinomas
- Pheochromocytomas
- Endolymphatic sac tumors of the middle ear
- Serous cystadenomas and neuroendocrine tumors of the pancreas
- Papillary cystadenomas of the epididymis and broad ligament

VHL disease can be broadly classified into two categories based on the likelihood of developing pheochromocytoma. Patients with type 1 disease have a lower risk of developing pheochromocytoma, whereas those with type 2 have a higher risk for it.

VHL disease results from a deletion or mutation in the *VHL* gene located on the short arm of chromosome 3. The normal *VHL* gene acts as a tumor-suppressor gene, with the function of preventing the formation of tumors. Incidence is 1 in 36,000 individuals and 20% of cases are due to de novo mutations.

Hemangioblastomas are the most common lesions associated with VHL disease, affecting 60% to 84% of patients, and typically occur in the cerebellum, spinal cord, or retina (Figure 9.35). Renal cell carcinomas (particularly the clear cell variant) are the second most common tumor, occurring in almost two-thirds of the patients. Patients with VHL disease also have a 25%–30% chance of developing pheochromocytoma. Pheochromocytomas seen in VHL disease usually present at a younger age, may be extra-adrenal, and are less likely to present with symptoms or biochemical evidence of catecholamine production compared with those occurring in patients without VHL.

Diagnosis is made by genetic testing to look for pathogenic variants in the *VHL* gene. Surveillance for the development of tumors, especially hemangioblastomas and pheochromocytomas, starts in childhood (Figures 9.36 and 9.37).

Treatment modalities include different surgical interventions based on tumor size and stage, and radiation therapy. Belzutifan is also used for the management of hemangioblastomas, renal cell carcinomas, and pancreatic tumors. Belzutifan specifically inhibits hypoxia-inducible factor-2 alpha (HIF-2 alpha), a key protein regulated by the VHL pathway.

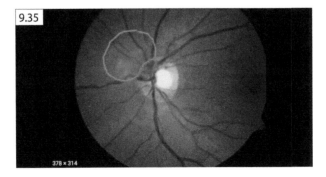

FIGURE 9.35   Retinal hemangioblastoma. (From Toth, Cynthia A., *Handbook of Pediatric Retinal OCT and the Eye–Brain Connection*, 2019, Elsevier Books. With permission.)

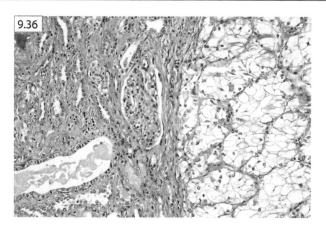

FIGURE 9.36   Histology of clear cell renal carcinoma. (From Nephron, CC BY-SA 3.0, via Wikimedia Commons.)

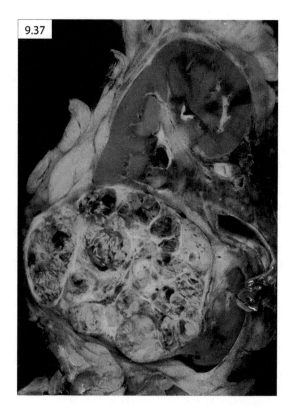

FIGURE 9.37   Gross specimen of clear cell renal carcinoma. (From Ed Uthman, MD (1953–), Public domain, via Wikimedia Commons.)

BIBLIOGRAPHY

Accardo, G., et al., Genetics of medullary thyroid cancer: An overview. *Int J Surg*, 2017. 41. suppl 1: p. S2–s6.

Adaway, J.E., et al., Serum and plasma 5-hydroxyindoleacetic acid as an alternative to 24-h urine 5-hydroxyindole-acetic acid measurement. *Ann Clin Biochem*, 2016. 53(5): p. 554–560.

Agarwal, S.K., Multiple endocrine neoplasia type 1. *Front Horm Res*, 2013. 41: p. 1–15.

Al-Salameh, A., C. Baudry, and R. Cohen, Update on multiple endocrine neoplasia Type 1 and 2. *Presse Med*, 2018. 47(9): p. 722–731.

Al-Salameh, A., et al., Clinical aspects of multiple endocrine neoplasia type 1. *Nat Rev Endocrinol*, 2021. 17(4): p. 207–224.

Alevizaki, M. and K. Saltiki, Primary hyperparathyroidism in MEN2 syndromes. *Recent Results Cancer Res*, 2015. 204: p. 179–186.

Amodru, V., et al., MEN2-related pheochromocytoma: Current state of knowledge, specific characteristics in MEN2B, and perspectives. *Endocrine*, 2020. 69(3): p. 496–503.

Aufforth, R.D., et al., Pheochromocytoma screening initiation and frequency in von Hippel-Lindau syndrome. *J Clin Endocrinol Metab*, 2015. 100(12): p. 4498–4504.

Baghai, M., et al., Pheochromocytomas and paragangliomas in von Hippel–Lindau disease: A role for laparoscopic and cortical-sparing surgery. *Arch Surg*, 2002. 137(6): p. 682–688; discussion 688–689.

Barzaghi, F., et al., Long-term follow-up of IPEX syndrome patients after different therapeutic strategies: An international multicenter retrospective study. *J Allergy Clin Immunol*, 2018. 141(3): p. 1036–1049.e5.

Bouma, G., et al., Niacin (vitamin B3) supplementation in patients with serotonin-producing neuroendocrine tumor. *Neuroendocrinology*, 2016. 103(5): p. 489–494.

Boutzios, G. and G. Kaltsas, Clinical syndromes related to gastrointestinal neuroendocrine neoplasms. *Front Horm Res*, 2015. 44: p. 40–57.

Boyce, A.M., et al., Fibrous dysplasia/McCune-Albright syndrome. In: *GeneReviews®*, Eds. M.P. Adam, et al. 1993, Seattle, WA: University of Washington.

Brandi, M.L., et al., CONSENSUS: Guidelines for diagnosis and therapy of MEN type 1 and type 2. *J Clin Endocrinol Metab*, 2001. 86(12): p. 5658–5671.

Buffet, A., et al., An overview of 20 years of genetic studies in pheochromocytoma and paraganglioma. *Best Pract Res Clin Endocrinol Metab*, 2020. 34(2): p. 101416.

Carlomagno, F., et al., The different RET-activating capability of mutations of cysteine 620 or cysteine 634 correlates with the multiple endocrine neoplasia type 2 disease phenotype. *Cancer Res*, 1997. 57(3): p. 391–395.

Carney, J.A. and B.C. Toorkey, Ductal adenoma of the breast with tubular features. A probable component of the complex of myxomas, spotty pigmentation, endocrine overactivity, and schwannomas. *Am J Surg Pathol*, 1991. 15(8): p. 722–731.

Castinetti, F., et al., A comprehensive review on MEN2B. *Endocr Relat Cancer*, 2018. 25(2): p. T29–T39.

Castinetti, F., et al., Outcomes of adrenal-sparing surgery or total adrenalectomy in phaeochromocytoma associated with multiple endocrine neoplasia type 2: An international retrospective population-based study. *Lancet Oncol*, 2014. 15(6): p. 648–655.

Correa, R., P. Salpea, and C.A. Stratakis, Carney complex: An update. *Eur J Endocrinol*, 2015. 173(4): p. M85–97.

Coyle, D., F. Friedmacher, and P. Puri, The association between Hirschsprung's disease and multiple endocrine neoplasia type 2a: A systematic review. *Pediatr Surg Int*, 2014. 30(8): p. 751–756.

Dalin, F., et al., Clinical and immunological characteristics of autoimmune Addison disease: A nationwide Swedish multicenter study. *J Clin Endocrinol Metab*, 2017. 102(2): p. 379–389.

Donovan, D.T., et al., Familial cutaneous lichen amyloidosis in association with multiple endocrine neoplasia type 2A: A new variant. *Henry Ford Hosp Med J*, 1989. 37(3–4): p. 147–150.

Dreijerink, K.M., et al., Breast-cancer predisposition in multiple endocrine neoplasia type 1. *N Engl J Med*, 2014. 371(6): p. 583–584.

Eisenbarth, G.S. and P.A. Gottlieb, Medical progress: Autoimmune polyendocrine Syndromes. *N Engl J Med*, 2004. 350(20): p. 2068–2079.

Eisenhofer, G., et al., Pheochromocytomas in von Hippel-Lindau syndrome and multiple endocrine neoplasia type 2 display distinct biochemical and clinical phenotypes. *J Clin Endocrinol Metab*, 2001. 86(5): p. 1999–2008.

Erichsen, M.M., et al., Clinical, immunological, and genetic features of autoimmune primary adrenal insufficiency: Observations from a Norwegian registry. *J Clin Endocrinol Metab*, 2009. 94(12): p. 4882–4890.

Feldman, J.M., Carcinoid tumors and the carcinoid syndrome. *Curr Probl Surg*, 1989. 26(12): p. 835–885.

Fisher, G.A., Jr., et al., Lanreotide therapy in carcinoid syndrome: Prospective analysis of patient-reported symptoms in patients responsive to prior octreotide therapy and patients naïve to somatostatin analogue therapy in the elect PHASE 3 study. *Endocr Pract*, 2018. 24(3): p. 243–255.

Golden, T. and J.A. Siordia, Osteochondromyxoma: Review of a rare carney complex criterion. *J Bone Oncol*, 2016. 5(4): p. 194–197.

Gomes-Porras, M., J. Cárdenas-Salas, and C. Álvarez-Escolá, Somatostatin analogs in clinical practice: A review. *Int J Mol Sci*, 2020. 21(5).

Grey, J. and K. Winter, Patient quality of life and prognosis in multiple endocrine neoplasia type 2. *Endocr Relat Cancer*, 2018. 25(2): p. T69–T77.

Guerin, C., et al., Looking beyond the thyroid: Advances in the understanding of pheochromocytoma and hyper-parathyroidism phenotypes in MEN2 and of non-MEN2 familial forms. *Endocr Relat Cancer*, 2018. 25(2): p. T15–T28.

Hassan, S.A., et al., Carcinoid heart disease. *Heart*, 2017. 103(19): p. 1488–1495.

Husebye, E.S., et al., Clinical manifestations and management of patients with autoimmune polyendocrine syndrome type I. *J Intern Med*, 2009. 265(5): p. 514–529.

Ito, T., L. Lee, and R.T. Jensen, Carcinoid-syndrome: Recent advances, current status and controversies. *Curr Opin Endocrinol Diabetes Obes*, 2018. 25(1): p. 22–35.

Javaid, M.K., et al., Best practice management guidelines for fibrous dysplasia/McCune-Albright syndrome: A consensus statement from the FD/MAS international consortium. *Orphanet J Rare Dis*, 2019. 14(1): p. 139.

Jensen, R., J. Norton, and K. Oberg, *Neuroendocrine Tumors in Sleisenger and Fordtran's Gastrointestinal and Liver Diseases*, 10th ed., Eds. M. Feldman, L.S. Friedman, L.J. Brandt. 2016, Philadelphia: Elsevier Saunders.

Jhiang, S.M., The RET proto-oncogene in human cancers. *Oncogene*, 2000. 19(49): p. 5590–5597.

Kamilaris, C.D.C. and C.A. Stratakis, Multiple endocrine neoplasia Type 1 (MEN1): An update and the significance of early genetic and clinical diagnosis. *Front Endocrinol (Lausanne)*, 2019. 10: p. 339.

Kloos, R.T., et al., Medullary thyroid cancer: Management guidelines of the American Thyroid Association. *Thyroid*, 2009. 19(6): p. 565–612.

Kornaczewski Jackson, E.R., et al., Utility of FDG-PET imaging for risk stratification of pancreatic neuroendocrine tumors in MEN1. *J Clin Endocrinol Metab*, 2017. 102(6): p. 1926–1933.

Lampasona, V., et al., Autoantibodies to harmonin and villin are diagnostic markers in children with IPEX syndrome. *PLOS ONE*, 2013. 8(11): p. e78664.

Lenders, J.W., et al., Phaeochromocytoma. *Lancet*, 2005. 366(9486): p. 665–675.

Li, S.R., et al., Clinical and biochemical features of pheochromocytoma characteristic of Von Hippel-Lindau syndrome. *World J Surg*, 2020. 44(2): p. 570–577.

Lonser, R.R., et al., Von Hippel-Lindau disease. *Lancet*, 2003. 361(9374): p. 2059–2067.

Luis, S.A. and P.A. Pellikka, Carcinoid heart disease: Diagnosis and management. *Best Pract Res Clin Endocrinol Metab*, 2016. 30(1): p. 149–158.

Maher, E.R. and W.G. Kaelin, Jr., Von Hippel-Lindau disease. *Med (Baltim)*, 1997. 76(6): p. 381–391.

Maher, E.R., et al., Clinical features and natural history of von Hippel-Lindau disease. *Q J Med*, 1990. 77(283): p. 1151–1163.

McDonnell, J.E., et al., Multiple endocrine neoplasia: An update. *Intern Med J*, 2019. 49(8): p. 954–961.

Mendelsohn, G., S.A. Wells, Jr., and S.B. Baylin, Relationship of tissue carcinoembryonic antigen and calcitonin to tumor virulence in medullary thyroid carcinoma. An immunohistochemical study in early, localized, and virulent disseminated stages of disease. *Cancer*, 1984. 54(4): p. 657–662.

Okafor, C., et al., Update on targeted therapy in medullary thyroid cancer. *Front Endocrinol (Lausanne)*, 2021. 12: p. 708949.

Powell, B.R., N.R.M. Buist, and P. Stenzel, An X-linked syndrome of diarrhea, polyendocrinopathy, and fatal infection in infancy. *J Pediatr*, 1982. 100(5): p. 731–737.

Raue, F. and K. Frank-Raue, Genotype-phenotype correlation in multiple endocrine neoplasia type 2. *Clin (S Paulo)*, 2012. 67 (Suppl 1): p. 69–75.

Rizzoli, R., J. Green, 3rd, and S.J. Marx, Primary hyperparathyroidism in familial multiple endocrine neoplasia type I. Long-term follow-up of serum calcium levels after parathyroidectomy. *Am J Med*, 1985. 78(3): p. 467–474.

Rubin de Celis Ferrari, A.C., J. Glasberg, and R.P. Riechelmann, Carcinoid syndrome: Update on the pathophysiology and treatment. *Clin (Sao Paulo)*, 2018. 73. suppl 1: p. e490s.

Russell, T.R. and R. Ho, Conversion of 3T3 fibroblasts into adipose cells: Triggering of differentiation by prostaglandin F2alpha and 1-methyl-3-isobutyl xanthine. *Proc Natl Acad Sci U S A*, 1976. 73(12): p. 4516–4520.

Sadowski, S.M., et al., Results of (68)gallium-DOTATATE PET/CT scanning in patients with multiple endocrine neoplasia Type 1. *J Am Coll Surg*, 2015. 221(2): p. 509–517.

Shetty Roy, A.N., et al., Familial recurrent atrial myxoma: Carney's complex. *Clin Cardiol*, 2011. 34(2): p. 83–86.

Shields, L.B., et al., Malignant psammomatous melanotic schwannoma of the spine: A component of Carney complex. *Surg Neurol Int*, 2011. 2: p. 136.

Soga, J., Y. Yakuwa, and M. Osaka, Carcinoid syndrome: A statistical evaluation of 748 reported cases. *J Exp Clin Cancer Res*, 1999. 18(2): p. 133–141.

Spencer, T., et al., The clinical spectrum of McCune-Albright syndrome and its management. *Horm Res Paediatr*, 2019. 92(6): p. 347–356.

Stratakis, C.A., Hereditary syndromes predisposing to endocrine tumors and their skin manifestations. *Rev Endocr Metab Disord*, 2016. 17(3): p. 381–388.

Stratakis, C.A., Carney complex: A familial lentiginosis predisposing to a variety of tumors. *Rev Endocr Metab Disord*, 2016. 17(3): p. 367–371.

Thakker, R.V., et al., Clinical practice guidelines for multiple endocrine neoplasia type 1 (MEN1). *J Clin Endocrinol Metab*, 2012. 97(9): p. 2990–3011.

Tonelli, F., et al., Surgical approach in hereditary hyperparathyroidism. *Endocr J*, 2009. 56(7): p. 827–841.

Torino, F., S.M. Corsello, and R. Salvatori, Endocrinological side-effects of immune checkpoint inhibitors. *Curr Opin Oncol*, 2016. 28(4): p. 278–287.

Uchino, S. Multiple endocrine neoplasia type 2 in Japan: Large-scale analysis of data from the MEN consortium of Japan. *Nihon Geka Gakkai Zasshi*, 2012. 113(4): p. 362–367.

Vinik, A., et al., ELECT: A phase 3 study of efficacy and safety of lanreotide autogel/depot (LAN) treatment for carcinoid syndrome in patients with neuroendocrine tumors (NETs). *J Clin Oncol*, 2014. 32(3): p. 268–268.

Voss, R.K., et al., Medullary thyroid carcinoma in MEN2A: ATA moderate- or high-risk RET mutations do not predict disease aggressiveness. *J Clin Endocrinol Metab*, 2017. 102(8): p. 2807–2813.

Waguespack, S.G., et al., Management of medullary thyroid carcinoma and MEN2 syndromes in childhood. *Nat Rev Endocrinol*, 2011. 7(10): p. 596–607.

Walther, M.M., et al., Clinical and genetic characterization of pheochromocytoma in von Hippel-Lindau families: Comparison with sporadic pheochromocytoma gives insight into natural history of pheochromocytoma. *J Urol*, 1999. 162(3 Pt 1): p. 659–664.

Wei, S., et al., Detection of molecular alterations in medullary thyroid carcinoma using next-generation sequencing: An institutional experience. *Endocr Pathol*, 2016. 27(4): p. 359–362.

Wells, S.A., Jr., et al., Revised American Thyroid Association guidelines for the management of medullary thyroid carcinoma. *Thyroid*, 2015. 25(6): p. 567–610.

Wildin, R.S., S. Smyk-Pearson, and A.H. Filipovich, Clinical and molecular features of the immunodysregulation, polyendocrinopathy, enteropathy, X linked (IPEX) syndrome. *J Med Genet*, 2002. 39(8): p. 537–545.

Wolin, E.M., et al., Phase III study of pasireotide long-acting release in patients with metastatic neuroendocrine tumors and carcinoid symptoms refractory to available somatostatin analogues. *Drug Des Devel Ther*, 2015. 9: p. 5075–5086.

Yip, L., et al., Multiple endocrine neoplasia type 2: Evaluation of the genotype-phenotype relationship. *Arch Surg*, 2003. 138(4): p. 409–416.

Zbar, B., et al., Germline mutations in the von Hippel-Lindau disease (VHL) gene in families from North America, Europe, and Japan. *Hum Mutat*, 1996. 8(4): p. 348–357.

Endocrinologic Care of Transgender Patients

10

Pranav Gupta, Mark Walsh,
Howa Yeung, and Mary O. Stevenson

ABSTRACT

The importance of providing comprehensive transgender care is increasingly recognized, with growing societal acceptance, destigmatization, and more transgender persons seeking medical care. Endocrinologists play an important role in providing gender-affirming hormonal therapy to help align secondary sex characteristics with the affirmed gender. For transgender adolescents, therapy can begin with medication to halt the progression of puberty followed by sex hormone therapy. Estradiol is the main hormone used for transgender females to induce feminizing characteristics in combination with antiandrogen therapy. For transgender males, testosterone is used to induce masculinizing characteristics. Fertility-preserving options should be discussed with all patients before initiation of gender-affirming hormone therapy. Patients on gender-affirming hormone therapy should be closely monitored to minimize the potential side effects and assess therapy progress. Assorted surgeries and procedures are available for transgender patients to help align their primary and secondary sex characteristics with their gender, which will be briefly reviewed.

INTRODUCTION AND TERMINOLOGY

Gender identity is defined as one's internal sense of being male, female, or something else. Transgender individuals are persons whose gender identity differs from their sex assigned at birth. Transgender men identify as male and were sex assigned female a birth. Transgender women identify as female and were sex assigned male at birth. Transgender individuals have always existed, but the fear of marginalization and social stigma have led to an underestimation of their numbers in the past. With more societal acceptance, the number of individuals publicly identifying as transgender is rising. Approximately 1 in every 250 adults, or almost 1.4 million Americans, identify as transgender (1). One avenue of gender affirmation that many, but not all, transgender persons will pursue is gender-affirming hormone therapy (GAHT). Additional methods may include social transition and/or gender-affirming surgeries. Endocrinologists play a pivotal role in providing gender-affirming care by prescribing and managing hormone therapy. This chapter will not discuss diagnosing or managing gender nonbinary or genderqueer patients.

DIAGNOSIS OF GENDER DYSPHORIA AND SPECIAL HEALTH CONSIDERATIONS

Gender dysphoria (GD) is the term used to describe the distress or impairment in social, occupational, or other important areas of functioning that can be caused when a person's biological sex and their gender identity are incongruent (2). Not all transgender persons experience gender dysphoria but articulate a gender identity that differs from their designated sex, known as gender incongruence (3). For adults, the criteria to start GAHT include persistent and well-documented GD/gender incongruence, full decision-making capacity and ability to provide informed consent, age of majority, and reasonable control of any mental health condition(s), if present (3).

Transgender persons are disproportionately affected by human immunodeficiency virus (HIV), depression, anxiety, substance use disorder, and risk of suicide, exacerbated by experiences of oppression, discrimination, and violence (4). In adults, GAHT can reduce symptoms of anxiety and depression, lower perceived and social distress, and improve quality of life and self-esteem (5). Therefore, access to GAHT is crucial for the well-being of transgender persons.

FERTILITY

For all patients wishing to start GAHT, clinicians should discuss possible permanent effects on fertility (6). This includes all adolescents seeking to initiate pubertal suppressant medications and patients of any age initiating sex hormone therapy. Techniques for fertility preservation should be addressed, which include cryopreservation of spermatozoa, oocytes, or embryos. Because the long-term outcomes of GAHT on reproductive ability have not been widely studied, it is ideal to offer fertility-preserving treatments prior to initiation of hormone therapy, but treatments may still be possible with or without interruption for those already on GAHT. Fertility-preserving procedures may be cost-prohibitive and can require examinations and invasive procedures that may be intolerable to patients.

Fertility potential may not be possible for adolescents that start pubertal suppression in early Tanner stages with subsequent initiation of hormones for the affirmed gender. This is due to impairment of spermatogenesis or oocyte maturation leading to gamete immaturity (3). Pubertal suppression can be delayed to later stages of puberty to allow for gamete maturation, but this is often not preferred by patients due to the development of secondary sexual characteristics associated with later stages of puberty.

PEDIATRIC AND ADOLESCENT GENDER CARE

The number of children and adolescents in the United States (U.S.) who identify as transgender continues to increase, with approximately 150,000 adolescents between the ages of 13 and 17 identifying as transgender (7). In adolescents, older age and later pubertal stage at the time of presentation for gender-affirming care are associated with increased rates of depression and anxiety (8). The Endocrine Society recommends a multidisciplinary team for the treatment of transgender children and adolescents, including a qualified mental health professional experienced in diagnosing GD (3). Parents or guardians need to consent to treatment as well as provide support throughout the transition process (3). Prepubertal children are not recommended to start medical treatment (3). Adolescents who meet diagnostic criteria for GD and express an understanding of the outcomes and side effects of treatment should initially undergo pubertal suppression using gonadotropin-releasing hormone (GnRH) analogues starting at Tanner stage 2 of puberty (3). Tanner stage 2 is discernable by breast budding in natal females (9), and penis and testicular enlargement in natal males (10). Pubertal suppression in transgender adolescents is associated with favorable mental health outcomes (11). Treatment with GnRH analogues is fully reversible with the return of pubertal progression after discontinuation of therapy.

Sex hormone therapy can be started once a multidisciplinary team has confirmed the persistence of GD and that an adolescent has sufficient capacity to give informed consent, which most adolescents have by age 16 (3). The impact of sex hormone initiation at 14 years of age is being studied due to possible detrimental effects on bone health and isolation from same-aged peers associated with delaying to 16 years of age (12). For adolescents presenting in later stages of puberty, GnRH analogues and sex hormone therapy may be started simultaneously. Sex hormone is initiated using gradually increasing doses with adjustments every 6 months. Clinical pubertal development should be monitored every 3–6 months; and laboratory parameters, including luteinizing hormone (LH), follicle-stimulating hormone (FSH), total testosterone or estradiol, and 25-hydroxy vitamin D levels, should be measured every 6–12 months (3). Due to the risk-impaired bone growth from GnRH analogues, bone mineral density (BMD) evaluation can be considered every 1–2 years (3, 13).

FEMINIZING HORMONE THERAPY, LONG-TERM MONITORING, AND ADVERSE OUTCOMES

Feminizing hormone therapy for transgender women includes both estradiol and antiandrogen therapy if testes are present. In the U.S., estradiol is prescribed as 17-beta estradiol in either oral, parenteral, or transdermal formulations. Oral estradiol is recommended at doses of 2–6 mg per day in twice-daily divided dosing, transdermal estradiol in 0.025–0.2 mg/day dosing with a new patch placed every 3–5 days, and intramuscular (IM) estradiol ester (either valerate or cypionate) at doses of 5–30 mg every 2 weeks or 2–10 mg every week (3). Weekly injections may cause less variation in hormone levels between injections. Spironolactone is the primary antiandrogen in the U.S. and acts principally as an androgen receptor antagonist. It is recommended in doses of 100–300 mg/day divided into twice-daily dosing (3). An alternative option for antiandrogen therapy is GnRH analogue therapy, recommended at doses of 3.75 mg subcutaneously (SQ) every month or 11.25 mg SQ every 3 months. Indications for GnRH analogue therapy may include failure to suppress testosterone level to goal at maximum doses, intolerable side effects, chronic kidney disease, or hyperkalemia limiting titration of doses.

Feminizing effects of therapy generally take 1–6 months to see the onset of changes, but some may take up to 12 months, and maximum feminizing effects can take up to 3 years (3). Feminizing changes include a redistribution of body fat from the abdomen to the gynoid (hips/buttocks) region; a decrease in muscle mass and strength; an increase in scalp hair growth; a decrease in terminal hair growth; decrease in oiliness and softening of skin; and decrease in testicular volume, sexual desire, and spontaneous erections (3).

The highest risk of adverse outcome from estradiol therapy is venous thromboembolism (VTE) (3). Additional risk factors, including tobacco smoking, immobilization, hypertension, hyperlipidemia, and baseline clotting disorders, likely amplify the possibility of VTE for transgender women on estradiol therapy (14). Transdermal formulations of estradiol may pose the least risk of VTE (15). The moderate risks of adverse outcomes include macroprolactinoma, coronary artery disease, cerebrovascular disease, hypertriglyceridemia, cholelithiasis, and breast cancer (3). There are currently conflicting data regarding breast cancer development risk, with some studies showing no increased signal for hormone-related cancers up to 10 years (14). However, a Dutch study in 2019 did find an increased risk of breast cancer in transgender women compared to cisgender men, but the risk was not increased compared to cisgender women (16). Transgender women may experience several dermatologic conditions, including hirsutism, pseudofolliculitis barbae, and melasma (17). Feminizing hormone therapy with estradiol has been shown to preserve or improve bone mineral density across studies (18–20).

Long-term monitoring should include clinical evaluation of patients every 3 months during the first year, as well as monitoring of laboratory values of estradiol and testosterone levels, and potassium and kidney function for individuals on spironolactone therapy (3, 21). The Endocrine Society recommends targeting estradiol levels of 100–200 pg/dL and testosterone <50 ng/dL (3). Estradiol levels should be measured halfway between injections or at peak/trough levels if patients are on parenteral therapy (3). Transgender females should have breast exams, mammograms, and prostate cancer screening, according to national cancer screening guidelines. BMD evaluation should be considered at baseline, as transgender females have been shown to have lower bone mineral density before starting GAHT as compared to cisgender males (13, 22), as well as for those patients who have been noncompliant with hormone therapy and have had a gonadectomy (3, 23).

MASCULINIZING HORMONE THERAPY, LONG-TERM MONITORING, AND ADVERSE OUTCOMES

For transgender men, testosterone is used to induce masculinizing secondary sex characteristics. Testosterone can be given as an injection in either IM or SQ form, or transdermally as a patch or gel. Testosterone enanthate or cypionate are recommended in doses of 100–200 mg IM every 2 weeks or half dose of 50–100 mg SQ every week (3). Subcutaneous injections are associated with less discomfort due to the smaller needle sizes used for SQ administration. Testosterone undecanoate is recommended at doses of 1000 mg every 12 weeks. For transdermal preparations, testosterone gel 1.6% is suggested at 50–100 mg/day and a testosterone patch of 2.5–7.5 mg/day (3). Testosterone gel can be transferred to intimate partners or children through skin-to-skin contact, and patients should be counseled on thorough handwashing and coverage of application sites. Testosterone patches may produce local contact dermatitis in areas of patch placement. Menstrual bleeding is expected to stop within 1–6 months of testosterone initiation, and progesterone can be initiated in either oral or parenteral formulation (as depot medroxyprogesterone) to halt menses before this time (24). Masculinizing changes of testosterone therapy include the redistribution of body fat from the hips and buttocks to the abdominal region, an increase in muscle mass and strength, an increase in facial/body hair growth, scalp hair loss, clitoral enlargement, vaginal atrophy, and deepening of the voice (3). The onset of changes can vary but typically are between 1 and 12 months, and maximum effects can be seen for up 5 years after initiation of therapy (3).

The highest risk of adverse outcome from testosterone therapy is erythrocytosis, defined as a hematocrit level >50% (3). The risk of erythrocytosis in transgender men on testosterone has been shown to increase with tobacco use, higher body mass index, underlying chronic obstructive pulmonary disease (COPD), sleep apnea, asthma (25), and longer-acting preparations of testosterone administration, particularly testosterone undecanoate (25, 26). Therefore, strategies to mitigate erythrocytosis include addressing underlying conditions that may be contributing to blood count elevations as well as changes to shorter-acting formulations of testosterone, including transdermal preparations. Clinicians should ensure testosterone levels are within the goal range outlined by the Endocrine Society (see later) and reduce dosages for supratherapeutic levels.

The moderate risks of testosterone therapy include liver dysfunction, coronary artery disease, cerebrovascular disease, hypertension, and breast or uterine cancer (3). The risk of severe liver dysfunction (transaminases >3-fold the upper limit of normal) was primarily associated with oral 17-alkylated testosterone use, which is not recommended due to this concern. To date, studies with approximately 10 years of follow-up have not shown an increase in cardiovascular outcomes, including myocardial infarction, ischemic stroke, or venous thromboembolism, in transgender men taking testosterone therapy (14, 27, 28). Similarly, no increased signal for hormone-related cancers has been seen in studies up to 10 years (14). Lipid profile changes may include increases in triglyceride and low-density lipoprotein levels and decreases in high-density lipoprotein cholesterol levels (28). Transgender men frequently experience acne vulgaris (see Figures 10.1 and 10.2) and androgenic alopecia (17). Finally, masculinizing therapy with testosterone resulted in stable or improved BMD across studies (13, 18, 20, 29).

Monitoring should include clinical evaluation every 3 months during the first year, including evaluation of weight and blood pressure, and laboratory values of testosterone, hemoglobin/hematocrit, liver function, and lipids (3). Recommended target testosterone levels are 400–700 ng/dL, measuring levels halfway between injections or peak/trough levels if patients are on parenteral therapy and at least 2 hours after transdermal administration (3). Annual breast exams, mammograms, and cervical cancer screening should be done according to national cancer screening guidelines. BMD testing should be considered for patients who are noncompliant with or discontinue hormone therapy after gonadectomy (3).

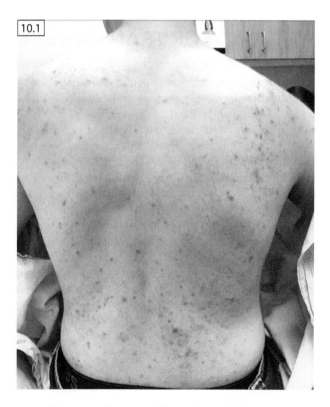

FIGURE 10.1   Eighteen-year-old transgender man with moderate inflammatory acne affecting the trunk.

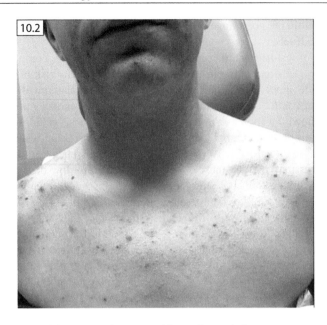

FIGURE 10.2   Eighteen-year-old transgender man with moderate inflammatory acne affecting the face and trunk.

SURGICAL OPTIONS FOR TRANSGENDER PATIENTS

Surgical procedures can be an important component of gender-affirming care. Some transgender patients will pursue surgeries to help further align either primary or secondary sexual characteristics with their gender identity. For both transgender men and women, special consideration should be paid to surgical procedures that have permanent effects on fertility and are further described later. The Endocrine Society recommends that for all surgical procedures that affect fertility, patients have persistent, well-documented GD; be the legal age of majority; have lived full-time in their affirmed gender; taken GAHT (if desired by the patient and not medically contraindicated) for 12 months; and demonstrate an understanding of the risks and benefits of surgery (3). Examples of surgical procedures that transgender women may seek include (but are not limited to) facial feminization, breast augmentation, orchiectomy, penectomy, and vaginoplasty (30). Surgical procedures that transgender men may undergo include bilateral mastectomy and reconstruction of the masculine chest (see Figures 10.3 and 10.4), hysterectomy and/or oophorectomy, phalloplasty, and metaoidioplasty (30).

Finally, for both transgender women and men, therapy with a speech language pathologist may be an additional resource to help patients align speech patterns with their gender identity.

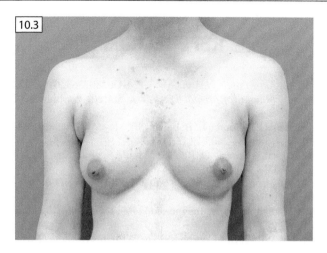

FIGURE 10.3 Nineteen-year-old transgender male who underwent double incision mastectomy with free nipple grafts, preoperative frontal view.

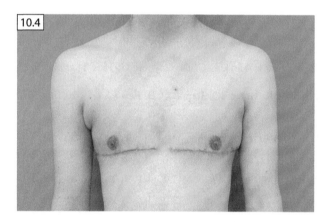

FIGURE 10.4 Nineteen-year-old transgender male who underwent double incision mastectomy with free nipple grafts, 3 months postoperative front view.

CONCLUSION

More individuals are now seeking GAHT. For transgender persons, GD can significantly improve on hormone therapy, and endocrinologists need to be aware of the current treatment guidelines, risks, and limitations of GAHT. Hormonal therapy is deemed safe when given in a clinical setting but should be monitored due to the risks and side effects. Fertility preferences should always be addressed prior to initiation of GAHT. Currently, there is limited but growing research on both the short- and long-term effects of GAHT on adolescents and adults. Most of the studies have been done in Western countries and higher socioeconomic groups, and therefore less is known about underrepresented populations. Transgender individuals have specific and unique needs during the journey of their transition. Therefore, GAHT should be done in a way that guidelines are followed but also aligns with patients' priorities and preferences.

REFERENCES

1. Meerwijk EL, Sevelius JM. *Am J Public Health* (2017). PMID: 28075632/DOI: 10.2105/ajph.2016.303578
2. *Diagnostic and Statistical Manual of Mental Disorders.* 5th ed. Washington, DC: American Psychiatric Association (APA); 2013.
3. Hembree WC, Cohen-Kettenis PT, Gooren L, Hannema SE, Meyer WJ, Murad MH, et al. *Endocr Pract* (2017). PMID: 29320642/DOI: 10.4158/1934-2403-23.12.1437
4. Winter S, Diamond M, Green J, Karasic D, Reed T, Whittle S, et al. *Lancet* (2016). PMID: 27323925/DOI: 10.1016/s0140-6736(16)00683-8
5. Nguyen HB, Chavez AM, Lipner E, Hantsoo L, Kornfield SL, Davies RD, et al. *Curr Psychiatry Rep* (2018). PMID: 30306351/DOI: 10.1007/s11920-018-0973-0
6. Mattawanon N, Spencer JB, Schirmer DA, Tangpricha V. *Rev Endocr Metab Disord* (2018). PMID: 30219984/DOI: 10.1007/s11154-018-9462-37
7. Herman JL FA, Brown TN, Wilson BD, Conron KJ. The Williams Institute (2017)
8. Sorbara JC, Chiniara LN, Thompson S, Palmert MR. *Pediatrics* (2020). PMID: 32958610/DOI: 10.1542/peds.2019-3600
9. Marshall WA, Tanner JM. *Arch Dis Child* (1969). PMID: 5785179/DOI: 10.1136/adc.44.235.291
10. Zachmann M, Prader A, Kind HP, Häfliger H, Budliger H. *Helv Paediatr Acta* (1974). PMID: 4838166
11. Turban JL, King D, Carswell JM, Keuroghlian AS. *Pediatrics* (2020). PMID: 31974216/DOI: 10.1542/peds.2019-1725
12. Rosenthal SM. *J Clin Endocrinol Metab* (2014). PMID: 25140398/DOI: 10.1210/jc.2014-1919
13. Stevenson MO, Tangpricha V. *Endocrinol Metab Clin North Am* (2019). PMID: 31027549/DOI: 10.1016/j.ecl.2019.02.006
14. Wierckx K, Elaut E, Declercq E, Heylens G, De Cuypere G, Taes Y, et al. *Eur J Endocrinol* (2013). PMID: 23904280/DOI: 10.1530/EJE-13-0493
15. Ott J, Kaufmann U, Bentz EK, Huber JC, Tempfer CB. *Fertil Steril* (2010). PMID:19200981/DOI: 10.1016/j.fertnstert.2008.12.017
16. de Blok CJM, Wiepjes CM, Nota NM, van Engelen K, Adank MA, Dreijerink KMA, et al. *BMJ* (2019). PMID: 31088823/DOI: 10.1136/bmj.l1652
17. Yeung H, Kahn B, Ly BC, Tangpricha V. *Endocrinol Metab Clin North Am* (2019). PMID: 31027550/DOI: 10.1016/j.ecl.2019.01.005
18. Wiepjes CM, de Jongh RT, de Blok CJ, Vlot MC, Lips P, Twisk JW, et al. *J Bone Miner Res* (2019). PMID: 30537188/DOI: 10.1016/j.ecl.2019.01.005
19. Van Caenegem E, Wierckx K, Taes Y, Schreiner T, Vandewalle S, Toye K, et al. *Osteoporos Int* (2015). PMID:25377496/DOI: 10.1530/EJE-14-0586
20. Singh-Ospina N, Maraka S, Rodriguez-Gutierrez R, Davidge-Pitts C, Nippoldt TB, Prokop LJ, et al. *J Clin Endocrinol Metab* (2017). PMID: 28945851/DOI: 10.1210/jc.2017-01642
21. Chantrapanichkul P, Stevenson MO, Suppakitjanusant P, Goodman M, Tangpricha V. *Endocr Pract* (2021). PMID: 33471729/DOI: 10.4158/ep-2020-0414
22. Van Caenegem E, Taes Y, Wierckx K, Vandewalle S, Toye K, Kaufman JM, et al. *Bone* (2013). PMID: 23369987/DOI: 10.1016/j.bone.2013.01.039
23. Rosen HN, Hamnvik OR, Jaisamrarn U, Malabanan AO, Safer JD, Tangpricha V, et al. *J Clin Densitom* (2019). PMID: 31327665/DOI: 10.1016/j.jocd.2019.07.004
24. T'Sjoen G, Arcelus J, Gooren L, Klink DT, Tangpricha V. *Endocr Rev* (2019). PMID: 30307546/DOI: 10.1210/er.2018-00011
25. Madsen MC, van Dijk D, Wiepjes CM, Conemans EB, Thijs A, den Heijer M. *J Clin Endocrinol Metab* (2021). PMID: 33599731/DOI: 10.210/clinem/dgab089
26. Nolan BJ, Leemaqz SY, Ooi O, Cundill P, Silberstein N, Locke P, et al. *Intern Med J* (2021). PMID: 32237098/DOI: 10.1111/imj.14839
27. Getahun D, Nash R, Flanders WD, Baird TC, Becerra-Culqui TA, Cromwell L, et al. *Ann Intern Med* (2018). PMID: 29987313/DOI: 10.7326/M17-2785
28. Maraka S, Singh Ospina N, Rodriguez-Gutierrez R, Davidge-Pitts CJ, Nippoldt TB, Prokop LJ, et al. *J Clin Endocrinol Metab* (2017). PMID: 28945852/DOI: 10.1210/jc.2017-01643
29. Van Caenegem E, Wierckx K, Taes Y, Schreiner T, Vandewalle S, Toye K, et al. *Eur J Endocrinol* (2015). PMID: 25550352/DOI: 10.1530/EJE-14-0586
30. Safer JD, Tangpricha V. *N Engl J Med* (2019). PMID: 31851801/DOI: 10.1056/NEJMcp1903650

Index

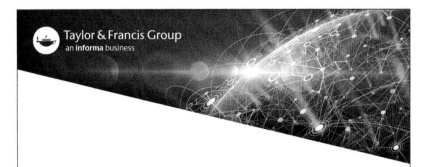

Printed and bound by CPI Group (UK) Ltd, Croydon, CR0 4YY

24/10/2024

01778292-0007